ACUTE AND
CHRONIC COUGH

LUNG BIOLOGY IN HEALTH AND DISEASE

Executive Editor

Claude Lenfant

Former Director, National Heart, Lung, and Blood Institute
National Institutes of Health
Bethesda, Maryland

The opinions expressed in these volumes do not necessarily represent the views of the National Institutes of Health.

ACUTE AND
CHRONIC COUGH

Edited by

Anthony E. Redington
Hammersmith Hospital
London, England

Alyn H. Morice
University of Hull
Hull, England

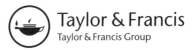

Taylor & Francis
Taylor & Francis Group

Boca Raton   London   New York   Singapore

Published in 2005 by
Taylor & Francis Group
6000 Broken Sound Parkway NW, Suite 300
Boca Raton, FL 33487-2742

International Standard Book Number-10: 0-8247-5958-3 (Hardcover)
International Standard Book Number-13: 978-0-8247-5958-2 (Hardcover)

This book contains information obtained from authentic and highly regarded sources. Reprinted material is quoted with permission, and sources are indicated. A wide variety of references are listed. Reasonable efforts have been made to publish reliable data and information, but the author and the publisher cannot assume responsibility for the validity of all materials or for the consequences of their use.

Library of Congress Cataloging-in-Publication Data

Catalog record is available from the Library of Congress

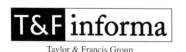

Taylor & Francis Group
is the Academic Division of T&F Informa plc.

Visit the Taylor & Francis Web site at
http://www.taylorandfrancis.com

Introduction

In 1833, the English essayist and poet Charles Lamb (1775–1834) wrote to one of his friends:

My bed fellows are cough and cramp, we sleep 3 in a bed.

Lamb was undoubtedly not alone in his gloomy view of coughing, especially if his cough happened to be a dry one. Indeed, another pessimistic assessment of coughing is reflected in an English proverb: "A dry cough is a trumpeter of death." Although the originator of this prognostication is unknown, it is unfortunately true that persistent dry cough is often caused by an endobronchial tumor. Other pathologies can lead to the opposite and arguably more welcome sort of cough—that is, the productive cough—which functions as a mode of self-cleaning and, in effect, protects the lung.

As pointed out by the editors of *Acute and Chronic Cough*, Dr. Anthony E. Redington and Prof. Alyn H. Morice, "the perception of cough as a symptom is now changing." Extensive research on the mechanisms of cough and on the sites of stimulation has improved understanding—for instance, the roles of receptors and neural pathways have been identified—and we can expect that this work will lead to better ways to control some types of coughing. On the other hand, it is recognized that drug-induced coughing can occur, leaving no alternative but to shift to different classes of medications.

To add to the complexity, coughing may have circulatory consequences such as posttussive syncope due to the very high intrapulmonary pressure that coughing sometimes creates.

Acute or chronic, dry or productive, annoying to the patient or virtually unnoticed—coughing is an important symptom that must not be ignored. This new monograph presented by the series Lung Biology in Health and Disease gives the readers a "timely, comprehensive, and authoritative summary of current understanding." The editors have called on experts from many countries to contribute their knowledge and perspectives. Coughing has surely been a bedfellow of man forever, but it is clear that this is still a relatively young research field. It is hoped that this volume will stimulate interest in exploring it further.

I want to thank the editors and contributors for the opportunity to include this monograph in the series.

Claude Lenfant, MD
Gaithersburg, Maryland

Preface

Cough is one of the most frequent complaints for which patients seek medical attention. Acute cough has massive health economic consequences and yet available treatments are at best of limited efficacy. Chronic cough is a common and debilitating symptom that in the past has frequently been poorly managed. Our perception of cough as a symptom is now changing. Progress has been made in defining the range of conditions responsible for persistent cough and scientific advances in understanding the biology of the cough reflex should in time lead to improved therapeutic strategies. In this volume, we have drawn on the expertise of a body of international opinion to present the current state of knowledge concerning the pathogenesis and treatment of acute and chronic cough.

The opening chapters address the basic science of the cough reflex. Dr. Hwang discusses the molecular biology of the putative cough receptor TRPV1, activation of this receptor by endogenous ligands, and molecular mechanisms that may operate to upregulate its function in the setting of pathologic cough. Dr. Canning and Dr. Mazzone discuss the conflicting work on afferent nerve pathways mediating cough and present evidence that a distinct and previously unrecognized subtype of afferent neuron may play a primary role in regulation of the cough reflex. Dr. Shannon and colleagues review central neuronal networks involved in generating the motor pattern of the cough reflex and present recent novel observations from their own laboratory. In chapter 4, Dr. Advenier and colleagues consider the evidence to support a role for tachykinins as important mediators of cough. They discuss the antitussive effects of tachykinin receptor antagonists in animal models, including recent work from their own laboratory, and consider their relevance to human disease. Angiotensin converting enzyme (ACE) inhibitors represent an important cause of chronic cough. In chapter 5, Dr. Morishima and colleagues review animal studies that provide insights into the mechanisms of ACE inhibitor-induced cough and also discuss the clinical management of this condition.

There is a need for more effective antitussive medications and the next chapters focus on recent developments in the pharmacology of cough. Dr. Geppetti and colleagues concentrate on the pharmacology of TRPV1 and other putative cough receptors: selective TRPV1 antagonists are now becoming available and it is likely these will play an important role in dissecting cough pathways in various settings. Dr. Chung appraises other agents that are under investigation as potential novel therapies in cough.

The third section concerns experimental methodologies. Dr. Earis and Dr. Smith describe their work on the acoustic properties of the cough sound and the development of automated cough recognition algorithms, studies that will be integral to the development of a robust, accurate, and clinically useful cough recorder. The remaining chapters in this section deal with the various sorts of inhalation cough challenge. The authors of these chapters critically appraise the various approaches that have been taken, make specific recommendations about how factors such as reproducibility can be improved, and consider the way forward in terms of increasing co-operation and standardization between different centers.

The final section addresses the more clinical aspects of cough in both the acute and chronic settings. The emphasis here is on helpful advice on appropriate investigation, avoiding pitfalls in diagnosis, and providing practical strategies for successful management. Prof. Eccles reviews the mechanisms of cough associated with acute upper respiratory tract infection and highlights the lack of evidence to support the various treatments that are widely used in this condition. Dr. Everett and Prof. Morice review the strategies that can be taken to investigate and manage patients with chronic cough and consider the relative merits of the different approaches. Chapters 14–19 are devoted to the major specific causes of chronic cough. The first two of these chapters are devoted to cough associated with gastroesophageal reflux disease (GERD). Dr. Ing discusses the pathogenesis of this condition in terms of a self-perpetuating cough-reflux cycle and also includes important recent information about hereditary autonomic neuropathies associated with cough. Dr. Allen concentrates on the effective management of GERD-related chronic cough, including assessment of nonacid reflux and the role of laparoscopic fundoplication. In chapter 16, Dr. Redington examines the epidemiology, pathophysiology, and pathology of cough-variant asthma with emphasis on how this differs from more typical asthma. Eosinophilic bronchitis has emerged as an important cause of chronic cough in some populations and Dr. Brightling and colleagues discuss the diagnosis, pathophysiology and management of this condition. Dr. Bartter and colleagues discuss the definition, differential diagnosis, and treatment of postnasal drip. Psychogenic cough is covered by Dr. Greenberger who offers practical advice on the diagnosis and management of this difficult condition. Prof. Morice discusses possible mechanisms that may be responsible for hypersensitivity of the cough reflex in disease states and speculates how this knowledge will allow rational drug design to normalize cough. In chapter 21, Dr. Fujimura reviews the evidence that chronic cough is more frequent in females and discusses possible mechanisms underlying this difference. Assessment of quality-of-life/health status is increasingly becoming an important outcome measure in many clinical studies. In chapter 22, Dr. Birring and Dr. Pavord describe the development of a validated cough-specific quality-of-life instrument, the Leicester Cough Questionnaire, and its use in clinical and research settings. Chronic cough in children differs in many aspects from that in adults. In the final chapter, Dr. Marchant and Dr. Chang describe the different approach that is necessary to diagnose and manage cough in children.

Our intention in co-editing this volume has been to produce a timely, comprehensive, and authoritative summary of current understanding, to suggest likely future developments, and to identify areas where knowledge is deficient and further research is required. We hope that this will be of interest to investigators, clinicians, and students.

Anthony E. Redington
Alyn H. Morice

Contributors

Charles Advenier U.F.R. Biomédicale des Saints Pères, Laboratoire de Pharmacologie, Paris, France

Christopher J. Allen Firestone Institute for Respiratory Health, St. Joseph's Healthcare—McMaster University, Hamilton, Ontario, Canada

David M. Baekey Department of Physiology and Biophysics, College of Medicine, University of South Florida, Tampa, Florida, U.S.A.

Thaddeus Bartter Division of Pulmonary and Critical Care Medicine, Robert Wood Johnson Medical School at Camden, Camden, New Jersey, U.S.A.

Mike A. Berry Respiratory Medicine, University Hospitals of Leicester NHS Trust, Glenfield Hospitals, Leicester, U.K.

Surinder S. Birring Respiratory Medicine, University Hospitals of Leicester NHS Trust, Glenfield Hospitals, Leicester, U.K.

Ziad C. Boujaoude Division of Pulmonary and Critical Care Medicine, Robert Wood Johnson Medical School at Camden, Camden, New Jersey, U.S.A.

Christopher E. Brightling Respiratory Medicine, University Hospitals of Leicester NHS Trust, Glenfield Hospitals, Leicester, U.K.

Brendan J. Canning Johns Hopkins Asthma and Allergy Center, Baltimore, Maryland, U.S.A.

Anne B. Chang Royal Children's Hospital, Herston Road, Herston, Queensland, Australia

K. F. Chung National Heart & Lung Institute, Imperial College and Royal Brompton & Harefield NHS Trust, London, U.K.

Peter V. Dicpinigaitis Albert Einstein College of Medicine and Montefiore Medical Center, Bronx, New York, U.S.A.

John Earis Aintree Chest Centre, University Hospital Aintree, Liverpool, U.K.

Ronald Eccles Common Cold Centre, Cardiff School of Biosciences, Cardiff University, Cardiff, U.K.

Caroline F. Everett Postgraduate Medical Institute, University of Hull, Castle Hill Hospital, Hull, U.K.

Giovanni A. Fontana Dipartimento di Area Critica Medico Chirurgica, Università di Firenze, Firenze, Italy

Masaki Fujimura Kanazawa Graduate University School of Medicine, Kanazawa, Japan

Pierangelo Geppetti Department of Critical Care Medicine and Surgery, Clinical Pharmacology Unit, Medical School, University of Florence, Florence, Italy

Paul A. Greenberger Department of Medicine, Northwestern University Feinberg School of Medicine, Chicago, Illinois, U.S.A.

Selena Harrison Department of Critical Care Medicine and Surgery, Clinical Pharmacology Unit, Medical School, University of Florence, Florence, Italy

Sun Wook Hwang College of Medicine, Korea University, Seoul, South Korea

Alvin J. Ing University of Sydney, Concord Hospital, Concord, New South Wales, Australia

Jack A. Kastelik Division of Academic Medicine, Postgraduate Medical Institute, University of Hull, Castle Hill Hospital, East Yorkshire, U.K.

Vincent Lagente Faculté des Sciences Pharmaceutiques et Biologiques, Université de Rennes, Rennes, France

Federico Lavorini Dipartimento di Area Critica Medico Chirurgica, Università di Firenze, Firenze, Italy

Bruce G. Lindsey Department of Physiology and Biophysics, College of Medicine, University of South Florida, Tampa, Florida, U.S.A.

Julie M. Marchant Royal Children's Hospital, Herston Road, Herston, Queensland, Australia

Stuart B. Mazzone Department of Neurobiology, Howard Florey Institute, University of Melbourne, Melbourne, Victoria, Australia

Alyn H. Morice Division of Academic Medicine, University of Hull, Hull, U.K.

Yuko Morishima Department of Pulmonary Medicine, Institute of Clinical Medicine, University of Tsukuba, Tsukuba, Japan

Kendall F. Morris Department of Physiology and Biophysics, College of Medicine, University of South Florida, Tampa, Florida, U.S.A.

Takashi Ohrui Department of Geriatric and Respiratory Medicine, Tohoku University School of Medicine, Sendai, Japan

Ian D. Pavord Respiratory Medicine, University Hospitals of Leicester NHS Trust, Glenfield Hospitals, Leicester, U.K.

Massimo Pistolesi Dipartimento di Area Critica Medico Chirurgica, Università di Firenze, Firenze, Italy

Melvin R. Pratter Division of Pulmonary and Critical Care Medicine, Robert Wood Johnson Medical School at Camden, Camden, New Jersey, U.S.A.

Anthony E. Redington Department of Respiratory Medicine, Hammersmith Hospital, London, U.K.

Hidetada Sasaki Department of Geriatric and Respiratory Medicine, Tohoku University School of Medicine, Sendai, Japan

Kiyohisa Sekizawa Department of Pulmonary Medicine, Institute of Clinical Medicine, University of Tsukuba, Tsukuba, Japan

Roger Shannon Department of Physiology and Biophysics, College of Medicine, University of South Florida, Tampa, Florida, U.S.A.

Jaclyn Smith Manchester Royal Infirmary, Manchester, U.K.

Marcello Trevisani Department of Critical Care Medicine and Surgery, Clinical Pharmacology Unit, Medical School, University of Florence, Florence, Italy

Contents

1

Molecular Biology of TRPV1 and Related Receptors

SUN WOOK HWANG

College of Medicine, Korea University,
Seoul, South Korea

Introduction

Vagal C-fibers form a large majority of the afferent nerves innervating the lungs and airways. These nerves show similar properties to those of the cutaneous C-fibers of somatic sensory populations (dorsal root ganglia neurons) studied in relation to functional and anatomical aspects of nociceptive transmission (1–3). The axons of C-fibers conducting nociceptive signals are unmyelinated and their cell bodies are small in size. Their peripheral terminals are specialized to detect painful (nociceptive) stimuli such as heat, mechanical insults, and inflammatory mediators, and are also referred to as nociceptors (4). Vagal C-fibers initiate bronchoconstriction and some types of cough reflex (5,6), and are closely involved in key aspects of airway diseases associated with hypersensitivity (2,7). The application of nociceptive stimuli to the airways results in excitation of airway C-fiber afferents leading to the subsequent release of tachykinins and neuropeptides from the fibers, thus causing local effects including smooth muscle contraction (8). Application of capsaicin, a potent activator of a major population of C-fibers, results in cough and neurogenic inflammation (1,9), and induces a functional desensitization of these afferents and depletion of neuropeptides and substance P (SP) in the periphery during disease states (10–12). Finally, large chronic doses of capsaicin reduce airway hypersensitivity to diverse external stimuli (13,14).

These phenomena led researchers to presume the existence of a capsaicin receptor on vagal neurons. A number of studies of these sensory neurons revealed that the receptor is a cation-selective ion channel present in the cell membrane and that capsaicin and other related vanilloids are able to activate this channel directly via a specific binding site (15,16). Activation of the channel results in sufficient Na^+ and Ca^{2+} influx to depolarize sensory nerve terminals, generate action potentials, transmit signals to the brain via ascending connections, and cause the antidromic release of tachykinins from the peripheral terminals. Excessive Ca^{2+} influx through the channel caused by chronic exposure to relevant stimuli desensitizes the afferent as well as the channel itself and sometimes leads to reversible degeneration of the nerve by complex mechanisms (7,17).

The molecular identity of the capsaicin-activated ion channel in sensory neurons was established in 1997 and initially termed the vanilloid receptor subtype 1 (18). To conform with the standardized nomenclature of the transient receptor potential (TRP) channel superfamily to which it belongs, its name was later changed to TRPV1 (Fig. 1) (21). Of the various kinds of ion channel expressed in sensory afferents, TRPV1 is probably the best known due to its physiologic importance in sensory mechanisms. The biophysical characteristics of the cloned TRPV1 channel are almost identical to those of the native capsaicin-activated channel (Figs. 2 and 3). TRPV1 shows a selective expression profile in the peripheral nervous system (16,18,25). It is believed to be the transducer of capsaicin-mediated responses in sensory nerves and is also activated by noxious high temperature or acidic pH (25), so that it is now accepted as a sensor of multiple harmful environmental and inflammatory conditions (26). Recent studies of molecular modulations of TRPV1 by diverse inflammatory signals not only confirmed the results of earlier studies performed on putative capsaicin receptors (27), but also suggest a plausible candidate for a link between the pathophysiologic signals and resultant biological phenomena related to airway hypersensitivity (7). Investigation of the molecular processes involved in activation and modulation of TRPV1 is therefore crucial to a detailed understanding of diseases associated with airway hyperresponsiveness.

The TRP Channel Superfamily

The first member of the TRP superfamily was identified in *Drosophila* where it functions as a key ion channel in fly phototransduction (28). An increasing number of TRP homologs have subsequently been cloned and are now

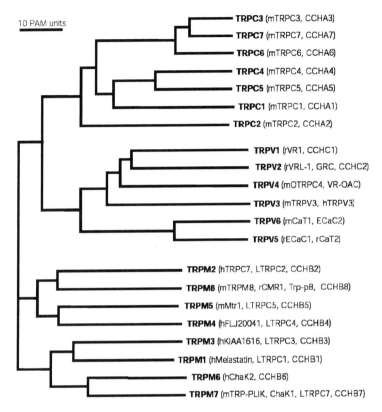

Figure 1 Phylogenetic relationship in the TRP protein superfamily. TRPML, TRPN, TRPP, and *Drosophila* TRP classes are omitted. The evolutionary tree is calculated by the neighbor-joining method (19). The evolutionary distance is shown by the total branch lengths in point accepted mutations (PAM) units, which is the mean number of substitutions per 100 residues. The corresponding GenBank accession numbers (*in parentheses*) for the proteins used are mTRPC3 (NP_062383), mTRPC7 (AAD42069), mTRPC6 (AAC06146), mTRPC4 (AAC05179), mTRPC5 (AAC13550), mTRPC1 (AAB50622), mTRPC2 (AAG29950), rVR1 (T09054), rVRL-1 (NP_035836), mOTRPC4 (AAG17543), mTRPV3 (AAM33069), mCaT1 (BAA99538), rECaC1 (BAA99541), LTRPC2 (NP_003298), mTRPM8 (AAL79553), mMtr1 (AAF98120), hFLJ20041 (NP_060106), hKIAA1616 (BAB13442), hMelastatin (NM_002420), hChaK2 (AAK31202), mTRP-PLIK (F376052). (From Ref. 20.)

being intensively investigated. Six mammalian subfamilies that share homology with *Drosophila* TRP have been described in this channel superfamily: the TRPC (canonical), TRPV (vanilloid), TRPM (melastatin), TRPN (nompc), TRPML (mucolipidin1), and TRPP (PKD2) subfamilies (Fig. 1). Members of the TRPV class are attracting great interest due to

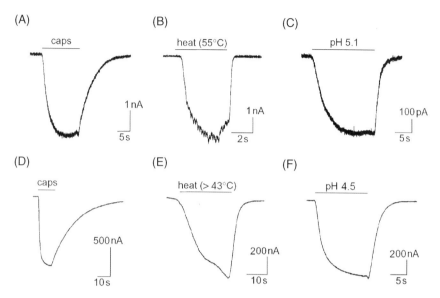

Figure 2 Whole-cell patch–clamp recordings from acutely isolated adult rat dorsal root ganglion neurons held at a membrane potential of $-80\,\text{mV}$ (**A, B, C**) and two-electrode voltage-clamp recording from *Xenopus laevis* oocytes heterologously expressing TRPV1 held at a membrane potential of $-25\,\text{mV}$ (**D, E, F**). Cation membrane currents were activated by capsaicin, noxious heat, and acidic solutions; agonists and hot saline were applied via a fast local perfusion system. (**A, D**) Current responses elicited by capsaicin (caps). (**B, E**) Current evoked by an increase in temperature from room temperature to noxious range. (**C, F**) Proton-activated current responses. The pH was reduced from a resting pH of 7.3 and 7.6 to a test pH of 5.1 and 4.5, respectively. [(A), (B), and (C) were modified from Ref. 22, and (D), (E), and (F) from Ref. 23.]

recent evidence that they have pivotal functions in peripheral sensory transmission.

TRPV1 is the prototype of the TRPV family of which six members have now been cloned, which share 30–75% identity (29). TRPV proteins are also ≈25% identical to TRPC proteins over the region spanning from the putative fifth transmembrane (TM) domain to the TRP box (see later). TRPV1 was cloned from sensory afferent neurons and is activated directly by noxious heat ($>43°C$) and acidic pH (<5.9) as well as by vanilloids (Fig. 2) (18). One stimulus can potentiate the response to another. For example, acidosis, as often occurs with inflammation or nerve injury (30), lowers the heat threshold of TRPV1. Endogenous substances such as 12-hydroperoxyeicosatetraenoic acid (12-HPETE), leukotrienes, anandamide, and N-arachidonoyl dopamine (NADA)—some of which are released during inflammatory processes—are also able to activate TRPV1 (31–34). On the

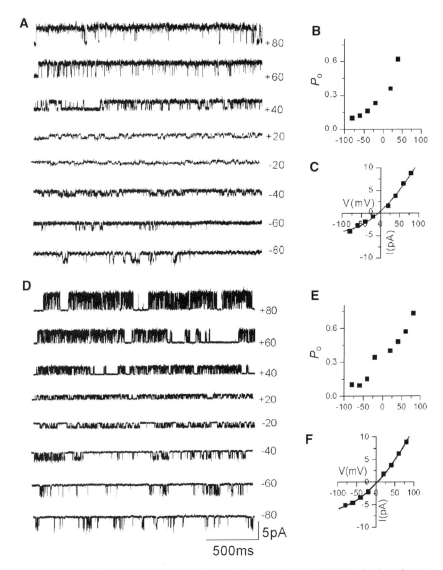

Figure 3 Single-channel current–voltage relationship of the TRPV1 in dorsal root ganglion neurons and in *Xenopus laevis* oocytes heterologously expressing TRPV1. (A) Single-channel current recorded at different membrane potentials from dorsal root ganglion neurons. Both single-channel open probability (Po) (B) and conductance (C) were reduced at hyperpolarized potentials. (D) Single-channel current recorded at different membrane potentials from an oocyte heterologously expressing TRPV1. (E) The channel shows progressive reduction in Po with hyperpolarization as similar to the native channels (B). (F) Current–voltage relationship showing that the single-channel conductance was smaller at negative potentials. (From Ref. 24.)

basis of its sensitivity to these stimuli and its relatively high level of expression in unmyelinated C- and thinly myelinated Aδ-populations of sensory afferent (18), a major physiologic role of TRPV1 appears to be the transduction of painful heat and inflammatory signals to the brain, enabling the perception of pain and consequent avoidance of harmful conditions by conscious and unconscious mechanisms (35).

TRPV2 is also a noxious heat-activated cation channel but it differs in temperature sensitivity ($> 52°C$) from TRPV1 and is expressed predominantly in heavily myelinated sensory fibers (36). TRPV2 is insensitive to vanilloids (36), as is TRPV3, the most recently cloned member of the TRPV family (37–39). TRPV3 responds to warm temperatures ($> 33°C$). TRPV4 has a similar temperature threshold ($> 34°C$) to TRPV3, and the prominent function of this channel is likely to be reflected by its sensitivity to hypotonicity (40,41). TRPV5 and TRPV6, previously termed ECaC1/CaT2 and ECaC2/CaT1, respectively, are constitutively active ion channels that show extremely high selectivity for Ca^{2+} compared with other TRPVs (42,43). These two members have been implicated in hormone-regulated active Ca^{2+} transport in nonneuronal tissues such as kidney epithelium and small intestine (44).

Molecular Characterization of TRPV1

In common with certain other voltage-activated Na^+, K^+, and Ca^{2+} channels, all members of the TRP superfamily have six TM domains, a putative pore region (G624–G645) for ion permeation, and intracellular N- and C-termini (Fig. 4). In addition to these common features, TRPV1 and other TRPVs uniquely possess three intracellular N-terminal ankyrin repeats, the role of which is not yet known. The TRP box, a conserved sequence of TRP channels that is also functionally uncharacterized, lies in the C-terminal region just after the TM6 segment of TRPV1 (21). It has been reported that four subunits of TRPV1 can associate to form a tetrameric complex (45,46), but there is no evidence of heteromultimer formation with other TRPVs.

Sensor Domains

Two groups have investigated capsaicin binding by TRPV1 and unexpectedly found that amino acid residues of the binding site are present on the intracellular side of the channel (47,48). Although the essential sequences reported in these studies were not identical, these results strongly suggest the presence of endogenous capsaicin-like ligands in the cytosol of sensory neurons, and indeed several promising candidates have now been identified (see later). Experiments using conventional deletion mutation methods suggested that R114 of the N-terminus and E761 of the C-terminus are important sites for capsaicin binding (48). In another study involving chimeric

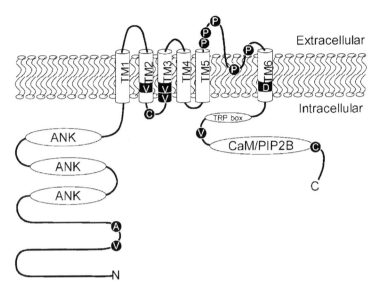

Figure 4 Putative transmembrane topology and domain structure of TRPV1 showing crucial amino acids subject to phosphorylation and ligand binding. White cylinders depict the six transmembrane domains (TM1–TM6). N-terminal, C-terminal, and linker regions between TM domains are shown as a thick curve. *Symbols*: A, substrates for PKA phosphorylation (S116;S502 is also subject to PKA); ANK, ankyrin repeat domains (K200–N232, F247–A279, K332–H364); C, substrates for PKC phosphorylation (S502;S800); CaM/PIP2B, binding sites for calmodulin and PIP2 (E767–T801 and L777–L792, respectively); P, binding sites for proton (E600, D601, E610, E636, D648); D, position particularly involved in Ca^{2+} permeability and external Ca^{2+}-dependent desensitization (Y671); TRP box, conserved sequences of members of TRP (I696–R701); V, binding sites for capsaicin (R114, R491, Y511, S512, E716).

constructs generated using avian TRPV1, which is responsive to heat but not to capsaicin, Y511 and some other lipophilic residues in the TM2–TM3 region as well as polar amino acids S512 and R491 were also implicated (47). Hydrophilic interactions involving N- and C-terminal regions and hydrophobic binding by a portion of TM2–TM3 both therefore appear involved in the activation of TRPV1 by capsaicin.

Phosphatidylinositol-4,5-biphosphate (PIP_2) acts as an intracellular inhibitor of TRPV1 under physiologic conditions. Bradykinin (BK) and nerve growth factor (NGF) release TRPV1 from PIP_2-mediated inhibition, the downstream signaling cascade occurring through the phospholipase C (PLC) pathway (49). Increased levels of BK or NGF in the vicinity of sensory neurons may therefore sensitize TRPV1. The binding site for PIP_2 has recently been localized to the intracellular C-terminal domain of TRPV1 (50).

Tissue acidosis occurs at sites of inflammation (1,51), and acidic pH is both a direct activator of TRPV1 and a potentiator of the heat response of the channel (Fig. 2). The proton-binding sites that mediate these actions are likely to be located mainly in the putative third extracellular loop (E600, D601, E610, and D648) and in E636 near the pore region (23,52). This is consistent with reports that extracellular, but not intracellular, acidic conditions activate both the native capsaicin-activated channel and TRPV1 expressed in heterologous systems (25,53).

Temperature-specific sensing domains of TRPV1 have not yet been identified, although the most basic role of the channel is in fact probably the detection of noxious heat.

Phosphorylation

Phosphorylation is involved in the downstream signaling cascades of typical inflammatory airway diseases (7), and several lines of evidence suggest that this is the most important mechanism of TRPV1 modulation. Among putative candidates, modification of two protein kinase C (PKC) substrates (S502 between TM2 and TM3, S800 in the C-terminal domain) and two protein kinase A (PKA) substrates (S116 on the intracellular N-terminal tail, S502 between TM2 and TM3) has produced the most significant changes in TRPV1 activity (54–56). It has been shown that activation of PKC is capable of directly activating TRPV1 and that ATP or BK, potent inflammatory mediators, are upstream of this signaling (54,57–60). Other groups have demonstrated that PKC activation augmented TRPV1 activity evoked by anandamide or capsaicin (57,58). The PKC activator PMA was also effective in the depolarization of airway C-fibers evoked by TRPV1 ligands (61), and PKC inhibitors selectively blocked its action. Prostaglandin E_2 (PGE_2) is one of the most potent inflammatory mediators (62,63). PKA, which is downstream of PGE_2 signaling through EP3C or EP4 receptors, was shown to strongly potentiate the activation of the native capsaicin-activated ion channel in sensory neurons in vagal bronchopulmonary C-fibers (64–67) and also of TRPV1 when expressed in heterologous systems (55,68). Indeed, it was reported in native sensory neurons that PKA, A-kinase anchor protein, and TRPV1 form a functional module responsive to Gs-protein activation that might mediate PGE_2-EP receptor signaling (56).

Desensitization of sensory afferents by capsaicin has provided a rationale for its development as an analgesic and also accounts for its reduction of airway hypersensitivity (5,12,69). Biophysical investigations in native sensory neurons have shown that the mechanism of capsaicin-evoked desensitization of TRPV1-mediated currents involves extracellular Ca^{2+} influx-dependent dephosphorylation (70). Activation of protein phosphatase 2B (calcineurin) was previously reported to be a strong candidate for this activity (71), although this hypothesis is still awaiting confirmation by molecular studies of TRPV1. An intracellular calmodulin-binding domain has been identified on a 35-amino acid segment in the C terminus of TRPV1 (72), overlapping the PIP_2 binding region (Fig. 4). Its ablation was shown to abolish Ca^{2+}-dependent desensitization, but it is still unknown whether calcineurin has an interaction with this binding site or with calmodulin itself. The Ca^{2+}/calmodulin-dependent kinase II, the only calmodulin-dependent enzyme known to be colocalized with TRPV1 in dorsal root ganglion neurons, is not likely to be involved in these phenomena (72,73).

An additional region proposed to participate in Ca^{2+}-dependent desensitization of TRPV1 is residue Y671 in the TM6 domain (74). Y671 does not seem to be affected by phosphorylation-related processes. However, mutations (Y671K or Y671R) may alter the gating properties of TRPV1 according to biophysical assessments including relative ratio of cation permeability, current–voltage relationship, and altered capsaicin sensitivity. In addition, it is likely that Y671 participates in pore formation together with the putative pore domain. The Y671K mutant exhibited prominently reduced Ca^{2+} permeability, although the lack of desensitization in the Y671K mutant did not appear due to this low relative Ca^{2+} permeability.

Recently, the Src family kinase Lyn was shown to mediate TRPV4 activation by hypotonic stimuli (75). It cannot therefore be definitively assumed that noxious heat—a physical stimulus like hypotonic stimuli-activates TRPV1 by direct physical distortion of the channel via a particular sensing unit. Additionally, it is likely that a beta-strand structure in the C-terminus acts to tune the specific thermal sensitivity of TRPV1 (76). Many aspects of TRPV1 modulation by phosphorylation remain to be explored, as the channel contains putative substrate sequences for other types of kinase and phosphatase in addition to those discussed here.

Endogenous Ligands

Under inflammatory conditions where protons are released from tissues in the vicinity of sensory afferents, a temperature of 36.5–37.5°C becomes a strong activator of TRPV1. Protons act on TRPV1 to lower its heat threshold (from 43°C to body temperature) via the extracellular proton-binding site of the channel, as described earlier. Several other kinds of ligands released endogenously from tissues or from sensory neurons themselves can also activate TRPV1.

Several types of unsaturated fatty acids activate TRPV1 selectively. Metabolic products of the phospholipase A2–lipoxygenase (PLA2–LO) pathway, such as arachidonic acid-derived 12-HPETE, result in the most potent activation of both native channels and TRPV1 when applied directly to the intracellular surface (32). The three-dimensional structure of 12-HPETE in an energy-minimized state is in fact quite similar to that of capsaicin, perhaps implying that capsaicin mimics the activation mechanism of this fatty acid. Single-channel currents evoked by 12-HPETE are blocked by capsazepine, which suggests that the fatty acid shares a binding site with capsaicin. These results are further supported by the fact that some other members of the TRP channel superfamily are activated by related lipids, such as arachidonic acid and linoleic acid (77). Recently, the proinflammatory actions of BK were found to be mediated by production of PLA2–LO metabolites in sensory neurons and their subsequent activation of TRPV1. This pathway has also been demonstrated in the airway (78,79). LO products such as leukotrienes released from nonneuronal tissues are increased under inflammatory conditions and are highly lipophilic or are transported. It is also possible, therefore, that these metabolites originate outside the afferent nerve and open the channels after penetrating the neuronal membrane (80).

Other lipids capable of activating TRPV1 include anandamide, characterized originally as a cannabinoid CB1 receptor agonist (31). Sensory afferents express both TRPV1 and CB1; activation of the latter induces the relaxation of nerves. The concentrations of anandamide necessary for CB1 activation are in a similar range to those required for TRPV1 activation, so that the consequence of anandamide action on sensory afferents may be complex (81–83). For example, a recent study showed that LO products and anandamide both depolarized guinea-pig airway C-fibers. These actions were antagonized not by the CB1 antagonist SR141716 but instead by the selective TRPV1 antagonist capsazepine (61).

NADA and *N*-oleoyl-dopamine also possess lipid-conjugated structures and activate TRPV1, but their actions are thought to be exerted in the central nervous system. They have mainly been detected in the striatum, hippocampus, and cerebellum, but have been difficult to identify in sensory afferents (33,34). Their sensory relevance will remain elusive until further studies determine whether they are sufficiently expressed in sensory afferents or in the surrounding tissues under pathophysiologic conditions.

PIP_2 is a plasma membrane component that has been identified as an important regulator of various kinds of ion transporters and channels, including members of the TRP superfamily (84,85). In the case of TRPV1, it is not a direct activator, but its dissociation from TRPV1 is required for sensitization of the channel to acid or heat (49). BK is not only an indirect activator of TRPV1 via PLA2–LO metabolism or PKC activation as mentioned above, but also a sensitizer of the channel via activation of PLC, which catalyses the hydrolysis (removal) of PIP_2 (Fig. 5). The group that isolated the specific PIP_2 binding unit in the TRPV1 sequences (50) also demonstrated that one mechanism of TRPV1 sensitization by NGF-TrkA signaling was the same as that of BK (49).

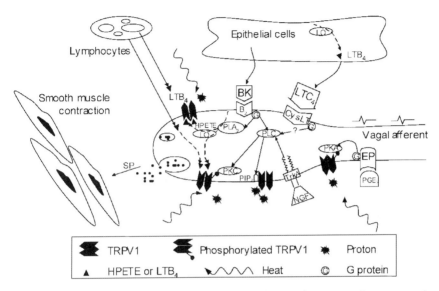

Figure 5 Schematic diagram of the signaling pathways that may activate or sensitize TRPV1 in an airway sensory neuron. BK can indirectly activate TRPV1 via the BK B2 receptor. The B2 receptor couples to a G protein to activate PLA2 and liberate arachidonic acid, which is then metabolized by LO to HPETE or LTB4, which in turn activates TRPV1. HPETE or LTB4 may also be released from lymphocytes or epithelial cells and penetrate the cell to act on TRPV1. These pathways, as well as direct activation by noxious heat or protons, activate the channel, allowing Na^+ and Ca^{2+} influx and generation of action potentials in these vagal sensory (afferent) fibers. In addition to activation of TRPV1, BK is capable of sensitizing TRPV1 via two possible pathways. First, a PLC–PKC cascade activated by BK B2 receptors, NGF TrkA receptors, and possibly CysLT receptors can phosphorylate and sensitize TRPV1. Second, activation of PLC removes constitutive inhibition of TRPV1 by PIP2. In the sensitized state the proton and heat sensitivity of the channel may be increased such that physiological pH and body temperature can activate the channel and allow Na^+ and Ca^{2+} influx. Once excited, for example, via TRPV1, action potentials are generated and propagated to the central nervous system, where transmitters are released from the central terminals of vagal afferents. Peripheral terminals of afferent fibers also release tachykinins such as SP when activated, which induces contraction of airway smooth muscle. (Modified from Ref. 7.)

Studies in TRPV1-Deficient Mice

The physiologic role of TRPV1 has been addressed in knockout experiments. In TRPV1-deficient mice generated by two independent groups, it has been shown that TRPV1 is essential for the development of thermal hyperalgesia induced by inflammation (86,87). Mice lacking TRPV1 exhibited reduced thermal hyperalgesia, consistent with previous studies on the sensitization of TRPV1 by inflammatory mediators such as acid, BK, pros-taglandins, and NGF. Sensory neurons isolated from knockout animals showed either a markedly reduced or a completely absent current response to capsaicin, acid, and heat in vitro. However, it is not clear that pain-related behavior in response to acidic stimuli is defective in TRPV1−/−animals (86,87). This is probably due to the presence of additional types of acid-activated channels, such as members of the acid-sensing ion channel (ASIC) gene family (88). These knockout experiments confirm that TRPV1 mediates certain modes of pain. Further studies are required to determine whether TRPV1-deficient mice show altered airway responses under inflam-matory states, although no significant changes in basal respiratory function are evident (on-line data supplements of Ref. 87).

Expression of TRPV1

In contrast to the original reports on TRPV1 cloning, which described exclusive expression by small-diameter sensory afferents, several groups have shown that this channel is also expressed in the central nervous system (89) and by urinary bladder epithelium, smooth muscle (90), and epidermal keratinocytes (91). Various putative functions in each region have been sug-gested. Although its role in these tissues remains to be fully defined, the function of TRPV1 may not show marked discrepancy with its originally characterized role (89,90,92,93). A valuable future approach may be to investigate possible functions of TRPV1 in the central nervous system from a viewpoint that considers its relationship with endogenous ligand candi-dates such as NADA. Despite the lack of data from jugular ganglia, it is rea-sonably certain that TRPV1 is significantly expressed in vagal afferent projecting to the airways. According to recent in situ hybridization and immunolocalization studies performed by several groups, TRPV1 mRNA or protein is present in nodose ganglia and vagal nerves (25,94,95).

TRPV1 is expressed in all parts of C-fiber afferents, including the plasma membrane, cell body, central or peripheral axon, and nerve ending (25,96–99). In some cell types, TRPV1 is also expressed on the ER mem-brane (100,101) and is thought to modify cytosolic Ca^{2+} levels (101). Inflammation and nerve injury frequently modulate the expression levels of ion channels, metabotropic receptors, enzymes, and the neuropeptide content of sensory neurons (102–106). TRPV1 expression is also markedly increased in neurons under inflammatory conditions, and this provides a mechanism to explain the chronic (within days) development of hyperalge-sia. In addition, acute sensitization of TRPV1 occurs within minutes (107). NGF appears to be a major factor mediating this change of expression in sensory neurons after inflammation (108–110), and previous studies have shown that production of NGF is increased in the asthmatic state and that it potentiates airway inflammatory reactions (111,112). It is well recognized that both the level of TRPV1 expression and the capsaicin sensitivity of cultured dorsal root ganglion neurons are highly dependent on the amount and duration of NGF treatment and that subsequent TrkA signaling is intimately involved (96,113–116). Woolf and colleagues (96) recently suggested that NGF did not affect TRPV1 mRNA levels but instead elevated TRPV1 protein, and that one downstream candidate for these NGF actions is p38 MAPK. Activated p38 appears to play its role via increased translation and peripheral transport of TRPV1 protein.

Functions of TRPV1 in the Airway

Many of the inflammatory mediators and intracellular signals that activate or modulate TRPV1 in the somatosensory system are known also to act on afferent nerves in the airways. In addition, TRPV1 is thought to be expressed by airway vagal afferents. Taken together, these characteristics of TRPV1 suggest that similar mechanisms of action are likely applicable to the pathogenesis of airway hypersensitivity and of cutaneous hyperalgesia (Fig. 5).

BK, a major mediator released in inflamed airways, might activate TRPV1 in bronchial afferents via the generation of PLA2–LO products and sensitization of TRPV1 through several pathways as described above. Sensitization of TRPV1 may also occur through PLC-dependent, PKC-dependent, or PIP2-dependent pathways. TRPV1 sensitization resulting from interactions between PLC and the NGF receptor TrkA probably underlies NGF-mediated hypersensitivity within the airway. LO products, such as 15-HPETE, and leukotriene B4 (LTB4), which are released from epithelial cells in the airways (117,118), may directly activate TRPV1, thus contributing to neuronal hypersensitivity. The role of anandamide, a candidate ligand for TRPV1, in mediating bronchospasm has been questioned recently by the finding that it counteracts the action of capsaicin on the airway (82). Actively released from the lung in vivo, anandamide blocks capsaicin-induced bronchospasm in a CB1 receptor-dependent manner, whereas this molecule produces bronchoconstriction in vagotomized animals. The TRPV1 receptor antagonist capsazepine fails to block anandamide-evoked bronchospasm (82). Thus, these results are somewhat contradictory with regard to whether anandamide is an endogenous activator of TRPV1. Since tissues become acidic when inflamed (51), low pH is a probable cause of TRPV1 activation in asthmatic inflammation and is also capable of potentiating TRPV1 responses to LO products. However, additional pathways such as an ASIC channel-related mechanism should be further investigated. The cysteinyl leukotrienes (CysLTs) LTC_4 and LTD_4 are potent bronchoconstrictors (80). Bronchospasm evoked by

CysLTs is thought to be mediated by the release of tachykinins such as SP from vagal afferent nerves (80,119,120). The biological effects of LTC_4 and LTD_4 are mediated by CysLT receptors, such as CysLT1 (121). The signaling pathways downstream of the CysLT receptors in the respiratory system are not known; however, LTD_4 has been shown to activate PLC in intestinal epithelial cells (122). Therefore, it is conceivable that PLC sensitization of TRPV1 via PKC-dependent or PIP_2-dependent pathways could underlie the bronchoconstrictor effects of CysLTs. However, this pathway is largely hypothetical because the presence of CysLT1 receptors or activation of PLC by the receptor in airway afferents has not yet been demonstrated.

It is difficult to single out one dominant molecular partner for TRPV1 among the signaling pathways suggested here, and it is highly likely that all these extracellular mediators act in concert upon TRPV1 via multiple pathways.

TRPs in Nonneuronal Cells of the Airway

TRPV1 expression by human bronchial epithelial cells was recently demonstrated by RT-PCR. It was suggested that airway epithelial TRPV1 may function as a sensor for negatively charged particulate matter of restricted size range and that it may subsequently initiate the release of cytokines from the cells (123,124). It was also proposed that epithelial TRPV1 may take part in vanilloid-induced airway inflammation and necrotic cell death. Epithelial cells and keratinocytes have in fact become regarded as strong expressers of other TRPVs (37,90,91,125). For instance, TRPV3, a warm temperature sensor, shows an exclusive pattern of expression in epidermal keratinocytes leading to the possibility that these cells are the primary detector immediately prior to dorsal root ganglia transmission (37). Therefore, epithelial TRPV1 might play a role in mediating cough or hypersensitivity qualitatively similar to that in the nerve, but this hypothesis awaits further examination. Additional studies are necessary to quantitatively define which of the various types of cell expressing TRPV1 is the major contributor to the development of pathophysiological states.

Few advances have been made in the identification of interrelationships between other TRP channel members and airway function. However, several groups have provided data to support the notion that some classes of this superfamily may be involved in specific physiological phenomena in the airways. TRPV4, which is not only a warm receptor like TRPV3 but also a hypo-osmosensor, is highly expressed in normal tracheal epithelial cells and bronchial cell lines. It is possible therefore that this channel could play a role in the airway response to hypotonic insult in asthma (2), although there are no reports that address this hypothesis to date. The recently cloned TRP members sensitive to cold temperature, TRPM8 and

ANKTM1, may participate in airway responses to cold (115,126,127). Polycystin 2, a member of the TRPP family, was found to mediate mechanotransduction in primary cilia of kidney epithelium in cooperation with polycystin 1 (128). Since polycystin 2 is also prominently expressed in stratified columnar epithelium in developing trachea, a similar action of removing particulates or mucus movement has been suspected but not yet identified (129). It is now accepted that TRPC1 and TRPC6 are largely involved in proliferation of pulmonary arterial smooth muscle cells (130,131) and TRPC1 and TRPC4 are likely to increase pulmonary vascular tone and permeability by store-operated mechanisms (132,133).

Conclusion

Many factors long recognized as airway inflammatory mediators also significantly affect the activity of TRPV1, a molecular sensor that detects multiple sorts of noxious environmental stimuli. Recent characterization of the molecular aspects of TRPV1 and related signaling pathways has provided insight into the mechanisms underlying the clinical symptoms associated with airway hypersensitivity. Many possible signaling pathways participate in the molecular modulations of TRPV1, and it is difficult to select a single pathway that is principally responsible for the excitation and sensitization of vagal afferent nerves in the airway. Future studies should be directed toward selective disruption of individual pathways to determine which is dominant in sensitizing airway C-fiber afferents via TRPV1. The role of TRPV1 may be relevant to mechanistic studies of airway nerve activation or sensitization. A focused study of TRPV1 might provide additional clues regarding the treatment or management of hypersensitivity.

Acknowledgment

I thank Gina M. Story, Ph.D. (The Scripps Research Institute) for critical reading of the manuscript.

References

1. Widdicombe J. Sensory mechanisms. Pulm Pharmacol 1996; 9:383–387.
2. Spina D, Shah S, Harrison S. Modulation of sensory nerve function in the airways. Trends Pharmacol Sci 1998; 19:460–466.
3. Joos GF, Germonpre PR, Pauwels RA. Neural mechanisms in asthma. Clin Exp Allergy 2000; 30(suppl 1):60–65.
4. Fields HL. Pain. New York: McGraw-Hill, 1987.
5. Karlsson JA. The role of capsaicin-sensitive C-fibre afferent nerves in the cough reflex. Pulm Pharmacol 1996; 9:315–321.

6. Canning BJ. Interactions between vagal afferent nerve subtypes mediating cough. Pulm Pharmacol Ther 2002; 15:187–192.

7. Hwang SW, Oh U. Hot channels in airways: pharmacology of the vanilloid receptor. Curr Opin Pharmacol 2002; 2:235–242.

8. Undem BJ, Carr MJ, Kollarik M. Physiology and plasticity of putative cough fibres in the guinea pig. Pulm Pharmacol Ther 2002; 15:193–198.

9. Saade NE, Massaad CA, Ochoa-Chaar CI, Jabbur SJ, Safieh-Garabedian B, Atweh SF. Upregulation of proinflammatory cytokines and nerve growth factor by intraplantar injection of capsaicin in rats. J Physiol 2002; 545:241–253.

10. Buck SH, Walsh JH, Davis TP, Brown MR, Yamamura HI, Burks TF. Characterization of the peptide and sensory neurotoxic effects of capsaicin in the guinea pig. J Neurosci 1983; 3:2064–2074.

11. Dickenson A, Ashwood N, Sullivan AF, James I, Dray A. Antinociception produced by capsaicin: spinal or peripheral mechanism? Eur J Pharmacol 1990; 187:225–233.

12. O'Neill TP. Mechanism of capsaicin action: recent learnings. Respir Med 1991; 85(suppl A):35–41.

13. Cadieux A, Springall DR, Mulderry PK, Rodrigo J, Ghatei MA, Terenghi G, Bloom SR, Polak JM. Occurrence, distribution and ontogeny of CGRP immunoreactivity in the rat lower respiratory tract: effect of capsaicin treatment and surgical denervations. Neuroscience 1986; 19:605–627.

14. Herd CM, Gozzard N, Page CP. Capsaicin pre-treatment prevents the development of antigen-induced airway hyperresponsiveness in neonatally immunised rabbits. Eur J Pharmacol 1995; 282:111–119.

15. Bevan S, Szolcsanyi J. Sensory neuron-specific actions of capsaicin: mechanisms and applications. Trends Pharmacol Sci 1990; 11:330–333.

16. Oh U, Hwang SW, Kim D. Capsaicin activates a nonselective cation channel in cultured neonatal rat dorsal root ganglion neurons. J Neurosci 1996; 16: 1659–1667.

17. Holzer P. Capsaicin: cellular targets, mechanisms of action, and selectivity for thin sensory neurons. Pharmacol Rev 1991; 43:143–201.

18. Caterina MJ, Schumacher MA, Tominaga M, Rosen TA, Levine JD, Julius D. The capsaicin receptor: a heat-activated ion channel in the pain pathway. Nature 1997; 389:816–824.

19. Saitou N, Nei M. The neighbor-joining method: a new method for reconstructing phylogenetic trees. Mol Biol Evol 1987; 4:406–425.

20. Clapham DE, Runnels LW, Strubing C. The TRP ion channel family. Nat Rev Neurosci 2001; 2:387–396.

21. Montell C. Physiology, phylogeny, and functions of the TRP superfamily of cation channels. Sci STKE 2001; 2001:RE1.

22. Kress M, Zeilhofer HU. Capsaicin, protons and heat: new excitement about nociceptors. Trends Pharmacol Sci 1999; 20:112–118.

23. Welch JM, Simon SA, Reinhart PH. The activation mechanism of rat vanilloid receptor 1 by capsaicin involves the pore domain and differs from the activation by either acid or heat. Proc Natl Acad Sci USA 2000; 97: 13889–13894.

24. Premkumar LS, Agarwal S, Steffen D. Single-channel properties of native and cloned rat vanilloid receptors. J Physiol 2002; 545:107–117.

25. Tominaga M, Caterina MJ, Malmberg AB, Rosen TA, Gilbert H, Skinner K, Raumann BE, Basbaum AI, Julius D. The cloned capsaicin receptor integrates multiple pain-producing stimuli. Neuron 1998; 21:531–543.

26. Cesare P, Moriondo A, Vellani V, McNaughton PA. Ion channels gated by heat. Proc Natl Acad Sci USA 1999; 96:7658–7663.

27. Caterina MJ, Julius D. The vanilloid receptor: a molecular gateway to the pain pathway. Annu Rev Neurosci 2001; 24:487–517.

28. Montell C, Jones K, Hafen E, Rubin G. Rescue of the Drosophila phototransduction mutation trp by germline transformation. Science 1985; 230: 1040–1043.

29. Gunthorpe MJ, Benham CD, Randall A, Davis JB. The diversity in the vanilloid (TRPV) receptor family of ion channels. Trends Pharmacol Sci 2002; 23:183–191.

30. Bevan S, Geppetti P. Protons: small stimulants of capsaicin-sensitive sensory nerves. Trends Neurosci 1994; 17:509–512.

31. Zygmunt PM, Petersson J, Andersson DA, Chuang H, Sorgard M, Di Marzo V, Julius D, Hogestatt ED. Vanilloid receptors on sensory nerves mediate the vasodilator action of anandamide. Nature 1999; 400:452–457.

32. Hwang SW, Cho H, Kwak J, Lee SY, Kang CJ, Jung J, Cho S, Min KH, Suh YG, Kim D, Oh U. Direct activation of capsaicin receptors by products of lipoxygenases: endogenous capsaicin-like substances. Proc Natl Acad Sci USA 2000; 97:6155–6160.

33. Huang SM, Bisogno T, Trevisani M, Al-Hayani A, De Petrocellis L, Fezza F, Tognetto M, Petros TJ, Krey JF, Chu CJ, Miller JD, Davies SN, Geppetti P, Walker JM, Di Marzo V. An endogenous capsaicin-like substance with high potency at recombinant and native vanilloid VR1 receptors. Proc Natl Acad Sci USA 2002; 99:8400–8405.

34. Chu CJ, Huang SM, De Petrocellis L, Bisogno T, Ewing SA, Miller JD, Zipkin RE, Daddario N, Appendino G, Di Marzo V, Walker JM. N-oleoyldopamine, a novel endogenous capsaicin-like lipid that produces hyperalgesia. J Biol Chem 2003; 278:13633–13639.

35. Wall PD, Melzack R. Textbook of Pain. 4th ed. London: Churchill Livingstone/ Harcourt Publisher Limited, 1999.

36. Caterina MJ, Rosen TA, Tominaga M, Brake AJ, Julius D. A capsaicin-receptor homologue with a high threshold for noxious heat. Nature 1999; 398: 436–441.

37. Peier AM, Reeve AJ, Andersson DA, Moqrich A, Earley TJ, Hergarden AC, Story GM, Colley S, Hogenesch JB, McIntyre P, Bevan S, Patapoutian A. A heat-sensitive TRP channel expressed in keratinocytes. Science 2002; 296:2046–2049.

38. Xu H, Ramsey IS, Kotecha SA, Moran MM, Chong JA, Lawson D, Ge P, Lilly J, Silos-Santiago I, Xie Y, DiStefano PS, Curtis R, Clapham DE. TRPV3 is a calcium-permeable temperature-sensitive cation channel. Nature 2002; 418:181–186.

39. Smith GD, Gunthorpe MJ, Kelsell RE, Hayes PD, Reilly P, Facer P, Wright JE, Jerman JC, Walhin JP, Ooi L, Egerton J, Charles KJ, Smart D, Randall AD, Anand P, Davis JB. TRPV3 is a temperature-sensitive vanilloid receptor-like protein. Nature 2002; 418:186–190.

40. Strotmann R, Harteneck C, Nunnenmacher K, Schultz G, Plant TD. OTRPC4, a nonselective cation channel that confers sensitivity to extracellular osmolarity. Nat Cell Biol 2000; 2:695–702.

41. Liedtke W, Choe Y, Marti-Renom MA, Bell AM, Denis CS, Sali A, Hudspeth AJ, Friedman JM, Heller S. Vanilloid receptor-related osmotically activated channel (VR-OAC), a candidate vertebrate osmoreceptor. Cell 2000; 103:525–535.

42. Hoenderop JG, van der Kemp AW, Hartog A, van de Graaf SF, van Os CH, Willems PH, Bindels RJ. Molecular identification of the apical Ca^{2+} channel in 1, 25-dihydroxyvitamin D3-responsive epithelia. J Biol Chem 1999; 274:8375–8378.

43. Peng JB, Chen XZ, Berger UV, Vassilev PM, Tsukaguchi H, Brown EM, Hediger MA. Molecular cloning and characterization of a channel-like transporter mediating intestinal calcium absorption. J Biol Chem 1999; 274: 22739–22746.

44. Nilius B, Prenen J, Hoenderop JG, Vennekens R, Hoefs S, Weidema AF, Droogmans G, Bindels RJ. Fast and slow inactivation kinetics of the Ca^{2+} channels ECaC1 and ECaC2 (TRPV5 and TRPV6). Role of the intracellular loop located between transmembrane segments 2 and 3. J Biol Chem 2002; 277:30852–30858.

45. Kedei N, Szabo T, Lile JD, Treanor JJ, Olah Z, Iadarola MJ, Blumberg PM. Analysis of the native quaternary structure of vanilloid receptor 1. J Biol Chem 2001; 276:28613–28619.

46. Kuzhikandathil EV, Wang H, Szabo T, Morozova N, Blumberg PM, Oxford GS. Functional analysis of capsaicin receptor (vanilloid receptor subtype 1) multimerization and agonist responsiveness using a dominant negative mutation. J Neurosci 2001; 21:8697–8706.

47. Jordt S-E, Julius D. Molecular basis for species-specific sensitivity to "hot" chili peppers. Cell 2002; 108:421–430.

48. Jung J, Lee S-Y, Hwang SW, Cho H, Shin J, Kang Y-S, Kim S, Oh U. Agonist recognition sites in the cytosolic tails of vanilloid receptor 1. J Biol Chem 2002; 277:44448–44454.

49. Chuang HH, Prescott ED, Kong H, Shields S, Jordt SE, Basbaum AI, Chao MV, Julius D. Bradykinin and nerve growth factor release the capsaicin receptor from PtdIns(4,5)P2-mediated inhibition. Nature 2001; 411:957–962.

50. Prescott ED, Julius D. A modular PIP2 binding site as a determinant of capsaicin receptor sensitivity. Science 2003; 300:1284–1288.

51. Reeh PW, Steen KH. Tissue acidosis in nociception and pain. Prog Brain Res 1996; 113:143–151.

52. Jordt S-E, Tominaga M, Julius D. Acid potentiation of the capsaicin receptor determined by a key extracellular site. Proc Natl Acad Sci USA 2000; 97: 8134–8139.

53. Jung J, Hwang SW, Kwak J, Lee S-Y, Kang C-J, Kim WB, Kim D, Oh U. Capsaicin binds to the intracellular domain of the capsaicin-activated ion channel. J Neurosci 1999; 19:529–538.

54. Numazaki M, Tominaga T, Toyooka H, Tominaga M. Direct phosphorylation of capsaicin receptor VR1 by protein kinase Cε and identification of two target serine residues. J Biol Chem 2002; 277:13375–13378.

55. Bhave G, Zhu W, Wang H, Brasier DJ, Oxford GS, Gereau RW 4th. cAMP-dependent protein kinase regulates desensitization of the capsaicin receptor (VR1) by direct phosphorylation. Neuron 2002; 35:721–731.

56. Rathee PK, Distler C, Obreja O, Neuhuber W, Wang GK, Wang SY, Nau C, Kress M. PKA/AKAP/VR-1 module: a common link of Gs-mediated signaling to thermal hyperalgesia. J Neurosci 2002; 22:4740–4745.

57. Premkumar LS, Ahern GP. Induction of vanilloid receptor channel activity by protein kinase C. Nature 2000; 408:985–990.

58. Vellani V, Mapplebeck S, Moriondo A, Davis JB, McNaughton PA. Protein kinase C activation potentiates gating of the vanilloid receptor VR1 by capsaicin, protons, heat and anandamide. J Physiol 2001; 534:813–825.

59. Tominaga M, Wada M, Masu M. Potentiation of capsaicin receptor activity by metabotropic ATP receptors as a possible mechanism for ATP-evoked pain and hyperalgesia. Proc Natl Acad Sci USA 2001; 98:6951–6956.

60. Olah Z, Karai L, Iadarola MJ. Protein kinase C(alpha) is required for vanilloid receptor 1 activation. Evidence for multiple signaling pathways. J Biol Chem 2002; 277:35752–35759.

61. Kagaya M, Lamb J, Robbins J, Page CP, Spina D. Characterization of the anandamide induced depolarization of guinea-pig isolated vagus nerve. Br J Pharmacol 2002; 137:39–48.

62. Kumazawa T, Mizumura K, Koda H, Fukusako H. EP receptor subtypes implicated in the PGE2-induced sensitization of polymodal receptors in response to bradykinin and heat. J Neurophysiol 1996; 75:2361–2368.

63. Southall MD, Vasko MR. Prostaglandin receptor subtypes, EP3C and EP4, mediate the prostaglandin E2-induced cAMP production and sensitization of sensory neurons. J Biol Chem 2001; 276:16083–16091.

64. Lopshire JC, Nicol GD. Activation and recovery of the PGE2-mediated sensitization of the capsaicin response in rat sensory neurons. J Neurophysiol 1997; 78:3154–3164.

65. Lopshire JC, Nicol GD. The cAMP transduction cascade mediates the prostaglandin E2 enhancement of the capsaicin-elicited current in rat sensory neurons: whole-cell and single-channel studies. J Neurosci 1998; 18:6081–6092.

66. De Petrocellis L, Harrison S, Bisogno T, Tognetto M, Brandi I, Smith GD, Creminon C, Davis JB, Geppetti P, Di Marzo V. The vanilloid receptor (VR1)-mediated effects of anandamide are potently enhanced by the cAMP-dependent protein kinase. J Neurochem 2001; 77:1660–1663.

67. Lee LY, Kwong K, Lin YS, Gu Q. Hypersensitivity of bronchopulmonary C-fibers induced by airway mucosal inflammation: cellular mechanisms. Pulm Pharmacol Ther 2002; 15:199–204.

68. Hu HJ, Bhave G, Gereau RW 4th. Prostaglandin and protein kinase A-dependent modulation of vanilloid receptor function by metabotropic

glutamate receptor 5: potential mechanism for thermal hyperalgesia. J Neurosci 2002; 22:7444–7452.

69. Szallasi A, Blumberg PM. Vanilloid (capsaicin) receptors and mechanisms. Pharmacol Rev 1999; 51:159–212.

70. Koplas PA, Rosenberg RL, Oxford GS. The role of calcium in the desensitization of capsaicin responses in rat dorsal root ganglion neurons. J Neurosci 1997; 17:3525–3537.

71. Docherty RJ, Yeats JC, Bevan S, Boddeke HW. Inhibition of calcineurin inhibits the desensitization of capsaicin-evoked currents in cultured dorsal root ganglion neurones from adult rats. Pflugers Arch 1996; 431:828–837.

72. Numazaki M, Tominaga T, Takeuchi K, Murayama N, Toyooka H, Tominaga M. Structural determinant of TRPV1 desensitization interacts with calmodulin. Proc Natl Acad Sci USA 2003; 100:8002–8006.

73. Carlton SM, Hargett GL. Stereological analysis of Ca^{2+}/calmodulin-dependent protein kinase II alpha -containing dorsal root ganglion neurons in the rat: colocalization with isolectin Griffonia simplicifolia, calcitonin gene-related peptide, or vanilloid receptor 1. J Comp Neurol 2002; 448: 102–110.

74. Mohapatra DP, Wang SY, Wang GK, Nau C. A tyrosine residue in TM6 of the Vanilloid Receptor TRPV1 involved in desensitization and calcium permeability of capsaicin-activated currents. Mol Cell Neurosci 2003; 23:314–324.

75. Xu H, Zhao H, Tian W, Yoshida K, Roullet JB, Cohen DM. Regulation of a transient receptor potential (TRP) channel by tyrosine phosphorylation. SRC family kinase-dependent tyrosine phosphorylation of TRPV4 on TYR-253 mediates its response to hypotonic stress. J Biol Chem 2003; 278: 11520–11527.

76. Vlachova V, Teisinger J, Suankova K, Lyfenko A, Ettrich R, Vyklicky L. Functional role of C-terminal cytoplasmic tail of rat vanilloid receptor 1. J Neurosci 2003; 23:1340–1350.

77. Chyb S, Raghu P, Hardie RC. Polyunsaturated fatty acids activate the Drosophila light-sensitive channels TRP and TRPL. Nature 1999; 397:255–259.

78. Shin J, Cho H, Hwang SW, Jung J, Shin CY, Lee SY, Kim SH, Lee MG, Choi YH, Kim J, Haber NA, Reichling DB, Khasar S, Levine JD, Oh U. Bradykinin-12-lipoxygenase-VR1 signaling pathway for inflammatory hyperalgesia. Proc Natl Acad Sci USA 2002; 99:10150–10155.

79. Carr MJ, Kollarik M, Meeker SN, Undem BJ. A role for TRPV1 in bradykinin-induced excitation of vagal airway afferent nerve terminals. J Pharmacol Exp Ther 2003; 304:1275–1279.

80. Montuschi P, Preziosi P, Ciabattoni G. Tachykinin-eicosanoid crosstalk in airway inflammation. Trends Pharmacol Sci 2000; 21:336–340.

81. Szolcsanyi J. Anandamide and the question of its functional role for activation of capsaicin receptors. Trends Pharmacol Sci 2000; 21:203–204.

82. Calignano A, Katona I, Desarnaud F, Giuffrida A, La Rana G, Mackie K, Freund TF, Piomelli D. Bidirectional control of airway responsiveness by endogenous cannabinoids. Nature 2000; 408:96–101.

83. Di Marzo V, Blumberg PM, Szallasi A. Endovanilloid signaling in pain. Curr Opin Neurobiol 2002; 12:372–379.

84. Hilgemann DW, Feng S, Nasuhoglu C. The complex and intriguing lives of PIP2 with ion channels and transporters. Sci STKE 2001; 2001:RE19.
85. Minke B, Cook B. TRP channel proteins and signal transduction. Physiol Rev 2002; 82:429–472.
86. Caterina MJ, Leffler A, Malmberg AB, Martin WJ, Trafton J, Petersen-Zeitz KR, Koltzenburg M, Basbaum AI, Julius D. Impaired nociception and pain sensation in mice lacking the capsaicin receptor. Science 2000; 288:306–313.
87. Davis JB, Gray J, Gunthorpe MJ, Hatcher JP, Davey PT, Overend P, Harries MH, Latcham J, Clapham C, Atkinson K, Hughes SA, Rance K, Grau E, Harper AJ, Pugh PL, Rogers DC, Bingham S, Randall A, Sheardown SA. Vanilloid receptor-1 is essential for inflammatory thermal hyperalgesia. Nature 2000; 405:183–187.
88. Waldmann R, Champigny G, Lingueglia E, De Weille JR, Heurteaux C, Lazdunski M. H(+)-gated cation channels. Ann NY Acad Sci 1999; 868: 67–76.
89. Mezey E, Toth ZE, Cortright DN, Arzubi MK, Krause JE, Elde R, Guo A, Blumberg PM, Szallasi A. Distribution of mRNA for vanilloid receptor subtype 1 (VR1), and VR1-like immunoreactivity, in the central nervous system of the rat and human. Proc Natl Acad Sci USA 2000; 97:3655–3660.
90. Birder LA, Kanai AJ, de Groat WC, Kiss S, Nealen ML, Burke NE, Dineley KE, Watkins S, Reynolds IJ, Caterina MJ. Vanilloid receptor expression suggests a sensory role for urinary bladder epithelial cells. Proc Natl Acad Sci USA 2001; 98:13396–13401.
91. Inoue K, Koizumi S, Fuziwara S, Denda S, Inoue K, Denda M. Functional vanilloid receptors in cultured normal human epidermal keratinocytes. Biochem Biophys Res Commun 2002; 291:124–129.
92. Birder LA, Nakamura Y, Kiss S, Nealen ML, Barrick S, Kanai AJ, Wang E, Ruiz G, De Groat WC, Apodaca G, Watkins S, Caterina MJ. Altered urinary bladder function in mice lacking the vanilloid receptor TRPV1. Nat Neurosci 2002; 5:856–860.
93. Marinelli S, Di Marzo V, Berretta N, Matias I, Maccarrone M, Bernardi G, Mercuri NB. Presynaptic facilitation of glutamatergic synapses to dopaminergic neurons of the rat substantia nigra by endogenous stimulation of vanilloid receptors. J Neurosci 2003; 23:3136–3144.
94. Helliwell RJ, McLatchie LM, Clarke M, Winter J, Bevan S, McIntyre P. Capsaicin sensitivity is associated with the expression of the vanilloid (capsaicin) receptor (VR1) mRNA in adult rat sensory ganglia. Neurosci Lett 1998; 250:177–180.
95. Michael GJ, Priestley JV. Differential expression of the mRNA for the vanilloid receptor subtype 1 in cells of the adult rat dorsal root and nodose ganglia and its downregulation by axotomy. J Neurosci 1999; 19:1844–1854.
96. Ji RR, Samad TA, Jin SX, Schmoll R, Woolf CJ. p38 MAPK activation by NGF in primary sensory neurons after inflammation increases TRPV1 levels maintains heat hyperalgesia. Neuron 2002; 36:57–68.
97. Guo A, Vulchanova L, Wang J, Li X, Elde R. Immunocytochemical localization of the vanilloid receptor 1 (VR1): relationship to neuropeptides, the P2X3 purinoceptor and IB4 binding sites. Eur J Neurosci 1999; 11:946–958.

98. Nakatsuka T, Furue H, Yoshimura M, Gu JG. Activation of central terminal vanilloid receptor-1 receptors and alpha beta-methylene-ATP-sensitive P2X receptors reveals a converged synaptic activity onto the deep dorsal horn neurons of the spinal cord. J Neurosci 2002; 22:1228–1237.

99. Doyle MW, Bailey TW, Jin YH, Andresen MC. Vanilloid receptors presynaptically modulate cranial visceral afferent synaptic transmission in nucleus tractus solitarius. J Neurosci 2002; 22:8222–8229.

100. Olah Z, Szabo T, Karai L, Hough C, Fields RD, Caudle RM, Blumberg PM, Iadarola MJ. Ligand-induced dynamic membrane changes and cell deletion conferred by vanilloid receptor 1. J Biol Chem 2001; 276:11021–11030.

101. Liu M, Liu MC, Magoulas C, Priestley JV, Willmott NJ. Versatile regulation of cytosolic Ca^{2+} by vanilloid receptor 1 in rat dorsal root ganglion neurons. J Biol Chem 2003; 278:5462–5472.

102. Noguchi K, Morita Y, Kiyama H, Ono K, Tohyama M. A noxious stimulus induces the preprotachykinin—a gene expression in the rat dorsal root ganglion: a quantitative study using in situ hybridization histochemistry. Brain Res 1988; 464:31–35.

103. Woolf CJ, Safieh-Garabedian B, Ma QP, Crilly P, Winter J. Nerve growth factor contributes to the generation of inflammatory sensory hypersensitivity. Neuroscience 1994; 62:327–331.

104. Ji RR, Zhang Q, Law PY, Low HH, Elde R, Hokfelt T. Expression of mu-, delta-, and kappa-opioid receptor-like immunoreactivities in rat dorsal root ganglia after carrageenan-induced inflammation. J Neurosci 1995; 15:8156–8166.

105. Ganju P, O'Bryan JP, Der C, Winter J, James IF. Differential regulation of SHC proteins by nerve growth factor in sensory neurons and PC12 cells. Eur J Neurosci 1998; 10:1995–2008.

106. Voilley N, de Weille J, Mamet J, Lazdunski M. Nonsteroid anti-inflammatory drugs inhibit both the activity and the inflammation-induced expression of acid-sensing ion channels in nociceptors. J Neurosci 2001; 21:8026–8033.

107. Shu XQ, Mendell LM. Neurotrophins and hyperalgesia. Proc Natl Acad Sci USA 1999; 96:7693–7696.

108. Lindsay RM, Harmar AJ. Nerve growth factor regulates expression of neuropeptide genes in adult sensory neurons. Nature 1989; 337:362–364.

109. Leslie TA, Emson PC, Dowd PM, Woolf CJ. Nerve growth factor contributes to the up-regulation of growth-associated protein 43 and preprotachykinin A messenger RNAs in primary sensory neurons following peripheral inflammation. Neuroscience 1995; 67:753–761.

110. Mannion RJ, Costigan M, Decosterd I, Amaya F, Ma QP, Holstege JC, Ji RR, Acheson A, Lindsay RM, Wilkinson GA, Woolf CJ. Neurotrophins: peripherally and centrally acting modulators of tactile stimulus-induced inflammatory pain hypersensitivity. Proc Natl Acad Sci USA 1999; 96:9385–9390.

111. Bonini S, Lambiase A, Bonini S, Angelucci F, Magrini L, Manni L, Aloe L. Circulating nerve growth factor levels are increased in humans with allergic diseases and asthma. Proc Natl Acad Sci USA 1996; 93:10955–10960.

112. Carr MJ, Hunter DD, Undem BJ. Neurotrophins and asthma. Curr Opin Pulm Med 2001; 7:1–7.
113. Winter J, Forbes CA, Sternberg J, Lindsay RM. Nerve growth factor (NGF) regulates adult rat cultured dorsal root ganglion neuron responses to the excitotoxin capsaicin. Neuron 1988; 1:973–981.
114. Winston J, Toma H, Shenoy M, Pasricha PJ. Nerve growth factor regulates VR-1 mRNA levels in cultures of adult dorsal root ganglion neurons. Pain 2001; 89:181–186.
115. Story GM, Peier AM, Reeve AJ, Eid SR, Mosbacher J, Hricik TR, Earley TJ, Hergarden AC, Andersson DA, Hwang SW, McIntyre P, Jegla T, Bevan S, Patapoutian A. ANKTM1, a TRP-like channel expressed in nociceptive neurons, is activated by cold temperatures. Cell 2003; 112:819–829.
116. Bonnington JK, McNaughton PA. Signalling pathways involved in the sensitisation of mouse nociceptive neurones by nerve growth factor. J Physiol. 2003; 551(pt 2):433–446.
117. Shelhamer JH, Levine SJ, Wu T, Jacoby DB, Kaliner MA, Rennard SI. NIH conference. Airway inflammation. Ann Intern Med 1995; 123:288–304.
118. Holtzman MJ. Arachidonic acid metabolism in airway epithelial cells. Annu Rev Physiol 1992; 54:303–329.
119. Drazen JM, Israel E, O'Byrne PM. Treatment of asthma with drugs modifying the leukotriene pathway. N Engl J Med 1999; 340:197–206.
120. Harrison S, Geppetti P. Substance P. Int J Biochem Cell Biol 2001; 33: 555–576.
121. Lynch KR, O'Neill GP, Liu Q, Im DS, Sawyer N, Metters KM, Coulombe N, Abramovitz M, Figueroa DJ, Zeng Z, Connolly BM, Bai C, Austin CP, Chateauneuf A, Stocco R, Greig GM, Kargman S, Hooks SB, Hosfield E, Williams DL Jr, Ford-Hutchinson AW, Caskey CT, Evans JF. Characterization of the human cysteinyl leukotriene CysLT1 receptor. Nature 1999; 399:789–793.
122. Thodeti CK, Adolfsson J, Juhas M, Sjolander A. Leukotriene D$_4$ triggers an association between gbetagamma subunits and phospholipase C-gamma1 in intestinal epithelial cells. J Biol Chem 2000; 275:9849–9853.
123. Reilly CA, Taylor JL, Lanza DL, Carr BA, Crouch DJ, Yost GS. Capsaicinoids cause inflammation and epithelial cell death through activation of vanilloid receptors. Toxicol Sci 2003; 73:170–181.
124. Veronesi B, Oortgiesen M, Carter JD, Devlin RB. Particulate matter initiates inflammatory cytokine release by activation of capsaicin and acid receptors in a human bronchial epithelial cell line. Toxicol Appl Pharmacol 1999; 154: 106–115.
125. Denda M, Fuziwara S, Inoue K, Denda S, Akamatsu H, Tomitaka A, Matsunaga K. Immunoreactivity of VR1 on epidermal keratinocyte of human skin. Biochem Biophys Res Commun 2001; 285:1250–1252.
126. McKemy DD, Neuhausser WM, Julius D. Identification of a cold receptor reveals a general role for TRP channels in thermosensation. Nature 2002; 416:52–58.
127. Peier AM, Moqrich A, Hergarden AC, Reeve AJ, Andersson DA, Story GM, Earley TJ, Dragoni I, McIntyre P, Bevan S, Patapoutian A. A TRP channel that senses cold stimuli and menthol. Cell 2002; 108:705–715.

128. Nauli SM, Alenghat FJ, Luo Y, Williams E, Vassilev P, Li X, Elia AE, Lu W, Brown EM, Quinn SJ, Ingber DE, Zhou J. Polycystins 1 and 2 mediate mechanosensation in the primary cilium of kidney cells. Nat Genet 2003; 33:129–137.

129. Ong AC, Ward CJ, Butler RJ, Biddolph S, Bowker C, Torra R, Pei Y, Harris PC. Coordinate expression of the autosomal dominant polycystic kidney disease proteins, polycystin-2 and polycystin-1, in normal and cystic tissue. Am J Pathol 1999; 154:1721–1729.

130. Sweeney M, Yu Y, Platoshyn O, Zhang S, McDaniel SS, Yuan JX. Inhibition of endogenous TRP1 decreases capacitative Ca^{2+} entry and attenuates pulmonary artery smooth muscle cell proliferation. Am J Physiol Lung Cell Mol Physiol 2002; 283:L144–L155.

131. Yu Y, Sweeney M, Zhang S, Platoshyn O, Landsberg J, Rothman A, Yuan JX. PDGF stimulates pulmonary vascular smooth muscle cell proliferation by upregulating TRPC6 expression. Am J Physiol Cell Physiol 2003; 284: C316–C330.

132. Tiruppathi C, Freichel M, Vogel SM, Paria BC, Mehta D, Flockerzi V, Malik AB. Impairment of store-operated Ca^{2+} entry in TRPC4($-/-$) mice interferes with increase in lung microvascular permeability. Circ Res 2002; 91: 70–76.

133. Tiruppathi C, Minshall RD, Paria BC, Vogel SM, Malik AB. Role of Ca^{2+} signaling in the regulation of endothelial permeability. Vascul Pharmacol 2002; 39:173–185.

2

Afferent Pathways Regulating the Cough Reflex

BRENDAN J. CANNING

Johns Hopkins Asthma and Allergy Center,
Baltimore, Maryland, U.S.A.

STUART B. MAZZONE

Department of Neurobiology, Howard Florey
Institute, University of Melbourne,
Melbourne, Victoria, Australia

Introduction

Coughing occurs as a consequence of aspiration, particulate matter, pathogens, accumulated secretions, inflammation, and mediators associated with inflammation. The elderly, newborns, lung transplant patients, and patients with paralysis or neuromuscular disorders have a poorly developed and/or compromised cough reflex and are rendered highly susceptible to lung infections and aspiration pneumonia (1–4). Under normal conditions, therefore, coughing serves an important protective role in the airways and lungs. In diseases such as asthma, chronic obstructive pulmonary disease, gastroesophageal reflux disease, and rhinitis, however, cough may become excessive and nonproductive, and is potentially harmful to the airway mucosa (4). These contrasting consequences of coughing highlight the difficulty associated with developing therapeutic strategies that prevent excessive and nonproductive cough, while preserving the important innate defensive role of this respiratory reflex.

A thorough understanding of the afferent neuronal pathways regulating cough would likely facilitate development of specific therapeutic interventions that reduce the excessive coughing associated with disease. Our current understanding of the afferent neuronal pathways regulating the cough reflex is derived almost entirely from studies in animals. In these studies, conclusive evidence that vagal afferent nerves are responsible for initiating the cough reflex has been provided (5–10). Afferent nerves innervating other viscera as well as somatosensory nerves innervating the chest wall, diaphragm, and abdominal musculature also likely play a less essential but important accessory role in regulating cough. In this chapter the classes of vagal afferent nerves innervating the airways and their role in regulating the cough reflex will be defined.

Classification of Airway Afferent Nerve Subtypes

Airway afferent nerve subtypes are abundant in the airway mucosa and in the airway wall and can be differentiated based on their physicochemical sensitivity, adaptation to sustained lung inflation, neurochemistry, origin, myelination, conduction velocity, and sites of termination in the airways (Fig. 1). The utility of each of these approaches for defining airway afferent nerve subtypes is limited in large part by the lack of specificity of the various characteristics studied (5–21). When used in combination, however, these attributes can be used in all species thus far studied to identify at least three broad classes of airway afferent nerves: rapidly adapting receptors (RARs), slowly adapting receptors (SARs), and unmyelinated C-fibers (Fig. 2). The attributes of these subtypes of airway afferent nerves are summarized in Table 1.

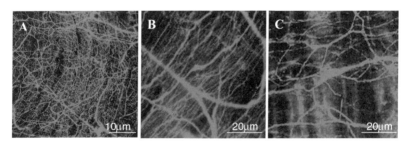

Figure 1   Wholemounts of (**A**) rat trachea, (**B**) guinea pig trachea, and (**C**) human bronchus stained immunohistochemically with antisera to the nonspecific neuronal marker protein gene product 9.5 (PGP 9.5). A dense neuronal plexus found beneath and within the airway epithelium of all species studied occupies this region of the airway mucosa. The afferent nerves regulating cough likely reside in this plexus.

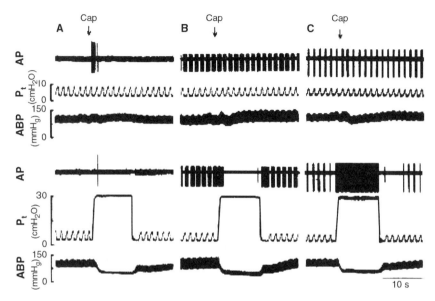

Figure 2 Representative traces of single-unit recordings from airway vagal afferent nerve subtypes in anesthetized rats. (**A**) Airway C-fibers are quiescent during tidal breathing and are relatively unresponsive to lung inflation. However, C-fibers respond vigorously to intravenously injected capsaicin. (**B**) RARs and (**C**) SARs are sporadically active during the respiratory cycle. Neither subtype of mechanoreceptor responds to capsaicin, but both respond intensely when the lungs are inflated. Note that RARs are easily differentiated from SARs by their rapid adaptation during sustained lung inflation. (Modified from Ref. 13.)

Properties of Airway Afferent Nerve Subtypes and Their Potential Role in Regulating Cough

Rapidly Adapting Receptors

The anatomical arrangement of RAR terminations in the airway wall is unknown. Functional studies suggest that RARs terminate within or beneath the epithelium and are localized to both intra- and extrapulmonary airways (11–17). RARs are differentiated from other airway afferent nerves by their rapid (1–2 sec) adaptation to sustained lung inflations (Fig. 2) (13–19). Other distinguishing properties of RARs include their sensitivity to lung collapse and/or lung deflation, their responsiveness to alterations in dynamic lung compliance (and thus their sensitivity to bronchospasm), and their conduction velocity (4–18 m/sec, suggestive of small myelinated axons) (11–21). The sustained activation of RARs produced by dynamic lung inflation, bronchospasm, or lung collapse indicates that the adaptation of RARs to sustained lung inflation is not attributable to an electrophysiological

Table 1 Properties of Vagal Afferent Nerve Subtypes Innervating the Airways

	RARs	SARs	C-fibers
Electrophysiological properties			
Conduction velocity (m/sec)	14–23	15–32	0.8–1.5
Myelination	Yes	Yes	No
Eupneic activity (impulses/sec)	0–20	10–40	0.3–1.5
Morphological properties			
Neuropeptide synthesis	No	No	Yes
Innervation of large airways[a]	Yes	Sparse	Yes
Innervation of small airways	Yes	Yes	Yes
Physical sensitivity			
Mechanical threshold	Low	Low	High
Lung deflation[a]	Activated	Inactivated	No effect
Edema	Increased	No effect	Increased
Chemical sensitivity[a]			
CO_2	No effect	Decreased	Increased
H^+	Increased	No effect	Increased
Capsaicin[a]	Increased[b]	No effect	Increased[c]
Bradykinin[a]	Increased[b]	No effect	Increased[c]
Reflex effects			
Parasympathetic	Excitatory	Inhibitory	Excitatory
Respiratory	Hyperpnea	Inhibit inspiration	Apnea
Axon reflex	No	No	Yes

[a]Typical attributes of the afferent nerve subtypes are listed. Species differences and subtypes of each class with distinct physiological properties and responsiveness have been reported.
[b]Activation of RARs by capsaicin and bradykinin is prevented by bronchodilator pretreatment, suggesting that activation occurs secondary to obstruction in the lung.
[c]C-fiber activation by bradykinin and capsaicin is enhanced by bronchodilators such as adrenaline, adenosine, and PGE, suggesting that agents directly stimulate C-fibers in the airways. See text for further details and references.

adaptation (11,13,20,21). Perhaps RARs are thus better defined as dynamic receptors that respond to changes in airway mechanical properties (e.g., diameter, length, interstitial pressures).

RARs are sporadically active throughout the respiratory cycle (Fig. 2), activated by the dynamic mechanical forces accompanying lung inflation and deflation and becoming more active as the rate and volume of lung inflation increase (13,20,21). It follows, therefore, that RAR activity during respiration correlates to respiratory rate and is higher in guinea pigs and rats (16–27 impulses/sec) and almost unmeasurable in larger animals such as dogs (<1–5 impulses/sec). It also follows that, at least in smaller animals, RAR-dependent reflexes require a heightened activity in the already active RARs.

RARs are generally insensitive to many "direct" chemical stimuli (Fig. 2). However, RAR activity can be increased by stimuli that evoke bronchospasm or obstruction resulting from mucus secretion or edema (11,14,15,19,22–27). Substances such as histamine, capsaicin, substance P, and bradykinin activate RARs in a way that can be markedly inhibited or abolished by preventing the local end-organ effects that these stimuli produce (e.g. mucus secretion, bronchospasm). This sensitivity of RARs to bronchospasm becomes critical when interpreting the ability of stimuli such as capsaicin or bradykinin to evoke coughing in animals and in human subjects (see later).

RARs respond to stimuli that evoke cough and fulfill many of the accepted criteria for mediating cough (5,8,14,17,28–30). Further evidence of their role in the cough reflex comes from studies of vagal cooling, which blocks cough at temperatures that selectively abolish activity in myelinated fibers (including RARs) while preserving C-fiber activity (14,29,30). Surprisingly, however, many stimuli that are extremely effective at activating RARs [e.g., thromboxane, leukotriene C_4 (LTC_4), histamine, neurokinins, and methacholine] are ineffective or only modestly effective at evoking cough (14,31–34). Moreover, it is difficult to reconcile the observation that RARs are spontaneously activate throughout the respiratory cycle in many species and yet cough is only induced under special circumstances and in response to very specific stimuli. This indicates that if RARs are indeed responsible for regulating cough, their pattern of activation must be changed or a specific subset of RARs must be recruited in response to a stimulus that results in coughing. Alternatively, RARs may act synergistically with other afferent nerve subtypes to induce coughing.

Slowly Adapting Stretch Receptors

SARs are highly sensitive to the mechanical forces put upon the lung during breathing. SAR activity increases sharply during the inspiratory phase and peaks just prior to the initiation of expiration (Fig. 2) (13,35). SARs are thus believed to be the primary afferent fibers involved in the Hering–Breuer reflex, which terminates inspiration and initiates expiration when the lungs are adequately inflated (35). SARs can be differentiated from RARs in some species based on action potential conduction velocity, and in most species by their lack of adaptation during sustained lung inflations.

SARs may also be differentially distributed throughout the airways (35). In cats, guinea pigs, and rats, few, if any, SARs but many RAR-like receptors and C-fibers can be found in the extrapulmonary airways. Rather, SARs appear to be associated with the smooth muscle of the intrapulmonary airways (in dogs, SARs may also be localized to extrapulmonary airways). SARs also differ from RARs with respect to the reflexes they precipitate. SAR activation results in central inhibition of respiration and inhibition of cholinergic drive to the airways, leading to decreased phrenic nerve activity and decreased airway smooth muscle tone (due to withdrawal of cholinergic nerve activity) (25,35,36).

Yu et al. (37) recently perfected a technique for morphologically defining the structure of electrophysiologically identified SARs innervating the intrapulmonary airways and lungs of rabbits. The sensory terminals of SARs assume a complex and varying position within the airway wall. Most of these SARs were found in the peripheral airways (associated with alveoli or bronchioles). Occasionally, but not uniformly, SAR dendritic arbors were associated with the bronchiolar smooth muscle. This contrasts with the SARs innervating the trachealis in dogs, which are intimately associated with the smooth muscle and are activated during bronchoconstriction (38). As mentioned before, however, cats, guinea pigs, rabbits, and rats appear to have few, if any, SARs in their extrapulmonary airways (35).

Single-unit recordings from the vagus nerve in rabbits suggest that SAR activity does not increase prior to or during ammonia-induced coughing (9). Although this suggests that SARs are unlikely to play a primary role in the cough reflex, their profound influence over respiratory pattern makes it likely that they influence coughing reflexes and other airway defensive reflexes. It has been proposed, for example, that enhancing baseline SAR activity with the loop diuretic furosemide may account for the reported antitussive effects of this agent in animals and in human subjects (39). In contrast, preloading, which will likely increase baseline SAR activity, has been reported to increase expiratory efforts during cough (40,41). Conversely, experiments performed on rabbits in which inhaled sulfur dioxide has been used in an attempt to selectively block SAR activity show that the cough reflex is coincidentally attenuated (8,42). However, it must be noted that the selectivity of sulfur dioxide for airway SARs is questionable since several reports indicate an excitatory action of sulfur dioxide on airway C-fibers (43,44). C-fiber activation may be inhibitory to cough (see later).

Studies of CNS processing also suggest that SARs may facilitate coughing. It has been proposed that a central cough network exists in which SARs facilitate cough via activation of brainstem second-order neurons (termed pump cells) of the SAR reflex pathway (6). In this model, SARs, through activation of pump cells, open an as yet unidentified "gate" in the brainstem that is thought to promote cough. However, an excitatory role for pump cells in cough is difficult to reconcile with studies showing that SARs (via pump cells) inhibit other RAR-mediated reflex pathways (25,45). Clearly, much about the role of SARs in coughing remains poorly defined.

C-Fibers

Unmyelinated afferent C-fibers are similar in many ways to the unmyelinated nociceptors of the somatic nervous system and comprise the majority of afferent nerves innervating the airways (18,46,47). In addition to their conduction velocity, afferent C-fibers are distinguished from RARs and SARs by their relative insensitivity to mechanical stimulation and lung inflation and their responsiveness to bradykinin and capsaicin (Fig. 2) (12,13,15,16,23,25,46). Afferent C-fibers are further distinguished from RARs by the observation that bradykinin- and capsaicin-evoked activation of their endings in the airways is not inhibited by pretreatment with bronchodilators. On the contrary, bronchodilators such as prostaglandin E_2 (PGE_2), adrenaline, and adenosine may enhance the excitability of airway C-fibers (46,48,49). Unlike their effects on RARs, then, substances such as bradykinin and capsaicin directly activate bronchopulmonary C-fibers.

Morphological studies in rats (Fig. 3) and in guinea pigs reveal that C-fiber afferent nerves innervate the airway epithelium as well as other effector structures within the airway wall (12,50–52). C-fibers may synthesize neuropeptides that are subsequently transported to their central and peripheral nerve terminals (12,50,52,53). This unique neurochemical property of bronchopulmonary C-fibers has been exploited to describe the distribution and peripheral nerve terminals of these unmyelinated airway afferent nerve endings. Although the expression of neuropeptides in their peripheral afferent nerve terminals may be species dependent, it seems likely that C-fibers innervating the airways of other species are morphologically (if not neurochemically) similar to those well characterized in guinea pigs and rats (51,54,55).

In dogs, airway afferent C-fibers may be further subdivided into bronchial and pulmonary C-fibers, a distinction based both on sites of termination and on responsiveness to chemical and mechanical stimuli (18). Notably, pulmonary C-fibers in dogs may be unresponsive to histamine, while bronchial C-fibers are activated by histamine. Whether similar physiological distinctions between bronchial and pulmonary afferent C-fibers can be defined in other species is not known. In guinea pigs, histamine appears to have no effect on bronchopulmonary C-fibers. Undem and colleagues (56,57) have recently described C-fiber subtypes innervating the intrapulmonary airways and lungs of mice and guinea pigs. In guinea pigs, C-fiber subtypes may be distinguished based on their ganglionic origin and sites of termination in the airways. C-fibers arising from the jugular ganglia in guinea pigs innervate

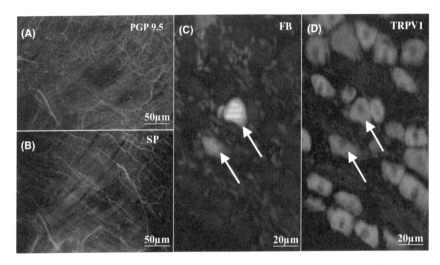

Figure 3 Neurokinin-containing C-fibers innervate the rat tracheal mucosa. Double-labeling immunohistochemistry with antisera for (**A**) the nonspecific neuronal marker PGP 9.5 and (**B**) substance P (SP) in wholemounts of rat trachea. Substance P-containing nerve fibers occupy a dense neuronal plexus beneath and within the airway epithelium. The majority of the nerves in this epithelial plexus in rats are C-fibers. (**C**) Retrograde neuronal tracing with fast blue (FB) indicates that the perikarya of the tracheal afferent nerves are located in vagal sensory ganglia. (**D**) Many of the retrogradely labeled neurons stain for TRPV1, the capsaicin receptor.

both intrapulmonary and extrapulmonary airways and almost uniformly express the neuropeptides substance P and calcitonin gene-related peptide (CGRP). These C-fibers are not activated by adenosine triphosphate (ATP), 5-hydroxytryptamine (5-HT), or adenosine but are readily activated by capsaicin, bradykinin, and acid. By contrast, C-fibers with cell bodies in the nodose ganglia terminate almost exclusively in the intrapulmonary airways. These C-fibers do not express substance P under normal conditions, and are activated by capsaicin, bradykinin, ATP, adenosine, and 5-HT. In mice, ATP activates all C-fibers, whereas capsaicin and bradykinin activate only a subset of the identified bronchopulmonary C-fibers. What if any differences exist in reflex effects initiated by activation of these C-fiber subtypes is not clear.

Afferent C-fibers likely play a key role in airway defensive reflexes. Although C-fiber endings are polymodal and thus respond to both chemical and mechanical stimulation, their threshold for mechanical activation is substantially higher then that of RARs and SARs (9,10). Accordingly, C-fibers are generally quiescent throughout the respiratory cycle but are activated by chemical stimuli such as capsaicin, bradykinin, citric acid, hypertonic saline, and sulfur dioxide (12,13,16,18,23,44,46). Reflex responses evoked by C-fiber activation include increased airway parasympathetic nerve activity and the chemoreflex, characterized by apnea (followed by rapid shallow breathing), bradycardia, and hypotension (18,25,46). In some species (particularly rats and guinea pigs) C-fiber activation evokes peripheral release of neuropeptides (via an axon reflex) leading to bronchospasm and neurogenic inflammation (46,58).

Several lines of evidence support the hypothesis that activation of airway C-fibers precipitates cough. Putatively selective stimulants of airway C-fibers such as capsaicin, bradykinin, and citric acid evoke cough in conscious animals and in humans (7,18,22,59–62). Capsaicin desensitization abolishes citric acid-induced coughing in conscious guinea pigs, but has no effect on cough evoked by mechanical probing of the airway mucosa in these same animals (59). Finally, pharmacological studies which take advantage of the unique expression of neurokinins by airway C-fibers have shown that bradykinin-, citric acid-, and capsaicin-induced cough in cats and guinea pigs is attenuated or abolished by neurokinin receptor antagonists (61,62; also see Chapter 4 in this volume).

Although the evidence summarized above supports a role for C-fibers in the cough reflex, there is also considerable evidence to indicate that airway C-fibers do not evoke cough and may actually inhibit cough evoked by RAR stimulation. In anesthetized animals, for example, C-fiber stimulation has consistently failed to evoke coughing, even though cough can be induced in these animals by mechanically probing the airway mucosa (5,10,28–30,47,63). Indeed, systemic administration of C-fiber stimulants has been shown to inhibit cough evoked by RAR stimulation in various species (5,28–30,63). The fact that vagal cooling to temperatures that can preserve C-fiber-dependent reflexes can abolish cough is further evidence against a role for C-fibers in cough (5,29,30).

It is unclear why so much conflicting evidence about C-fibers in cough has been reported. Perhaps general anesthesia selectively disrupts the ability of C-fibers to evoke cough in animals without adversely affecting cough induced by RAR stimulation. General anesthesia has a profound influence over the cough reflex (64). Alternatively, since coughing in anesthetized animals is typically studied following tracheotomy with stimuli delivered to lower airways, larynx, and trachea, perhaps C-fiber-dependent coughing is evoked from or requires airflow through the bypassed airways. It is unlikely, however, that anesthesia prevents C-fiber activation and C-fiber-mediated reflex effects entirely. C-fibers are readily activated in anesthetized animals and can precipitate profound cardiopulmonary reflexes (18,23,25), (65–68). Rather, anesthesia must selectively inhibit cough-related neural pathways or may act by accentuating the inhibitory effects of C-fiber activation on cough. Alternatively, general anesthesia may interfere with the conscious perception of airway irritation and the resulting urge to cough. In this context, it is interesting that capsaicin-evoked cough can be consciously suppressed in human subjects (69). Yet an equally viable hypothesis is that C-fiber stimulation alone is simply insufficient to evoke cough but depends upon airway afferent nerve interactions both in the periphery and at the level of the central nervous system (see later).

Other Airway Afferent Nerve Subtypes

Not all airway afferent nerves fit into the three classes of nerves just described. In guinea pigs (commonly used to study cough), a second type of nociceptor-like afferent nerve has been described in vitro (12,20,52,53,63). Extracellular recording in the vagal sensory ganglia of guinea pigs indicates that about half of the tracheal afferent nerves responsive to both bradykinin and capsaicin are small myelinated $A\delta$-fibers (12). Physiologically, these myelinated airway nociceptors resemble the myelinated nociceptors described in somatic tissues (70). The guinea pig tracheal $A\delta$-nociceptors have their cell bodies in the jugular ganglia and are distinguished from RAR-like $A\delta$-fibers innervating the guinea pig trachea, which have their cell bodies in the nodose ganglia. Compared with the jugular $A\delta$-fibers, nodose-derived RARs are utterly unresponsive to direct stimulation by either capsaicin or bradykinin in vitro and are 15-fold more sensitive to mechanical stimulation. The adaptation index (a measurement of afferent responsiveness to sustained mechanical stimulation) of these fibers also differs considerably. McAlexander et al. (20) reported that the nodose-derived RARs had an adaptation index that averaged 95 ± 2, whereas the adaptation index of the jugular $A\delta$-fibers was comparable to the adaptation index of tracheal/bronchial C-fibers in the preparation, averaging 46 ± 8. Histological analyses reveal that, like C-fibers, $A\delta$-nociceptors innervating the guinea pig trachea express the capsaicin receptor TRPV1 (VR1) but, unlike airway C-fibers, do not synthesize neuropeptides (12,52,53). These myelinated nociceptors likely innervate the epithelium but are confined almost exclusively to the extrapulmonary airways.

The role of $A\delta$-nociceptors in airway homeostatic and defensive reflexes, and whether these afferent nerve subtypes are unique to the guinea pig trachea, is not known. No such fibers have been described in rats or dogs. Whether this is reflective of their peculiarity to the guinea pig or that myelinated, nociceptor-like fibers innervating the airways of other species have been excluded from published analyses is also not known. It is interesting, however, that about half of the RARs studied in other species are responsive to capsaicin (16,22).

Subtypes of RARs and SARs have also been proposed (13–15,18,35,71,72). Differences in the airway segments innervated and not differences in the physiological properties of the SARs and RARs likely account in part for some of the subtypes described. In other instances, it could be argued that the evidence for SAR and RAR subtypes is more an argument of semantics than physiology. For example, Bergren and Peterson (72) and Ho et al. (13) both described a population of myelinated afferent nerves innervating the airways of rats that were activated vigorously by lung deflation yet adapted rapidly to sustained lung inflation. These afferent nerves, which were active throughout the respiratory cycle, appeared to be physiologically identical in every way and yet Bergren and Peterson (72) classified these fibers as SARs while Ho et al. (13) called them RARs. Such divergent interpretations of essentially identical data by experienced investigators highlight the importance of establishing universal criteria for identifying airway afferent nerve subtypes.

Evidence for a "Cough Receptor"

The conflicting evidence that either C-fibers or RARs regulate the cough reflex makes it reasonable to hypothesize that a previously unrecognized subtype of airway afferent nerve—cough receptors—plays the primary role in regulating this defensive reflex. Studies in guinea pigs support this notion. Selective nerve cuts and a comprehensive analysis of the stimuli that evoke coughing and afferent nerve activation in guinea pigs indicate that tracheal, laryngeal, and bronchial afferent nerves primarily responsible for regulating the cough reflex arise from the nodose ganglia (63). These afferent nerves are polymodal, being activated by punctate mechanical stimuli, acid, and the potassium channel blocker 4-aminopyridine (12,73,74). However, they are unresponsive to capsaicin, bradykinin, or hypertonic saline and do not express TRPV1, the capsaicin receptor (12,53,73,74; also see Chapter 1). These putative cough receptors are myelinated and do not synthesize and express neuropeptides under normal conditions (12,53).

Their myelination and insensitivity to capsaicin clearly differentiate the putative cough receptors from bronchopulmonary C-fibers. Because they are myelinated and adapt rapidly to a punctate mechanical stimulation, it is tempting to conclude that the cough receptors are merely RARs that innervate the extrapulmonary airways. However, there are a number of attributes and observations that clearly distinguish the cough receptors from the classically defined RARs. Unlike RARs, the putative cough receptors are utterly unresponsive to a wide variety of spasmogens and autacoids that induce airway smooth muscle contraction, including methacholine, histamine, LTC$_4$, substance P, neurokinin A, 5-HT, ATP, and adenosine (12,53). All of these stimuli have been shown to activate RARs and yet none of them are effective or only modestly effective at inducing cough (11,14,31–34). Cough receptors, unlike RARs (13,14), are also unresponsive to changes in luminal pressure, even pressures changes exceeding -100 to $100\,\mathrm{cm}$ H$_2$O. The cough receptors may also be distinguished from RARs based on conduction velocity. Cough receptors innervating the larynx, trachea, and bronchus of guinea pigs conduct action potentials at 5 m/sec, whereas intrapulmonary RARs in guinea pigs conduct action potentials at a much faster rate, upward of 15 m/sec (11,12).

Using the styryl dye FM2-10 (75), we have identified the receptive fields of putative cough receptors innervating the guinea pig tracheal and bronchial mucosa in situ in living tissue (Fig. 4). The putative cough receptors assume a stereotypical position in the airway wall, with complex dendritic arbors that are invariably arranged in a circumferential pattern in the airway mucosa. These endings (approximately four per tracheal ring, approximately 150–200 along the entire length of the guinea pig trachea) are located in the mucosa, above the smooth muscle (which likely accounts for their insensitivity to smooth muscle constriction) but below the

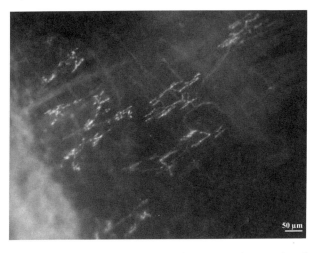

Figure 4 Intravital labeling of putative cough receptors innervating the bronchial mucosa of guinea pigs using the styryl dye FM2-10. The cough receptors are selectively labeled by FM2-10 (compare the unique structure of these afferent nerve endings with the nerve fibers in Figs. 1 and 3). These endings arise from the nodose ganglia and are readily activated by punctate mechanical stimuli and acid but are insensitive to stretch, smooth muscle constriction, capsaicin, or bradykinin (24). The receptive fields of the cough receptors assume a characteristic position in the mucosa, above the smooth muscle and below the epithelium (note the intact epithelium in the living wholemount in the bottom left corner of the photomicrograph). Approximately four to six receptive fields per cartilage ring are labeled using the styryl dye (200–300 receptors over the entire trachea and mainstem bronchi of guinea pigs). Comparable staining of rat airways reveals that this rodent species has few if any cough receptors (less than 10 in the entire trachea) in the tracheal or bronchial mucosa. Not surprisingly then, neither electrical ($n = 5$) nor mechanical ($n = 5$) stimulation of the tracheal or laryngeal mucosa of rats evokes coughing while both of these stimuli readily initiate coughing in guinea pigs. See text for further details.

epithelium. The left and right vagus nerves contribute approximately equal numbers of these receptors, with terminals located primarily ipsilateral to their vagal origin. The terminal adhesions of the cough receptors and the characteristic orientation within the tissue indicate that they have attached to components in the extracellular matrix comprising the basement membrane. Comparable structures have been identified in the airway mucosa of fixed tissue using the osmium tetroxide staining method (76). Given that remodeling of the basement membrane occurs in disease (77), it is tempting to speculate that alterations in the composition and/or structure of the basement membrane may confer an altered responsiveness to tussive stimuli to the putative cough receptors.

FM2-10 labeling of the putative cough receptors has facilitated identification of a key regulatory mechanism of the excitability of these afferent nerves. We found that labeling with FM2-10 was absolutely dependent upon Na^+–K^+–ATPase activity. Subsequent immunohistochemical analyses revealed that the putative cough receptors, but not C-fibers, express an isozyme of the sodium pump containing the $\alpha 3$ subunit. This unique expression of this isozyme is of interest, given its association with mechanoreceptors and not C-fibers in the somatic nervous system (78). The intense and brilliant labeling of the cough receptors with FM2-10, which does not distinguish among sodium pump isozymes, indicates that sodium pump activity is particularly high in the putative cough receptor endings, suggesting an essential role in regulating their excitability. Indeed, ouabain potently and selectively inhibited coughing evoked by citric acid, mechanical stimulation, or electrical stimulation of the tracheal and laryngeal mucosa in anesthetized guinea pigs while having no effect on C-fiber-dependent reflexes evoked from the trachea. In vitro electrophysiological recordings confirm the potent and selective inhibitory effects of ouabain on the putative cough receptor. This inhibitory effect of ouabain on the cough receptors contrasts sharply with the ability of this compound to greatly enhance the excitability of SARs in the lung, baroreceptors, and mechanoreceptors innervating the renal artery (79–81).

Interactions Between Afferent Nerve Subtypes Evoking Cough

Peripheral Interactions

Activation of airway C-fibers, particularly by capsaicin, evokes axon reflex-dependent peripheral release of the neuropeptides substance P, neurokinin A, and CGRP (58). Axon reflexes in the airways and lungs induce bronchospasm, vasodilatation, edema, leukocyte recruitment, mucus secretion, altered parasympathetic nerve activity, and stimulation of endothelial and epithelial cells (82–88) (Fig. 5). Peripheral neuropeptide release in the

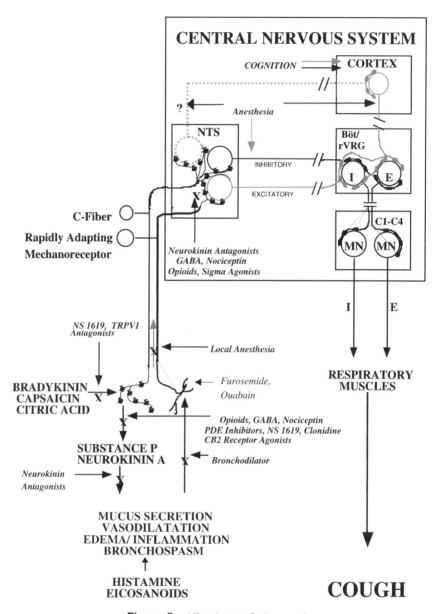

Figure 5   (*Caption on facing page*)

airways or administration of exogenous substance P has also been shown to activate RARs in rabbits and in guinea pigs (26,27,89). The neuropeptide-evoked RAR activation probably occurs secondary to actions on structural cells in the airway wall that in turn indirectly activate RARs (17,23,28). Capsaicin- and bradykinin-induced stimulation of RARs in anesthetized guinea pigs correlates with the increases in pulmonary insufflation pressure evoked by these agents. The associated increases in RAR activity can be substantially reduced or abolished by pretreating animals with isoprotere-nol, thereby preventing the obstruction produced by these agents (23). Not surprisingly, therefore, preventing the axon reflex with β-agonists, inhaled neurokinin receptor antagonists, or inhaled neutral endopeptidase (which enzymatically inactivates neurokinins and bradykinin) is effective at preventing cough evoked by capsaicin, cigarette smoke, bronchospasm, or the neutral endopeptidase inhibitor phosphoramidon (90–94).

It is not clear whether axon reflexes or any peripheral interactions between C-fibers and RARs play any role in defensive reflex responses in the airways of humans or in the airways of any species other than guinea pigs. In cats and dogs, bradykinin and capsaicin evoke bronchospasm, bronchial vasodilatation, and mucus secretion, but these responses can be prevented entirely with atropine or by vagotomy, indicating a CNS-depen-dent parasympathetic reflex, not an axon reflex (18,95,96). Similar findings have been reported in humans (97). Morphological and functional studies also indicate that the axon reflex is unlikely to play a prominent role in humans, as there are few substance P-containing nerve fibers in human air-ways and EFS-induced responses of human airway preparations in vitro have never been shown to be mediated by neurokinins (51,55,98–100).

Figure 5 (*Facing page*) Potential actions of and interactions between the afferent nerves mediating cough. RARs and capsaicin-sensitive C-fibers likely play an impor-tant role in regulating cough. C-fibers might initiate cough secondary to axon reflex-dependent activation of RARs. C-fibers might also mediate cough by acting syner-gistically with RARs at the level of the brainstem. C-fiber-mediated cough, but apparently not cough mediated by RAR activation, is highly sensitive to general anesthesia. Indeed, C-fiber activation under general anesthesia is inhibitory to cough reflexes initiated by RAR activation. Dashed lines indicate potential pathways and mechanisms regulating cough for which supporting or opposing evidence is limited. Likely sites of action for antitussive agents are indicated with in. Excitatory path-ways regulating cough are highlighted in gray; inhibitory pathways regulating cough are highlighted. See text for further details. *Abbreviations*: Böt/rVRG, Bötzinger complex/pre-Bötzinger complex/rostral ventral respiratory group; C1–C4, cervical spinal cord; CB, cannabinoid; E, expiratory related; GABA, gamma aminobutyric acid; I, inspiratory related; MN, motor neuron; NTS, nucleus tractus solitarii; PDE inhibitor, phosphodiesterase inhibitor (e.g., theophylline, rolipram). (Modified from Ref. 28.)

The apparent lack of the axon reflex in humans (and other species) notwithstanding, there are considerable data indicating that C-fiber activation is extremely effective at evoking cough. This would indicate that other mechanisms must underlie C-fiber-dependent coughing. It is possible that peripheral interactions between C-fibers and RARs may also proceed independent of axon reflexes (Fig. 2). For example, C-fiber activation evokes CNS-dependent parasympathetic reflex-induced bronchospasm, vasodilatation, and mucus secretion (18,25,46,65–67,95–97). These end-organ effects are mediated in large part by acetylcholine released from airway parasympathetic nerves and may be sufficient to activate RARs in the airway wall. That inhaled anticholinergics have some antitussive properties in animals and in human subjects is consistent with this notion (101,102).

Central Interactions

Central integration of airway afferent nerve input is poorly understood. Insights into how C-fibers and RARs might interact in the brainstem may be gained from studies in other systems, particularly the somatic nervous system. C-fibers and mechanoreceptors arising from somatic tissues interact in the spinal cord in a process known as central sensitization (47,103). The consequence of this central interaction manifests as a heightened reflex responsiveness and exaggerated sensations of pain following cutaneous stimulation. Studies of central sensitization in the spinal cord have revealed two features of the somatosensory system that facilitate this hyperreflexia. First, C-fiber and mechanoreceptor reflex pathways appear to converge through common integrative circuits in the spinal cord. Second, this convergent input can amplify afferent signaling following the coincident activation of both afferent nerve subtypes. The synergy and resulting hyperreflexia is often dependent on neurokinins released from the central terminals of somatosensory C-fibers, producing a long-lasting hyperexcitability of spinal integrative neurons (47,103).

Several lines of evidence suggest that a process similar to central sensitization may play a role in airway defensive reflexes (Fig. 5). The morphological, electrophysiological, and pharmacological properties of airway C-fibers and mechanoreceptors are similar to those in the somatic nervous system (12,13,18,47,103). Anatomical and functional studies have also shown considerable convergence of vagal afferents at sites of brainstem integration, particularly in the nucleus tractus solitarii (NTS) (104–106). As mentioned above, lung mechanoreceptors are sporadically active throughout the respiratory cycle, whereas C-fibers are typically quiescent, even during large lung inflations (13–18). The central processing of C-fiber afferent nerve activity must therefore be integrated into a reflex pathway that is continually receiving input from airway mechanoreceptors. C-fiber activation, via central interactions with RARs, may promote coughing by facilitating synaptic transmission at RAR relay neurons in the brainstem (Fig. 2). Indeed, substance P can facilitate synaptic transmission between lung afferents and NTS neurons in guinea pigs (107,108).

Direct evidence for central interactions between airway C-fibers and RARs in the regulation of airway parasympathetic tone has been documented (106). Activation of C-fibers in the lung evokes profound increases in cholinergic tone in the airways by facilitating airway mechanoreceptor activity in the brainstem. In the absence of airway mechanoreceptor activity, C-fibers are ineffective at evoking reflex responses. The facilitating effects of C-fibers on RAR reflex pathways in the brainstem appear to be mediated by neurokinins, since the central synergistic interactions are prevented entirely by neurokinin receptor antagonists administered intracerebroventricularly. The sensitizing effect of nociceptor stimulation can also be mimicked, in the absence of C-fiber stimulation, by administering substance P to the brainstem (106). Importantly, a comparable interaction between cough receptors and C-fibers has been documented in studies of coughing. Thus, in anesthetized guinea pigs, C-fiber activation does not evoke cough but greatly sensitizes the cough reflex evoked by activating the cough receptors. This sensitizing effect is prevented by neurokinin receptor antagonists (109).

Concluding Remarks

Studies carried out in animals provide clear evidence that vagal afferent nerves regulate coughing. It remains unclear, however, what relative role the identified afferent nerve subtypes play in mediating cough. Evidence both for and against the role of C-fibers and RARs has been reported. These conflicting data suggest that activation of both afferent nerve subtypes may be required to induce coughing, or that a previously unrecognized airway afferent nerve subtype subserves a primary role in cough. Recent studies in guinea pigs and circumstantial evidence gathered from the existing literature suggest that a cough receptor quite distinct from either C-fibers or RARs may exist. Moreover, these afferent nerve subtypes may interact to produce cough and heightened sensitivity to tussive stimuli. It seems imperative that future studies identify mechanisms of integration of afferent nerve input in the CNS, the role of consciousness and perception in coughing, and the mechanisms by which afferent nerves are activated.

References

1. Fleming PJ, Bryan AC, Bryan MH. Functional immaturity of pulmonary irritant receptors and apnea in newborn preterm infants. Pediatrics 1978; 61:515–518.

2. Schramm CM. Current concepts of respiratory complications of neuromuscular disorders in children. Curr Opin Pediatr 2000; 12:203–207.

3. Mosconi P, Langer M, Cigada M, Mandelli M. Epidemiology and risk factors of pneumonia in critically ill patients. Intensive care unit for infection control. Eur J Epidemiol 1991; 7:320–327.

4. Irwin RS, Boulet LP, Cloutier MM, Fuller R, Gold PM, Hoffstein V, Ing AJ, McCool FD, O'Byrne P, Poe RH, Prakash UB, Pratter MR, Rubin BK. Managing cough as a defense mechanism and as a symptom. A consensus panel report of the American College of Chest Physicians. Chest 1998; 114(suppl 2): 133S–181S.

5. Widdicombe JG. Afferent receptors in the airways and cough. Respir Physiol 1998; 114:5–15.

6. Shannon R, Baekey DM, Morris KF, Lindsey BG. Ventrolateral medullary respiratory network and a model of cough motor pattern generation. J Appl Physiol 1998; 84:2020–2035.

7. Karlsson JA. The role of capsaicin-sensitive C-fibre afferent nerves in the cough reflex. Pulm Pharmacol 1996; 9:315–321.

8. Sant'Ambrogio G, Sant'Ambrogio FB, Davies A. Airway receptors in cough. Bull Eur Physiopathol Respir 1984; 20:43–47.

9. Matsumoto S. The activities of lung stretch and irritant receptors during cough. Neurosci Lett 1988; 90:125–129.

10. Deep V, Singh M, Ravi K. Role of vagal afferents in the reflex effects of capsaicin and lobeline in monkeys. Respir Physiol 2001; 125:155–168.

11. Bergren DR, Sampson SR. Characterization of intrapulmonary, rapidly adapting receptors of guinea pigs. Respir Physiol 1982; 47:83–95.

12. Riccio MM, Kummer W, Biglari B, Myers AC, Undem BJ. Interganglionic segregation of distinct vagal afferent fibre phenotypes in guinea-pig airways. J Physiol 1996; 496:521–530.

13. Ho CY, Gu Q, Lin YS, Lee LY. Sensitivity of vagal afferent endings to chemical irritants in the rat lung. Respir Physiol 2001; 127:113–124.

14. Widdicombe J. Functional morphology and physiology of pulmonary rapidly adapting receptors (RARs). Anat Rec 2003; 270A(1):2–10.

15. Widdicombe J. Airway receptors. Respir Physiol 2001; 125:3–15.

16. Armstrong DJ, Luck JC. A comparative study of irritant and type J receptors in the cat. Respir Physiol 1974; 21:47–60.

17. Sant'Ambrogio G, Widdicombe J. Reflexes from airway rapidly adapting receptors. Respir Physiol 2001; 125:33–45.

18. Coleridge JC, Coleridge HM. Afferent vagal C fibre innervation of the lungs and airways and its functional significance. Rev Physiol Biochem Pharmacol 1984; 99:1–110.

19. Jonzon A, Pisarri TE, Coleridge JC, Coleridge HM. Rapidly adapting receptor activity in dogs is inversely related to lung compliance. J Appl Physiol 1986; 61:1980–1987.

20. McAlexander MA, Myers AC, Undem BJ. Adaptation of guinea-pig vagal airway afferent neurones to mechanical stimulation. J Physiol 1999; 521: 239–247.

21. Pack AI, DeLaney RG. Response of pulmonary rapidly adapting receptors during lung inflation. J Appl Physiol 1983; 55:955–963.

22. Mohammed SP, Higenbottam TW, Adcock JJ. Effects of aerosol-applied capsaicin, histamine and prostaglandin E2 on airway sensory receptors of anaesthetized cats. J Physiol 1993; 469:51–66.

23. Bergren DR. Sensory receptor activation by mediators of defense reflexes in guinea-pig lungs. Respir Physiol 1997; 108:195–204.

24. Morikawa T, Gallico L, Widdicombe J. Actions of moguisteine on cough and pulmonary rapidly adapting receptor activity in the guinea pig. Pharmacol Res 1997; 35:113–118.

25. Canning BJ, Reynolds SM, Mazzone SB. Multiple mechanisms of reflex bronchospasm in guinea pigs. J Appl Physiol 2001; 91:2642–2653.

26. Joad JP, Kott KS, Bonham AC. Nitric oxide contributes to substance P-induced increases in lung rapidly adapting receptor activity in guinea-pigs. J Physiol 1997; 503:635–643.

27. Bonham AC, Kott KS, Ravi K, Kappagoda CT, Joad JP. Substance P contributes to rapidly adapting receptor responses to pulmonary venous congestion in rabbits. J Physiol 1996; 493:229–238.

28. Canning BJ. Interactions between vagal afferent nerve subtypes mediating cough. Pulm Pharmacol Ther 2002; 15:187–192.

29. Tatar M, Webber SE, Widdicombe JG. Lung C-fibre receptor activation and defensive reflexes in anaesthetized cats. J Physiol 1988; 402:411–420.

30. Tatar M, Sant'Ambrogio G, Sant'Ambrogio FB. Laryngeal and tracheobronchial cough in anesthetized dogs. J Appl Physiol 1994; 76:2672–2679.

31. Barnes NC, Piper PJ, Costello JF. Comparative effects of inhaled leukotriene C4, leukotriene D4, and histamine in normal human subjects. Thorax 1984; 39:500–504.

32. Joos GF, Pauwels RA, Van Der Straeten ME. Effect of inhaled substance P and neurokinin A on the airways of normal and asthmatic subjects. Thorax 1987; 42:779–783.

33. Fujimura M, Sakamoto S, Kamio Y, Matsuda T. Effects of methacholine induced bronchoconstriction and procaterol induced bronchodilation on cough receptor sensitivity to inhaled capsaicin and tartaric acid. Thorax 1992; 47:441–445.

34. Shinagawa K, Kojima M, Ichikawa K, Hiratochi M, Aoyagi S, Akahane M. Participation of thromboxane A(2) in the cough response in guinea-pigs: antitussive effect of ozagrel. Br J Pharmacol 2000; 131:266–270.

35. Schelegle ES, Green JF. An overview of the anatomy and physiology of slowly adapting pulmonary stretch receptors. Respir Physiol 2001; 125:17–31.

36. Richardson CA, Herbert DA, Mitchell RA. Modulation of pulmonary stretch receptors and airway resistance by parasympathetic efferents. J Appl Physiol 1984; 57:1842–1849.

37. Yu J, Wang YF, Zhang JW. Structure of slowly adapting pulmonary stretch receptors in the lung periphery. J Appl Physiol 2003; 95:385–393.

38. Sant'Ambrogio FB, Sant'Ambrogio G, Mathew OP, Tsubone H. Contraction of trachealis muscle and activity of tracheal stretch receptors. Respir Physiol 1988; 71:343–353.

39. Sudo T, Hayashi F, Nishino T. Responses of tracheobronchial receptors to inhaled furosemide in anesthetized rats. Am J Respir Crit Care Med 2000; 162:971–975.

40. Hanacek J, Korpas J. Modification of the intensity of the expiration reflex during short-term inflation of the lungs in rabbits. Physiol Bohemoslov 1982; 31:169–174.

41. Nishino T, Sugimori K, Hiraga K, Hond Y. Influence of CPAP on reflex responses to tracheal irritation in anesthetized humans. J Appl Physiol 1989; 67:954–958.

42. Hanacek J, Davies A, Widdicombe JG. Influence of lung stretch receptors on the cough reflex in rabbits. Respiration 1984; 45:161–168.

43. Atzori L, Bannenberg G, Corriga AM, Lou YP, Lundberg JM, Ryrfeldt A, Moldeus P. Sulfur dioxide-induced bronchoconstriction via ruthenium red-sensitive activation of sensory nerves. Respiration 1992; 59:272–278.

44. Wang AL, Blackford TL, Lee LY. Vagal bronchopulmonary C-fibers and acute ventilatory response to inhaled irritants. Respir Physiol 1996; 104:231–239.

45. Ezure K, Tanaka I. Lung inflation inhibits rapidly adapting receptor relay neurons in the rat. Neuroreport 2000; 11:1709–1712.

46. Lee LY, Pisarri TE. Afferent properties and reflex functions of bronchopul-monary C-fibers. Respir Physiol 2001; 125:47–65.

47. Ma QP, Woolf CJ. Involvement of neurokinin receptors in the induction but not the maintenance of mechanical allodynia in rat flexor motoneurones. J Physiol 1995; 486:769–777.

48. Ho CY, Gu Q, Hong JL, Lee LY. Prostaglandin E(2) enhances chemical and mechanical sensitivities of pulmonary C fibers in the rat. Am J Respir Crit Care Med 2000; 162:528–533.

49. Gu Q, Lee LY. Epinephrine enhances chemical stimulation evoked calcium transients in cultured rat vagal sensory neurons (abstract). Am J Respir Crit Car Med 2003; 167:A150.

50. Baluk P, Nadel JA, McDonald DM. Substance P-immunoreactive sensory axons in the rat respiratory tract: a quantitative study of their distribution and role in neurogenic inflammation. J Comp Neurol 1992; 319:586–598.

51. Lundberg JM, Hokfelt T, Martling CR, Saria A, Cuello C. Substance P-immunoreactive sensory nerves in the lower respiratory tract of various mammals including man. Cell Tissue Res 1984; 235:251–261.

52. Hunter DD, Undem BJ. Identification and substance P content of vagal affer-ent neurons innervating the epithelium of the guinea pig trachea. Am J Respir Crit Care Med 1999; 159:1943–1948.

53. Myers AC, Kajekar R, Undem BJ. Allergic inflammation-induced neuropep-tide production in rapidly adapting afferent nerves in guinea pig airways. Am J Physiol Lung Cell Mol Physiol 2002; 282:L775–L781.

54. Dey RD, Altemus JB, Zervos I, Hoffpauir J. Origin and colocalization of CGRP- and SP-reactive nerves in cat airway epithelium. J Appl Physiol 1990; 68:770–778.

55. Lamb JP, Sparrow MP. Three-dimensional mapping of sensory innervation with substance p in porcine bronchial mucosa: comparison with human airways. Am J Respir Crit Care Med 2002; 166:1269–1281.

56. Kollarik M, Dinh QT, Fischer A, Undem BJ. Capsaicin-sensitive and -insensitive vagal bronchopulmonary C-fibres in the mouse. J Physiol 2003; 551(Pt 3):869–879.
57. Undem BJ, Oh EJ, Lee M, Weinreich D. Subtypes of vagal nociceptive C-fibers in guinea pig lungs. Am J Respir Crit Care Med 2003:A708.
58. Barnes PJ. Neurogenic inflammation in the airways. Respir Physiol 2001; 125:145–154.
59. Forsberg K, Karlsson JA. Cough induced by stimulation of capsaicin-sensitive sensory neurons in conscious guinea-pigs. Acta Physiol Scand 1986; 128:319–320.
60. Choudry NB, Fuller RW, Pride NB. Sensitivity of the human cough reflex: effect of inflammatory mediators prostaglandin E2, bradykinin, and histamine. Am Rev Respir Dis 1989; 140:137–141.
61. Mazzone SB, Mori N, Canning BJ. Bradykinin-induced cough in conscious guinea pigs (abstract). Am J Respir Crit Care Med 2002; 165:A773.
62. Bolser DC, DeGennaro FC, O'Reilly S, McLeod RL, Hey JA. Central antitussive activity of the NK1 and NK2 tachykinin receptor antagonists, CP-99,994 and SR 48968, in the guinea-pig and cat. Br J Pharmacol 1997; 121:165–170.
63. Canning BJ, Mazzone SB, Meeker SN, Mori N, Reynolds SM, Undem BJ. Identification of the tracheal and laryngeal afferents neurones mediating cough in anaesthetized guinea-pigs. J Physiol 2004; 557(Pt 2):543–558.
64. Nishino T, Tagaito Y, Isono S. Cough and other reflexes on irritation of airway mucosa in man. Pulm Pharmacol 1996; 9:285–292.
65. Roberts AM, Kaufman MP, Baker DG, Brown JK, Coleridge HM, Coleridge JC. Reflex tracheal contraction induced by stimulation of bronchial C-fibers in dogs. J Appl Physiol 1981; 51:485–493.
66. Davis B, Roberts AM, Coleridge HM, Coleridge JC. Reflex tracheal gland secretion evoked by stimulation of bronchial C-fibers in dogs. J Appl Physiol 1982; 53:985–991.
67. Pisarri TE, Coleridge JC, Coleridge HM. Capsaicin-induced bronchial vasodilation in dogs: central and peripheral neural mechanisms. J Appl Physiol 1993; 74:259–266.
68. Bergren DR. Enhanced lung C-fiber responsiveness in sensitized adult guinea pigs exposed to chronic tobacco smoke. J Appl Physiol 2001; 91:1645–1654.
69. Hutchings HA, Morris S, Eccles R, Jawad MS. Voluntary suppression of cough induced by inhalation of capsaicin in healthy volunteers. Respir Med 1993; 87:379–382.
70. Szolcsányi J. Actions of capsaicin on sensory receptors. In: Wood JN, ed. Capsaicin in the Study of Pain. London: Academic Press, 1993.
71. Yu J. Spectrum of myelinated pulmonary afferents. Am J Physiol Regul Integr Comp Physiol 2000; 279:R2142–R2148.
72. Bergren DR, Peterson DF. Identification of vagal sensory receptors in the rat lung: are there subtypes of slowly adapting receptors? J Physiol 1993; 464:681–698
73. Pedersen KE, Meeker SN, Riccio MM, Undem BJ. Selective stimulation of jugular ganglion afferent neurons in guinea pig airways by hypertonic saline. J Appl Physiol 1998; 84:499–506.

74. McAlexander MA, Undem BJ. Potassium channel blockade induces action potential generation in guinea-pig airway vagal afferent neurones. J Auton Nerv Syst 2000; 78:158–164.
75. Mazzone SB and Canning BJ. Identification of the afferent nerves mediating cough in guinea pigs (abstract). FASEB J 2003; 17:A822.
76. Baluk P, Gabella G. Afferent nerve endings in the tracheal muscle of guinea-pigs and rats. Anat Embryol (Berl) 1991; 183:81–87.
77. Jeffery PK. Remodeling in asthma and chronic obstructive lung disease. Am J Respir Crit Care Med 2001; 164(10 Pt 2):S28–S38.
78. Dobretsov M, Hastings SL, Sims TJ, Stimers JR, Romanovsky D. Stretch receptor-associated expression of alpha 3 isoform of the Na^+, K^+-ATPase in rat peripheral nervous system. Neuroscience 2003; 116:1069–1080.
79. Matsumoto S, Takahashi T, Tanimoto T, Saiki C, Takeda M. Effects of ouabain and flecainide on CO(2)-induced slowly adapting pulmonary stretch receptor inhibition in the rabbit. Life Sci 2000; 66:441–448.
80. Chapleau MW, Lu J, Hajduczok G, Abboud FM. Mechanism of baroreceptor adaptation in dogs: attenuation of adaptation by the K^+ channel blocker 4-aminopyridine. J Physiol 1993; 462:291–306.
81. Kopp UC, Smith LA, Pence AL. Na(+)-K(+)-ATPase inhibition sensitizes renal mechanoreceptors activated by increases in renal pelvic pressure. Am J Physiol 1994; 267:R1109–R1117.
82. Lundberg JM, Saria A, Brodin E, Rosell S, Folkers K. A substance P antagonist inhibits vagally induced increase in vascular permeability and bronchial smooth muscle contraction in the guinea pig. Proc Natl Acad Sci USA 1983; 80:1120–1124.
83. Kuo HP, Rohde JA, Tokuyama K, Barnes PJ, Rogers DF. Capsaicin and sensory neuropeptide stimulation of goblet cell secretion in guinea-pig trachea. J Physiol 1990; 431:629–641.
84. Manzini S. Bronchodilatation by tachykinins and capsaicin in the mouse main bronchus. Br J Pharmacol 1992; 105:968–972.
85. Piedimonte G, Hoffman JI, Husseini WK, Snider RM, Desai MC, Nadel JA. NK1 receptors mediate neurogenic inflammatory increase in blood flow in rat airways. J Appl Physiol 1993; 74:2462–2468.
86. Baluk P, Bertrand C, Geppetti P, McDonald DM, Nadel JA. NK1 receptors mediate leukocyte adhesion in neurogenic inflammation in the rat trachea. Am J Physiol 1995; 268:L263–L269.
87. Ricciardolo FL, Rado V, Fabbri LM, Sterk PJ, Di Maria GU, Geppetti P. Bronchoconstriction induced by citric acid inhalation in guinea pigs: role of tachykinins, bradykinin, and nitric oxide. Am J Respir Crit Care Med 1999; 159:557–562.
88. Canning BJ, Reynolds SM, Anukwu LU, Kajekar R, Myers AC. Endogenous neurokinins facilitate synaptic neurotransmission in guinea pig airway parasympathetic ganglia. Am J Physiol Regul Integr Comp Physiol 2002; 283:R320–R330.
89. Matsumoto S, Takeda M, Saiki C, Takahashi T, Ojima K. Effects of tachykinins on rapidly adapting pulmonary stretch receptors and total lung resistance

in anesthetized, artificially ventilated rabbits. J Pharmacol Exp Ther 1997; 283:1026–1031.

90. Ujiie Y, Sekizawa K, Aikawa T, Sasaki H. Evidence for substance P as an endogenous substance causing cough in guinea pigs. Am Rev Respir Dis 1993; 148:1628–1632.

91. Bolser DC, DeGennaro FC, O'Reilly S, Hey JA, Chapman RW. Pharmacological studies of allergic cough in the guinea pig. Eur J Pharmacol 1995; 277:159–164.

92. Sekizawa K, Ebihara T, Sasaki H. Role of substance P in cough during bronchoconstriction in awake guinea pigs. Am J Respir Crit Care Med 1995; 151:815–821.

93. Yasumitsu R, Hirayama Y, Imai T, Miyayasu K, Hiroi J. Effects of specific tachykinin receptor antagonists on citric acid-induced cough and bronchoconstriction in unanesthetized guinea pigs. Eur J Pharmacol 1996; 300: 215–219.

94. Kohrogi H, Nadel JA, Malfroy B, Gorman C, Bridenbaugh R, Patton JS, Borson DB. Recombinant human enkephalinase (neutral endopeptidase) prevents cough induced by tachykinins in awake guinea pigs. J Clin Invest 1989; 84:781–786.

95. Russell JA, Lai-Fook SJ. Reflex bronchoconstriction induced by capsaicin in the dog. J Appl Physiol 1979; 47:961–967.

96. Ichinose M, Inoue H, Miura M, Yafuso N, Nogami H, Takishima T. Possible sensory receptor of nonadrenergic inhibitory nervous system. J Appl Physiol 1987; 63:923–929.

97. Fuller RW, Dixon CM, Barnes PJ. Bronchoconstrictor response to inhaled capsaicin in humans. J Appl Physiol 1985; 58:1080–1084.

98. Baker B, Peatfield AC, Richardson PS. Nervous control of mucin secretion into human bronchi. J Physiol 1985; 365:297–305.

99. Rogers DF, Barnes PJ. Opioid inhibition of neurally mediated mucus secretion in human bronchi. Lancet 1989; 1:930–932.

100. Ellis JL, Sham JS, Undem BJ. Tachykinin-independent effects of capsaicin on smooth muscle in human isolated bronchi. Am J Respir Crit Care Med 1997; 155:751–755.

101. Jia YX, Sekizawa K, Sasaki H. Cholinergic influence on the sensitivity of cough reflex in awake guinea-pigs. J Auton Pharmacol 1998; 18:257–261.

102. Lowry R, Wood A, Johnson T, Higenbottam T. Antitussive properties of inhaled bronchodilators on induced cough. Chest 1988; 93:1186–1189.

103. Woolf CJ, Salter MW. Neuronal plasticity: increasing the gain in pain. Science 2000; 288:1765–1769.

104. Kubin L, Davies RO. Central pathways of pulmonary and airway vagal afferents. In: Hornbein TF, ed. Regulation of Breathing. New York: Marcel Dekker 1995:79:219–284.

105. Jordan D. Central nervous pathways and control of the airways. Respir Physiol 2001; 125:67–81.

106. Mazzone SB, Canning BJ. Synergistic interactions between airway afferent nerve subtypes mediating reflex bronchospasm in guinea pigs. Am J Physiol Regul Integr Comp Physiol 2002; 283:R86–R98.

107. Mutoh T, Bonham AC, Joad JP. Substance P in the nucleus of the solitary tract augments bronchopulmonary C fiber reflex output. Am J Physiol 2000; 279:R1215–R1223.
108. Bonham AC, Coles SK, McCrimmon DR. Pulmonary stretch receptor afferents activate excitatory amino acid receptors in the nucleus tractus solitarii in rats. J Physiol 1993; 464:725–745.
109. Mazzone SB, Canning BJ. Central interactions between airway afferent nerve subtypes mediating cough (abstract). Am J Respir Crit Care Med 2003; 167:A146.

3

Central Cough Mechanisms: Neuroanatomy and Neurophysiology

ROGER SHANNON, DAVID M. BAEKEY, KENDALL F. MORRIS, and
BRUCE G. LINDSEY

Department of Physiology and Biophysics, College of Medicine,
    University of South Florida,
Tampa, Florida, U.S.A.

Introduction

Substantial progress has been made in our laboratory toward identifying brainstem regions and understanding neural network mechanisms involved in the control of coughing and the laryngeal expiration reflex (1–7). These advances, as well as contributions by other groups, have been summarized in recent reviews (8–10).

It is now well documented that the ventrolateral medullary respiratory neuronal network (Bötzinger, pre-Bötzinger, and ventral respiratory group, or "Böt-VRG") that generates the basic breathing rhythm and motor pattern also participates in configuration of motor patterns during cough (1–5,11–15). The emphasis of this chapter will be on the role of neural networks in other regions of the brainstem in the production of the cough motor pattern by the Böt-VRG network. These regions include the nucleus tractus solitarii, midline raphe nuclei and lateral tegmental field in the medulla, and the pontine respiratory group and cerebellum (Fig. 1). There is a general consensus that these networks are linked and essential for the

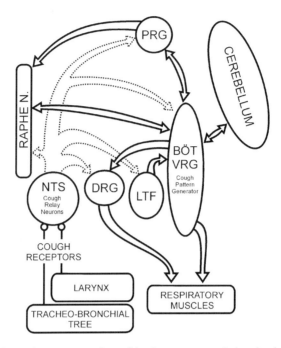

Figure 1 Schematic representation of brainstem network involved in the generation and modulation of cough. Arrows represent hypothesized (*dotted*) and known (*solid*) interactions. *Abbreviations*: Böt-VRG, Bötzinger, pre-Bötzinger, ventral respiratory group; DRG, dorsal respiratory group; LTF, lateral tegmental field; NTS, nucleus tractus solatarii; PRG, pontine respiratory group.

production of a normal (eupnic) breathing pattern and ventilatory responses to respiratory reflexes.

This review includes some recent findings from our laboratory and relevant observations from other investigators. We have taken some liberty with speculation on selected mechanisms, with the intent to stimulate future research on this complicated issue.

Cough is elicited by stimulation of central airway receptors that project to relay neurons in the nucleus tractus solitarii (NTS) (16,17). It is generally accepted that "cough receptors" are a subtype of rapidly adapting "irritant" receptors (18). The location, properties, and specific projections of NTS cough relay neurons are unknown. It is well known that stimulation of tracheobronchial or laryngeal irritant receptors have pronounced effects on the respiratory pattern, which is most likely through widely distributed polysynaptic pathways (17,19). Based on our studies discussed in the following text, we propose that NTS cough relay neurons have a similar widespread effect on the brainstem respiratory network (Fig. 1).

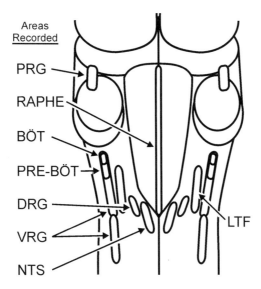

Areas
Recorded

PRG

RAPHE

BÖT

PRE-BÖT

DRG

VRG

NTS

LTF

Figure 2 Schematic of the dorsal view of the brainstem illustrating regions from which we have recorded neuron activity during fictive cough (excluding the LTF).

We have recorded simultaneous and sequential changes in the discharge patterns of many respiratory modulated neurons in various brainstem sites (Fig. 2) during fictive cough in decerebrated, neuromuscular blocked, phrenic driven ventilated cats. Cough-like inspiratory and expiratory motor patterns were elicited by mechanical stimulation of the intrathoracic trachea. Figure 3 illustrates alterations in the patterns of respiratory modulated neurons in the rostral and caudal ventral respiratory group, pontine respiratory group, and midline raphe nuclei during a cough episode. The responses are consistent with these networks being involved in the production and modulation of cough motor patterns.

Bötzinger, Pre-Bötzinger, Ventral Respiratory Group

Our previous studies support a network model for the participation of Böt-VRG neurons in the generation of the cough motor patterns of respiratory pump (diaphragm, intercostals, and abdominal) and laryngeal muscles (3–5). A comprehensive model can be found in a recent review (8). There are still gaps in our understanding and the model.

Dorsal Respiratory Group

Although not involved in the generation of the cough motor pattern, premotor neurons in the medullary dorsal respiratory group (DRG) provide

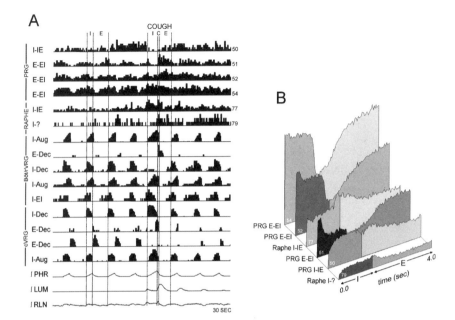

Figure 3 (A) Firing rate histograms of simultaneous responses of respiratory modulated neurons in the pontine respiratory group, midline raphe nuclei, and rostral (Böt-VRG) and caudal ventral respiratory groups during a cough episode. Numbers to right of spike trains represent recording channel. The fictive cough cycle is indicated by the large increase in phrenic and subsequent lumbar nerve activities. (B) Cycle-triggered histograms of selected neuron activities from the PRG and midline raphe nuclei. Inspiratory and expiratory phases, as determined from phrenic activity, are indicated by shading. *Abbreviations*: E, neuron with peak activity during the expiratory phase; I, neuron with peak activity during the inspiratory phase; EI, activity spans the expiratory–inspiratory transition; IE, activity spans the inspiratory–expiratory transition; Aug, augmenting—peak firing rates in the last half of the phase; Dec, decrementing—peak firing rates in the first half of the phase; ?, could not determine discharge pattern; ∫PHR, LUM, and RLN, integrated (time-moving average, 200 msec time constant) of phrenic, lumbar, and recurrent laryngeal nerve motor activities; COUGH I, C, and E, neural inspiratory, compressive, and expulsive phases of cough.

excitatory drive to phrenic and inspiratory intercostal motoneurons during cough (11,16,20). The DRG corresponds to the ventral lateral nucleus of the solitarii tract and adjoining reticular formation. Inspiratory modulation of the neurons is due primarily to excitatory and inhibitory inputs from Böt-VRG neurons (21,22). The increase in inspiratory neuron activity during cough results most likely from inspiratory drive from the Böt-VRG; input from NTS cough receptor relay neurons cannot be discounted.

Pontine Respiratory Group

Neurons located in the medial parabrachial and Kolliker–Fuse nuclei and the lateral pons/mesencephalic junction constitute the pontine respiratory group (PRG) and are known to modulate the eupnic breathing pattern (21,23–25). Most PRG neurons are tonically active with various superimposed respiratory modulated discharge patterns; the "respiratoriness" of their patterns is much less than cells in the medullary dorsal and ventral respiratory groups. We have presented evidence that PRG neuron activity is altered during fictive cough (26). A sample of four simultaneously recorded phase spanning (IE, EI) neurons is shown in Fig. 3. The control discharge patterns of the neurons are shown in the cycle-triggered histograms in Fig. 3B. Peak firing rates of these neurons were altered during the cough cycle; the inspiratory neuron decreased and three expiratory neurons increased firing rates (Fig. 3A). We postulate that observed changes in PRG neuron activity reflect inputs from the NTS (19), interactions among PRG neurons (27), and reciprocal interactions with the Böt-VRG (21,23–25) (Fig. 1). Whether there are direct influences of the raphe nuclei, lateral tegmental field, or cerebellum on the respiratory modulated activity in the PRG is unknown.

Kainic acid inactivation of neurons in the PRG region of cats demonstrated they were essential for the expression of the cough reflex (28). The control breathing pattern was also altered in these experiments, reflecting the importance of the PRG in the generation of a eupnic pattern by the Böt-VRG and its ability to respond to reflexes. The pathways and mechanisms by which the PRG interacts with the Böt-VRG to modulate cough are unknown.

Medullary Raphe Nuclei

The medullary midline raphe nuclei contain respiratory modulated neurons, with discharge patterns similar to the PRG, as well as nonrespiratory modulated neurons; neurons in both categories change activity during cough episodes (6). Two inspiratory modulated cells are shown in Fig. 3A and B. Possible sources of input that alter raphe neuron activity include the Böt-VRG (29), PRG (30), and NTS (6) (Fig. 1). If NTS cough afferent information is relayed to the raphe network, it is most likely through unknown polysynaptic pathways. Anatomical tracing studies suggest there are no direct connections from NTS to the raphe network (31). DRG inspiratory neurons are not considered to be inputs; they do not project to the raphe nuclei (22). Whether there are interactions of raphe neurons with the cerebellum is unknown.

As is the case with PRG lesions, kainic acid destruction of cells in the medullary raphe nuclei alters the control respiratory pattern and eliminates cough patterns in spinal respiratory motoneurons (32). The mechanism by which midline neurons influence the cough reflex is unknown. There is substantial evidence for action of neurons in the raphe nuclei on the Böt-VRG (29,33–35), but the effects do not appear to be on the short-term, breath-to-breath pattern. They have been proposed to have a permissive or enabling role in respiratory rhythmogenesis.

Nucleus Tractus Solitarii

We conducted experiments to characterize NTS neurons involved in the cough reflex (16,36). Approximately 25% of the neurons recorded from the commissural nucleus region (caudal to obex), which contains most of the tracheobronchial irritant receptor second-order relay neurons (17,37), increased activity coincident with tracheal stimulation; 10% decreased activity. The duration of the changes varied from brief periods associated with the stimulus to several breaths following stimulation. The responsive cells included neurons with weak inspiratory and expiratory modulation and cells with no respiratory modulation; other neurons, silent during control periods, were recruited. The respiratory modulated units were determined to be neurons, as opposed to fibers projecting through from the DRG or VRG. We concluded that the respiratory input to the neurons is most likely from the DRG and/or Böt-VRG, and not airway stretch or irritant receptors. Some respiratory modulated cells increased activity during one or more of the respiratory phases during cough, suggesting that some of these cells also receive feedback from the cough pattern generator (Böt-VRG).

Similar responsive cells were also recorded from the NTS/DRG region (rostral to obex). In addition, DRG inspiratory bulbospinal cells increased activity during cough with a pattern like the altered phrenic motor activity, as reported previously by others (11,20). We did not determine whether the responsive cells (putative relay neurons) in this region were second- or third-order neurons. Tracheobronchial irritant receptors do not project directly to the DRG (17,37). If "cough receptor" fibers have similar projection patterns to the NTS as other irritant receptors, then it is likely that the responsive cells near the DRG are at least third-order neurons.

We had hypothesized that airway "cough receptors" and their NTS relay neurons would be silent during normal breathing. The varied responses of tonically active cells suggested that the processing of cough afferent information in the NTS and its transmission to other areas also includes a network of active neurons.

The response of neurons in the commissural nucleus region to mechanical stimulation of the larynx (16) was also examined; these experiments gave us the opportunity to assess possible convergence of cough afferent stimuli from the trachea and larynx in this region. Most laryngeal receptor afferent fibers project to regions of the NTS rostral to the obex and medial to the DRG (38,39). We observed some neurons that were excited or inhibited by only one of the stimuli, while others were excited or inhibited by both stimuli. These results suggested that some putative interneurons in cough reflex pathways receive convergent afferent information related to both laryngeal and tracheobronchial cough.

We also obtained simultaneous recordings of cough responsive NTS and Böt-VRG neurons to test for functional connections using cross-correlation analysis of spike-trains (unpublished). The data included 732 pairs of neurons; each pair was composed of a cell from each domain. There were no short-latency offset features in the correlograms suggestive of direct excitatory or inhibitory influences in either direction. These results are consistent with, but do not prove, the absence of direct connections; they do suggest the existence of interneurons in the pathways. Bolser and colleagues (8,40) have proposed the existence of a functional "gate" through which cough afferent information passes (see subsequent section).

There are challenges to studying rapidly adapting receptor (RAR) (irritant, cough) relay neurons in the NTS. It is difficult to isolate spikes and record single NTS cells for long periods (19, personal observation). The cell bodies are small (8–15 µm), compacted, near the dorsal surface, and subject to brainstem movement (19).

Cerebellum

The deep cerebellar nuclei (i.e., fastigial, interposed and infracerebellar/lateral) modulate breathing, particularly during respiratory stresses (41). The interposed and lateral nuclei appear to be involved in pulmonary reflexes, while the fastigial nucleus is important in the facilitation of the respiratory response to chemical challenges. These nuclei contain cells with respiratory modulated firing rates due to afferent information from pulmonary stretch receptors and presumably Böt-VRG neurons (42). Whether there are respiratory modulated inputs from the PRG and respiratory muscle proprioceptors is unknown. Specific connections and pathways between the cerebellum and the Böt-VRG are also unknown. The effect of the fastigial nucleus on the VRG involves relay neurons in the medullary gigantocellular nucleus (43), and not the PRG or the red and paramedian reticular nuclei (44). Interactions between the interposed or infracerebellar/lateral nuclei and the PRG are unknown, although likely because both regions are involved in the response of the brainstem respiratory network during pulmonary reflexes.

In a collaborative study with Xu and Frazier (7), we demonstrated in cats that the cerebellum was important for the expression of cough motor patterns. The primary alteration in cough responsiveness following cerebellectomy was a reduction in the number of coughs generated by a maximum stimulus (cough frequency). There was also a reduction in the peak discharge rate in abdominal expiratory motor nerves. A decreased cough frequency, but not lumbar nerve amplitude, was also observed following electrical lesioning of the interposed nucleus region. Whether the change in cough frequency caused by the interposed nucleus lesion was due to destruction of cells or fibers of passage is unknown. Destruction of the fastigial nucleus had no effect on cough responsiveness. The cerebellar effect on a single cough was not studied.

Coughing is a complex motor act and other cerebellar nuclei may be involved. The infracerebellar nucleus influences medullary expiratory neuron activity, spinal nerve expiratory activity, and respiratory frequency (45). Furthermore, the cerebellum receives pulmonary stretch receptor input (42) and appears to attenuate the pulmonary stretch receptor facilitatory effect on expiratory muscles during increased lung volume (46). This observation raises the question of cerebellar involvement in the essential, permissive role of pulmonary stretch receptors in the production of cough (47).

The stimulation of cough-like motor patterns in neuromuscular blocked animals indicates that feedback from mechanoreceptors in contracting muscles or postural muscle is not essential for cough. The cough pattern in intact, awake, spontaneously breathing animals may be further influenced by the cerebellum, due to processing and modulation of muscle proprioreceptor reflexes. During cough, there would be substantial alteration in mechanoreceptor activity in both respiratory and thoracic cage postural muscles.

The mechanisms and pathways by which the cerebellar and brainstem respiratory neural networks interact to modulate cough patterns needs further study. One hypothesis for the multiple cough cycles following a stimulus is that the first cycle is produced by the Böt/rVRG which then sends an efference copy to the cerebellum; feedback from the cerebellum stimulates an oscillation in cough patterns by the Böt-VRG which is ultimately damped out. Cerebellar output to the Böt-VRG could also be modulated by "cough" receptor and pulmonary stretch receptor second-order neuron inputs from the NTS.

A role of the cerebellum in cough is consistent with its known functions of sensory-motor integration, motor coordination, motor learning and timing.

Lateral Tegmental Field

The lateral tegmental field (LTF) is considered generally to integrate and modulate a variety of reflexes, including those involved in respiratory and cardiovascular control. There is evidence that LTF neurons in the medulla are involved in the modulation of the eupnic breathing pattern and essential for the expression of cough and expiration reflexes (48). Kainic acid destruction of cells in the nucleus reticularis ventralis and the adjacent parts of the rostral medullary LTF altered the eupnic breathing pattern and elimi- nated cough and expiration reflex motor responses. There was also a decrease in systemic arterial pressure. The critical injection site for suppres- sion of the reflexes was located between the DRG and VRG (Fig. 2).

Further support for participation of this region in breathing and reflex responses includes the presence of weakly modulated respiratory neurons (49). Also, non-respiratory modulated neurons with projections to the spinal cord have been shown to increase activity during the laryngeal expiration reflex (50). That medial LTF neurons may increase activity during coughing was suggested by C-fos expression during fictive coughing, and its elimination with codeine (51).

Changes in the control breathing pattern and the elimination of cough and expiration reflex responses by destruction of LTF neurons suggests that they have an important role in maintaining the responsiveness of the Böt- VRG network to afferent inputs, in a manner similar to the PRG and raphe networks. Of course, the LTF could also be a critical relay network for afferent information to the eupnic/cough generation network (Böt-VRG). The mechanisms and pathways by which the medial LTF influences breath- ing and cough reflexes are unknown.

Cough Gating Mechanism/Process

Bolser et al. (8,40) have proposed a functional model regulating the central production of cough by the Böt-VRG network. The model is based on observations from antitussive drug studies. They showed in cats that cen- trally acting antitussive drugs do not inhibit tracheobronchial cough by a generalized suppression of the Böt-VRG; rather they had very specific effects on various components of the cough motor pattern. Low doses of antitussive drugs (administered via the vertebral artery) decreased the num- ber of coughs elicited per stimulus trial without changes in inspiratory and expiratory phase durations. There were also decreases in expiratory muscle electromyogram burst amplitude without changes in inspiratory burst amplitude. At higher doses, expiratory muscle bursts, but not the inspira- tory bursts, could be eliminated. At doses just sufficient to eliminate both inspiratory and expiratory changes during airway stimulation, there was no alteration in the eupnic motor pattern.

They concluded that central antitussive drugs acted "upstream" from the cough network (Böt-VRG), on elements designated as a functional "gate." It was also suggested that laryngeal and tracheobronchial coughs are controlled by separate gates, with the laryngeal one being less sensitive to central antitussive drugs than the tracheobronchial one. The gate modulates afferent inputs from cough receptors and pulmonary stretch receptors. The mechanism is unknown, but is proposed to consist of, in part, unidentified neurons active only during cough.

Laryngeal Expiration Reflex

The expiration reflex is a distinct airway defensive response characterized by a brief, intense expiratory effort in the pump muscles and coordinated closure and opening of the laryngeal folds. The reflex prevents entry of foreign materials into the lower airways and removes mucus from the subglottal region, and is considered distinct from cough because there is no preceding large inspiratory effort (10,52).

Previous studies have suggested that neurons in the ventral lateral medulla participate in coordinating the reflex (50,53–56). We conducted a comprehensive study of Böt-VRG neurons to test this hypothesis (57,58). Figure 4 shows responses of various types of simultaneously recorded respiratory neurons following mechanical stimulation of the laryngeal folds to elicit the reflex. In general, most Böt-VRG expiratory neurons are excited and inspiratory neurons inhibited. In addition to the response data, neurons were further tested for axonal projections to the spinal cord (premotor) using antidromic stimulation methods, and for functional connectivity with laryngeal motoneurons utilizing spike-triggered averaging of recurrent laryngeal nerve efferent activity. Increased firing rates of bulbospinal expiratory premotor neurons and expiratory laryngeal premotor and motoneurons during the expiratory burst in abdominal muscle nerves were accompanied by changes in the firing patterns of other neurons within the respiratory network. The concurrent responses and inferred connectivity supported the proposal that elements of both the rostral ventral respiratory group, including the Bötzinger and pre-Bötzinger complexes, and the caudal ventral respiratory group are involved in configuring respiratory motor patterns during the expiration reflex.

The schematic model in Fig. 5 and the following paragraphs present a summary of hypotheses, supported by the results, regarding mechanisms by which antecedent neurons in the Böt-rVRG network excite bulbospinal expiratory premotor neurons and laryngeal motoneurons during the expiration reflex. This model does not include proposed mechanisms for the

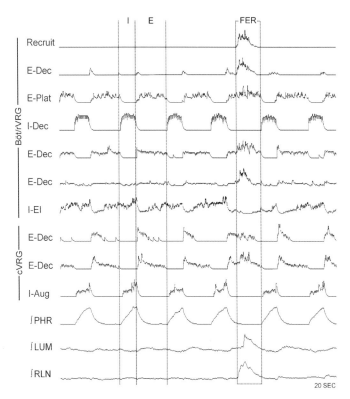

Figure 4 Integrated spike trains showing simultaneous responses of respiratory modulated neurons in the rostral (Böt-VRG) and caudal ventral respiratory groups (cVRG) during fictive expiration reflex (FER). Spike train integrated signals are time-moving averages with a 100 msec time constant.

brief excitation of inspiratory laryngeal motoneuron activity reported by Poliacek et al. (59).

Expiration reflex receptors in the larynx excite second-order neurons in the NTS that, in turn, act through unknown pathways on network neurons. Neurons that are excited could receive direct input from NTS relay neurons. The increase in firing rates of caudal VRG bulbospinal premotor expiratory neurons (E-Aug), which drive intercostal and abdominal expiratory muscles, is due to excitation and reduced inhibition from different subsets of Böt-rVRG expiratory neurons with augmenting (E-Aug) and decrementing (E-Dec) discharge patterns (Fig. 5, connections 1–3). Arrows in the neuron balls indicate firing rate changes during the expiration reflex.

The increased firing rates of expiratory laryngeal motoneurons (ELMs), leading to closure of the glottis, result primarily from excitation by rostral VRG premotor E-Dec neurons (Fig. 5, connection 4). Other

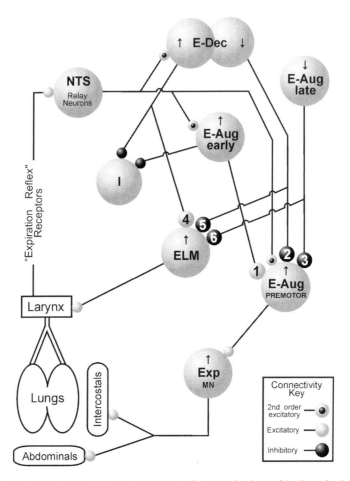

Figure 5 Network model for the control of the excitation of bulbospinal expiratory premotor neurons (E-Aug) and laryngeal motoneurons (ELM) during the expiration reflex. See text for details.

factors that may promote this burst of activity include disinhibition by a different group of E-Dec neurons and E-Aug neurons (Fig. 5, connections 5 and 6).

Subpopulations of E-Dec and E-Aug neurons inhibit inspiratory neurons during the reflex. Other neurons, with discharge patterns different from those described previously, also changed activity during the expiration reflex indicating that the entire Böt-VRG network is affected. As with cough, the Böt-VRG network cannot express the expiration reflex following inactivation of neurons in the LTF (48), midline raphe nuclei (32), or PRG (28).

Summary

There is convincing evidence that the ventrolateral medullary respiratory neuronal network (Böt-VRG) that generates the basic breathing rhythm and motor pattern also produces the cough and expiration reflex motor patterns. The dorsal respiratory group, which is associated with the NTS, also transmits premotor drive to spinal inspiratory motoneurons. Cough receptor relay neurons are located in NTS. The midline raphe nuclei, lateral tegmental field and pontine respiratory group are essential for expression of cough and expiration reflexes, and the cerebellum modulates the cough reflex. Very little is known about the interaction of these various brainstem neural networks during airway defensive reflexes. This is understandable since the pathways and connectivity among neurons of the NTS, Böt-VRG, midline raphe nuclei, lateral tegmental field, pontine respiratory group, and cerebellum are unknown. It would not be surprising if other areas of the brainstem found to alter the eupnic respiratory pattern also influence the responsiveness of cough and other respiratory reflexes. Considerable work is needed to completely understand the neural network mechanisms involved in airway defensive reflexes.

Acknowledgment

This work was supported by grant HL49813 from the National Heart, Lung and Blood Institute.

References

1. Shannon R, Bolser DC, Lindsey BG. Neural control of coughing and sneezing. In: Miller AD, Bianchi AL, Bishop BP, eds. Neural Control of Breathing. Boca Raton, FL: CRC Press, 1996:215–224.
2. Shannon R, Baekey DM, Morris KF, Lindsey BG. Brainstem respiratory networks and cough. Pulm Pharmacol 1997; 9:343–347.
3. Shannon R, Morris KF, Lindsey BG. Ventrolateral medullary respiratory network and a model of cough motor pattern generation. J Appl Physiol 1998; 84:2020–2035.
4. Shannon R, Baekey DM, Morris KF, Li Z, Lindsey BG. Functional connectivity among ventrolateral medullary respiratory neurons and responses during fictive cough in the cat. J Physiol 2000; 525:207–224.
5. Baekey DM, Morris KF, Gestreau C, Lindsey BG, Shannon R. Medullary respiratory neurones and control of laryngeal motoneurones during fictive eupnoea and cough in the cat. J Physiol 2001; 534:565–581.
6. Baekey DM, Morris KF, Gestreau C, Lindsey BG, Shannon R. Medullary raphe neuron activity is altered during fictive cough in the decerebrate cat. J Appl Physiol 2003; 94:93–100.

7. Xu F, Frazier DT, Zhang Z, Baekey DM, Shannon R. Influence of the cerebellum on the cough motor pattern. J Appl Physiol 1997; 83:391–397.
8. Bolser DC, Davenport PW, Golder FJ, Baekey DM, Morris KF, Lindsey BG, Shannon R. Neurogenesis of cough. In: Boushey H, Chung KF, Widdicombe JG, eds. Cough: Causes, Mechanisms and Therapy. Oxford: Blackwell Science, 2003:173–180.
9. Pantaleo T, Bongianni F, Donatella D. Central nervous mechanisms of cough. Pulm Pharmacol 2002; 15:227–233.
10. Korpas J, Jakus J. The expiration reflex from the vocal folds. Acta Physiol Hung 2000; 87:201–215.
11. Engelhorn R, Weller E. Zentrale represenation hustenwirksamer afferenzen in der medulla oblongata der katze. Pflugers Arch 1965; 284:224–239.
12. Jakus J, Tomori Z, Stransky A, Boselova L. Bulbar respiratory activity during defensive airways reflexes in cats. Acta Physiol Hung 1987; 70:245–254.
13. Dawid-Milner MS, Lara JP, Milan A, Gonzalez-Baron S. Activity of inspiratory neurons of the ambiguous complex during cough in the spontaneously breathing decerebrate cat. Exp Physiol 1993; 78:835–838.
14. Oku Y, Tanaka I, Ezure K. Activity of bulbar respiratory neurons during fictive coughing and swallowing in the decerebrate cat. J Physiol 1994; 480:309–384.
15. Bongianni F, Mutolo D, Fontana GA, Pantaleo T. Discharge patterns of Bötzinger complex neurons during cough in the cat. Am J Physiol 1998; 274:R1015–R1024.
16. Bolser DC, Baekey DM, Morris KF, Nuding SC, Lindsey BG, Shannon R. Responses of putative nucleus tractus solitarius (NTS) interneurons in cough reflex pathways during laryngeal and tracheobronchial cough. FASEB J 2000; 14:A644.
17. Kubin L, Davies RO. Central pathways of pulmonary and airway vagal afferents. In: Dempsey JA, Pack AI, eds. Regulation of Breathing: Lung Biology in Health and Disease. New York: Marcel Dekker 1995:79:219–284.
18. Widdicombe JG. Neuroregulation of cough: implications for drug therapy. Curr Opin Pharmacol 2002; 2:256–263.
19. Ezure K, Otake K, Lipski J, Wong She RB. Efferent projections of pulmonary rapidly adapting receptor relay neurons in the cat. Brain Res 1991; 564:268–278.
20. Gestreau C, Milano S, Bianchi AL, Grelot L. Activity of dorsal respiratory group inspiratory neurons during laryngeal-induced fictive coughing and swallowing in decerebrate cats. Exp Brain Res 1996; 108:247–256.
21. Bianchi AL, Denavit-Saubie M, Champagnat J. Central control of breathing in mammals: neuronal circuitry, membrane properties, and neurotransmitters. Physiol Rev 1995; 75:1–45.
22. Ezure K. Synaptic connections between medullary respiratory neurons and considerations on the genesis of respiratory rhythm. Prog Neurobiol 1990; 35:429–450.
23. Fung M, St. John WM. Neuronal activities underlying inspiratory termination by pneumotaxic mechanisms. Respir Physiol 1994; 98:267–281.
24. Dick TE, Bellingham MC, Richter DW. Pontine respiratory neurons in anesthetized cats. Brain Res 1994; 636:259–269.

25. Segers LS, Shannon R, Lindsey BG. Interactions between rostral pontine and ventral medullary respiratory neurons. J Neurophysiol 1985; 54:318–334.
26. Baekey DM, Morris KF, Li Z, Nuding SC, Lindsey BG, Shannon R. Concurrent changes in pontine respiratory group neuron activities during fictive coughing. FASEB J 1999; 13:A824.
27. Morris KF, Baekey DM, Nuding SC, Segers LS, Shannon R, Lindsey BG. Pontine cardiorespiratory network interactions. Soc Neurosci Abstr 2003; Program No. 503. 8.
28. Poliacek I, Jakus J, Stransky A, Barani H, Halasova E, Tomori Z. Cough, expiration and aspiration reflexes following kainic acid lesions to the pontine respiratory group in anaesthetized cats. Physiol Res 2004; 53:155–163.
29. Lindsey BG, Segers LS, Morris KF, Hernandez YM, Saporta S, Shannon R. Distributed actions and dynamic associations in respiratory-related neuronal assemblies of the ventrolateral medulla and brain stem midline: evidence from spike train analysis. J Neurophysiol 1994; 72:1830–1851.
30. Gang S, Mizuguchi A, Aoki M. Axonal projections from the pontine pneumotaxic region to the nucleus raphe magnus in cats. Respir Physiol 1991; 85: 329–339.
31. Ter Horst GJ, Streefland C. Ascending projections of the solitary tract nucleus. In: Robin I, Barraco A, eds. Nucleus of the Solitary Tract. Boca Raton, FL: CRC Press, 1994:93–104.
32. Jakus A, Stransky A, Poliacek I, Barani H, Boselova L. Effects of medullary midline lesions on cough and other airway reflexes in anaesthetized cats. Physiol Res 1998; 47:203–213.
33. Lalley PM, Benacka R, Bischoff AM, Richter DW. Nucleus raphe obscurus evokes 5-HT-1A receptor-mediated modulation of respiratory neurons. Brain Res 1997; 747:156–159.
34. Lovick TA. The medullary raphe nuclei: a system for integration and gain control in autonomic and somatomotor responsiveness? Exp Physiol 1997; 82:31–41.
35. Smith JC, Morrison DE, Ellenberger HH, Otto MR, Feldman JL. Brain stem projections to the major respiratory neuron populations in the medulla of the cat. J Comp Neurol 1989; 281:69–96.
36. Shannon R, Morris KF, Lindsey BG. Nucleus tractus solitarius neuronal responses during fictive cough. FASEB J 1995; 9:A667.
37. Lipski JK, Ezure K, Wong She RB. Identification of neurons receiving input from pulmonary rapidly adapting receptors in the cat. J Physiol 1991; 443:55–77.
38. Kalia M, Mesulum MM. Brain stem projections of sensory and motor components of the vagus complex in the cat: II. Laryngeal, tracheobronchial, pulmonary, cardiac, and gastrointestinal branches. J Comp Neuro 1980; 193:467–508.
39. Lucier GE, Egizil R, Destrovsky JO. Projections of the internal branch of the superior laryngeal nerve in the cat. Brain Res Bull 1986; 16:713–721.
40. Bolser DC, Davenport PW. Functional organization of the central cough generation mechanism. Pulm Pharmacol Ther 2002; 15:221–225.
41. Xu F, Frazier DT. Role of the cerebellar deep nuclei in respiratory modulation. Cerebellum 2002; 1:35–40.

42. Xu F, Frazier DT. Respiratory-related neurons of the fastigial nucleus in response to chemical and mechanical changes. J Appl Physiol 1997; 82: 1177–1184.

43. Xu F, Zhou T, Gibson T, Frazier DT. Fastigial nucleus-mediated respiratory responses depend on the medullary gigantocellular nucleus. J Appl Physiol 2001; 91:1713–1722.

44. Zhang Z, Xu F, Frazier DT. Role of the Botzinger complex in fastigial nucleus-mediated respiratory responses. Anat Rec 1999; 254:542–548.

45. Huang Q, Zhou D, St. John WM. Cerebellar control of expiratory activities of medullary neurons and spinal nerves. J Appl Physiol 1993; 74:1934–1940.

46. Xu F, Frazier DT. Role of the cerebellum in expiratory loading. J Appl Physiol 1994; 77:1232–1238.

47. Hanacek J. Reflex inputs to cough. Eur Respir Rev 2002; 12(85):259–263.

48. Jakus J, Stransky A, Poliacek I, Barani H, Boselova L. Kainic acid lesions to the lateral tegmental field of medulla: effects on cough, expiration and aspiration reflexes in anesthetized cats. Physiol Res 2000; 49:387–398.

49. Fung ML, Tomori Z, St. John WM. Medullary neuronal activities in gasping induced by pharyngeal stimulation and hypoxia. Respir Physiol 1995; 100: 195–202.

50. D'iachenko I, Preobrazhenkii N. Responses of bulbo-spinal neurons during the expiration reflex in cats [in Russian]. Neirofiziologiia 1991; 23:88–98.

51. Gestreau C, Bianchi AL, Grelot L. Differential brainstem fos-like iummunoreactivity after laryngeal-induced coughing and its reduction by codeine. J Neurosci 1997; 17:9340–9352.

52. Korpas J, Tomori Z. The expiration reflex. In: Herzog H, ed. Cough and Other Respiratory Reflexes. Basel: VEDA, 1979:189–217.

53. Hanacek J, Korpas J, Kulik AM, Kondrateva LN. Changes of electrical activity in the respiratory centre during the expiration reflex in cats. Physiol Bohemoslovaca 1977; 26:253.

54. Jakus J, Stransky A, Poliacek I, Barani H. Laryngeal patency and expiration reflex following focal cold block of the medulla in the cat. Physiol Res 1996; 45:107–116.

55. Jakus J, Tomori Z, Stransky A. Activity of bulbar respiratory neurones during cough and other respiratory tract reflexes in cats. Physiol Bohemoslovaca 1985; 34:128–136.

56. Jakus J, Tomori Z, Stransky A, Boselova L. Bulbar respiratory activity during defensive airways reflexes in cats. Acta Physiol Hung 1987; 70:54–254.

57. Baekey DM, Morris KF, Nuding SC, Segers LS, Li Z, Lindsey BG, Shannon R. Involvement of ventral respiratory group neurons in the fictive expiration reflex. FASEB J 2001; 15(5):A798.

58. Baekey DM. Brainstem Control of Cough and Expiration Reflex in the Cat. Ph.D. dissertation, University of South Florida, Tampa, FL, 2003.

59. Poliacek I, Stransky A, Jakus J, Barani H, Tomori Z, Halasova E. Activity of the laryngeal abductor and adductor muscles during cough, expiration and aspiration reflexes in cats. Physiol Res 2003; 52:749–762.

4

Role of Tachykinins in Cough

CHARLES ADVENIER

U.F.R. Biomédicale des Saints Pères,
Laboratoire de Pharmacologie,
Paris, France

VINCENT LAGENTE

Faculté des Sciences Pharmaceutiques et
Biologiques, Université de Rennes,
Rennes, France

BRENDAN J. CANNING

Johns Hopkins Asthma and Allergy Center,
Baltimore, Maryland, U.S.A.

Introduction

Tachykinins—namely, substance P (SP), neurokinin A (NKA), and neuro-kinin B (NKB)—are members of a family of neuropeptides that are widely distributed in sensory nerves and in the central nervous system (CNS). They play a pivotal role in airway neurogenic inflammation, bronchocon-striction, immunomodulation, and cough.

Our understanding of the role of tachykinins in the neuroregulation of cough has recently been improved by (i) studies of the electrophysiological properties of sensory nerves, (ii) better knowledge of the plasticity of these fibers during inflammatory processes, and (iii) analysis of the pharmacological profiles of selective antagonists of various tachykinin receptors. The present review reports on all of these different aspects.

Tachykinins and Tachykinin Receptors in the Airways

Members of the tachykinin family of peptides are colocalized with other neuropeptides such as calcitonin gene-related peptide and dynorphin in the sensory unmyelinated C-fibers that innervate all compartments of the airways (1–4). Tachykinins have also been found in autonomic ganglia neurons and in neurons in the spinal cord and elsewhere in the CNS (5–7). Moreover, studies in animals and in humans suggest that inflammatory cells including eosinophils, monocytes, macrophages, dendritic cells, and lymphocytes may also produce tachykinins and/or express tachykinin receptors (8–10).

Tachykinins cause local neurogenic inflammation including bronchoconstriction, increases in vascular permeability, vasodilatation, hypersecretion of mucus, epithelial cell activation, facilitation of cholinergic neurotransmission, and recruitment and activation of inflammatory cells (4,11,12). Tachykinins are also involved in airway hyperresponsiveness (12,13) and play an important role in cough.

The biological actions of tachykinins are mediated via three types of receptors, denoted neurokinin receptors 1–3 (NK_1, NK_2, and NK_3), which have the highest affinity for SP, NKA, and NKB, respectively. This receptor classification has been established from receptor binding and functional studies using specific agonists (14). Over the past decade, a number of potent and selective nonpeptide neurokinin receptor antagonists have become available for the NK_1, NK_2, and NK_3 receptors (Table 1). Tachykinin receptors have been cloned and shown to belong to the seven transmembrane-spanning G protein-coupled receptor superfamily. Each

Table 1 Mammalian Tachykinins: Receptors, Agonists, and Antagonists

Receptor	Endogenous agonist	Selective agonist	Selective antagonists used in cough studies
NK_1	SP > NKA > NKB	$Sar^9(MetO_2)^{11}$-SP	CP-99,994
			FK 888
			R 116301
			SR 140333
			(nolpitantium)
			SR 240600
			GR 205171
NK_2	NKA > NKB > SP	$[Nle^{10}]$-NKA (4–10)	SR 48968
			(saredutant)
		$[\beta\ Ala^8]$-NKA (4–10)	SR 144190
			MEN 10627
NK_3	NKA > NKB > SP	$[Mephe^7]$-NKB	SB 235375
			SR 142801
			(osanetant)
			SSR 146977

receptor subtype is present in the airways. Receptors types involved in the effects of tachykinins are shown in Table 2. Although some species differences are apparent, it is accepted that NK_1 receptors are predominantly distributed on epithelial cells, on vascular endothelium, and within mucus glands, NK_2 receptors are primarily associated with airway smooth muscle (11–13), and NK_3 receptors are considered to be more important in nerve

Table 2 Receptors Involved in the Pharmacological Effects of Tachykinins in the Airways

Target	Effects	Receptors		
		NK_1	NK_2	NK_3
Cholinergic nerve	Increase in ganglionic transmission	+		+++
	Increase in release of Ach	++	+	
NTS	Respiratory changes	++	+	++
	Reflex integration	++	++	++
Bronchial smooth muscle	Contraction of human bronchus or guinea pig trachea	+	+++	
	Relaxation of rat and mouse trachea	++		
	Airway smooth muscle proliferation	++		
Vascular permeability	Plasma protein extravasation	+++	+	
Recruitment and activation of inflammatory cells	Chemotaxis	+++		
	Lymphocyte proliferation	+++	+	
	Increase in neutrophil motility	+++	+	
	Monocyte/macrophage stimulation	++	+	
	Mast cell activation[a]	++	+	
Mucus glands	Increased secretion	+++	±	
Epithelium	Increased chloride secretion	+++	±	
	PG/NO release	+++	±	
Airway hyperresponsiveness	Increase	+++	+++	++
Cough	Increase	++	+++	+++

Receptor involvement: +++, very strong; ++, strong; +, moderate; ±, doubtful.
[a]A nonreceptor effect has also been reported in some preparations.

transmission especially in parasympathetic ganglia (15,16) and in the nucleus tractus solitarii (NTS) (17,18). Recent studies suggest that all three types are expressed by inflammatory cells that reside in the airways or infiltrate lungs in inflammatory diseases, and are involved in airway hyperresponsiveness. Finally, all three types of tachykinin receptors are also involved in cough.

Involvement of Tachykinins in Cough

Stimulation of C-Fibers with Capsaicin or Citric Acid Elicits Cough

The involvement of tachykinins and of C-fiber receptors in cough is supported by experiments with capsaicin or citric acid, which can both stimulate bronchial C-fiber receptors (19–21) and induce the release of tachykinins through activation of the TRPV1 (VR1) receptor and/or acid-sensing ion channels (22,23).

When administered by aerosol, capsaicin and citric acid are powerful tussigenic agents in humans and other animals and are used as standard methods to investigate cough in preclinical and clinical studies (24,25). The concept that C-fiber receptor activation and tachykinin release may cause cough was proposed by Forsberg et al. (20) who studied cough induced in guinea pigs by inhalation of citric acid, capsaicin, nicotine, and mechanical stimulation of the trachea. Prior administration of large doses of capsaicin, which induced the release of tachykinins and sensory nerve degeneration, blocked the cough reflex due to citric acid and capsaicin, but not that due to nicotine or mechanical stimulation. These authors concluded that citric acid and capsaicin activate C-fiber receptors and induce tachykinin release, whereas nicotine and mechanical stimulation activate rapidly adapting receptors (RARs).

Despite the evidence in favor of the role of C-fibers in cough, there is also evidence against their role in regulating this defensive reflex. The selectivity of both capsaicin and citric acid for C-fiber activation has also been questioned (22,23,26; also see Chapter 2). However, the data summarized in the previous sections, and the ability of tachykinin receptor antagonists to markedly inhibit or abolish cough in guinea pigs, cats, and pigs, provide strong evidence in favor of the hypothesis that C-fibers are important in regulating or modulating the cough reflex.

Ability of Exogenous Tachykinins to Induce Cough

Controversial reports have proposed that tachykinins act as tussive agents by themselves in guinea pigs. Kohrogi et al. (27) reported that SP could induce a cough reflex in guinea pigs at very low concentrations

$(10^{-18}-10^{-14} M)$ but several groups have been unable to reproduce these results. Takahama et al. (28) and Fox et al. (29) found that SP given at concentrations up to $10^{-4} M$ did not evoke cough in guinea pigs. Similar negative data have been reported in pigs (30). In humans, SP aerosols given to healthy subjects or to patients with asthma did not cause cough, but did evoke a sensation of tightness in the chest of asthmatics, possibly secondary to bronchoconstriction, indicating that some sensory nerves were being stimulated (31). In another study, aerosolized SP caused cough in patients with upper respiratory tract infection but not in healthy subjects (32). It is thus possible that both SP and NKA could evoke cough secondary to their ability to evoke bronchospasm and/or activate RARs (see later).

Tachykinins Elicit a Marked Sensitizing Effect on Cough

While tachykinins might not themselves induce cough, they may elicit a marked sensitizing effect on the cough reflex through enhanced activation of RARs (Fig. 1) (see also Chapters 2 and 3). Such an action was established in vivo by recording the activity of single RAR fibers in rabbits (33,34). In these experiments, systemic SP not only caused reflex changes characteristic of stimulation of lung RARs but also increased the impulse frequency in single vagal fibers coming from RARs. In electrophysiological studies in guinea pigs in vitro, Fox (35) have reported that SP applied directly onto receptive fields in the trachea did not activate either single C-fibers or Aδ-fibers. In contrast, in vivo, prior exposure of guinea pigs to SP markedly enhanced citric acid-induced cough (35). Similar enhancement of citric acid-induced cough by SP was reported in vivo in pigs (30). This direct sensitizing effect of SP on fibers coming from RARs can be amplified by increased release of tachykinins under the influence of inflammatory mediators such as prostaglandin (PGE$_2$, PGF2α, and bradykinin (36,37), of agents such as ozone (38), eosinophil cationic protein (39), or in inflammatory diseases (viral infections, asthma) (40,41).

Tachykinins can also lead to indirect activation of RAR fibers through airway obstruction, particularly by stimuli that decrease dynamic lung compliance, and by accumulation of mucus in the airway lumen (42,43).

The sensitizing effect of tachykinins on RAR fibers has also been demonstrated in the vagal ganglia and in the CNS (37), especially in the NTS where bronchopulmonary C-fiber and RAR termination sites overlap considerably (44). It has been shown that SP can facilitate synaptic transmission between bronchopulmonary afferent nerve endings and NTS neurons (45). This pharmacological and morphological evidence suggests that C-fibers might act synergistically with cough reflexes. Direct evidence for such a synergism in cough and reflex bronchospasm has been reported in anesthetized guinea pigs by Mazzone and Canning (18,46). Cough was induced by electrical stimulation of the tracheal mucosa and the threshold

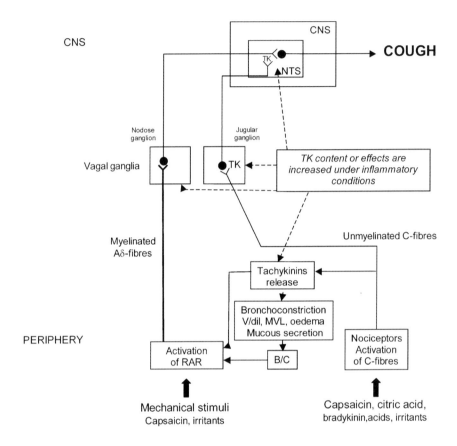

Figure 1 Tachykinins and cough. *Abbreviations*: B/C, bronchoconstriction; CNS, central nervous system; MVL, microvascular leakage; NTS, nucleus tractus solitarii; RAR, rapidly adapting receptor; TK, tachykinins; V/dil, vasodilatation. (Adapted from Refs. 7,22, and 23.)

voltage for evoking cough was recorded. Application of capsaicin to the trachea or microinjection of capsaicin into the commissural NTS did not by itself evoke cough but reduced the threshold voltage for cough. This enhanced cough sensitivity produced by capsaicin could be prevented by tracheal administration of capsazepine, a specific antagonist of vanilloid VR1 receptors, or by the tachykinin NK_3 receptor antagonist SB 223412, or the NK1 receptor antagonist CP99994 administered by intracerebroventricular (i.c.v.) infusion (46).

Tachykinins and Plasticity of the Cough Reflex

The sensitizing effect of tachykinins on cough may be amplified by the increased levels of neuropeptides localized in airway tissues and nerves under inflammatory conditions (23). Fischer et al. (6) have shown that in guinea pigs sensitized to ovalbumin, there was a three- to fourfold enhancement of tissue concentrations of NKA and SP in the lungs 24 hr after allergen exposure. They also observed that 12 hr after antigen stimulation, preprotachykinin mRNA was increased by 20% in nodose ganglia, but they did not detect a significant quantitative change in jugular ganglia. Myers et al. (40) have also reported such a phenotypic switch in neuropeptide production in neurons following allergic inflammation. Carr et al. (41) reported comparable effects on airway innervation following respiratory virus infection. Finally, long-term facilitatory interactions between RARs and C-fiber receptors have been reported in the NTS, suggesting that CNS plasticity results in enhanced cough in chronic airway conditions (18,47).

Tachykinin Receptor Antagonists and Cough

Tachykinin Receptor Antagonists Inhibit Cough

It is now clearly established that tachykinin receptor antagonists inhibit cough in several experimental conditions in animals (Table 3).

Antitussive effects of tachykinin NK_2 receptor antagonists have been reported using various compounds. SR 48968 was shown to inhibit citric acid- (48,50,52) and capsaicin- (53,63) induced cough in unanesthetized guinea pigs or pigs (30). It also blocked cough induced by mechanical stimulation of the intrathoracic trachea in anesthetized cats (53). MEN 10627, a peptide tachykinin NK_2 receptor antagonist, inhibits cough induced by allergen challenge in ovalbumin-sensitized guinea pigs (59). In contrast, Lalloo et al. (55) reported that the compound SR 48968 had a nonsignificant effect in naive guinea pigs but abolished the enhancement of citric acid-induced cough in animals previously exposed to ozone, suggesting an effect of tachykinin receptor antagonists on the sensitizing effect of ozone on C-fibers.

When administered by the intraperitoneal route, the NK_2 receptor antagonist SR 48968 was approximately 150 times more potent than codeine in inhibiting citric acid-induced cough in guinea pigs (52). In contrast to codeine, this effect was not reversed by naloxone. SR 48968 was also effective when administered by aerosol, but the difference in potency between SR 48968 and codeine was slightly lower under these conditions (48). It may also be important to note that both SR 48968 and codeine only partially inhibited the cough response (approximately 60–70%) (50,52). The inhibitory effect of SR 48968 on citric acid-induced cough has been reported to be independent of its inhibitory effect on citric acid-induced

Table 3 Tachykinin Receptor Antagonists in Experimental Models of Cough

Species	Cough induced by	Tachykinin receptor antagonists	Response	References
Guinea pig	Citric acid or capsaicin	NK$_1$	SR 140333,	0	(48)
			CP-99,994	0	(35)
			SSR 240600,	↓	(49)
			GR 205171	↓	(49)
			FK 888	↓	(50,51)
		NK$_2$	SR 48968,	↓	(48,52–54)
			SR 144190	↓	(54)
			SR 48968	0	(55)
		NK$_3$	SR 142801,	↓	(56,57)
			SR 146977	↓	(57)
			SB 235375	↓	(58)
	Tobacco smoke, phosphoramidon, SP	NK$_1$	FK 888	↓	(50)
	Allergen challenge	NK$_2$	MEN 10627	↓	(59)
	[β Ala^8] NKA (4–10)	NK$_1$	R116301	0	(60)
Cat	Mechanical stimulation of the trachea	NK$_1$	CP-99,994	↓	(53)
		NK$_2$	SR 48968	↓	(53)
		NK$_3$	SR 142801	↓	(53)
Pig	Citric acid	NK$_1$	SR 140333	↓	(30)
		NK$_2$	SR 48968	↓	(30)
		NK$_3$	SR 142801	↓	(30)
Asthmatic patients	Hypertonic saline	NK$_1$	CP-99,994	0	(61)
	Bradykinin	NK$_1$	FK 888	↓	(62)

bronchoconstriction in guinea pigs, since SR 48968 blocked cough in guinea pigs pretreated with bronchodilator doses of salbutamol that did not reduce cough (48).

The antitussive effect of tachykinin NK$_1$ receptor antagonists has also been studied. CP-99,994 and SR 140333 have been shown to be ineffective on citric acid-induced cough in unanesthetized guinea pigs (35,48). No inhibitory activity of CP-99,994 was observed on cough induced by inhalation of hypertonic saline in asthmatic patients (61). In contrast, FK 888 has been shown to inhibit cough induced by various agents (phosphoramidon, tobacco smoke, SP, citric acid) in unanesthetized guinea pigs (50,51) and cough evoked by bradykinin in asthmatic patients (62). Moreover, Bolser et al. (53) have observed that CP-99,994 was able to inhibit cough induced by capsaicin in guinea pigs or cough induced by mechanical stimulation of the trachea in anesthetized cats. Finally, SSR 240600, a potent and centrally active NK_1 antagonist was able to inhibit cough induced by citric acid in guinea pigs (49).

On the other hand, SR 140333 has been reported to potentiate, in terms of maximal effect, the antitussive activity of a tachykinin NK_2 receptor antagonist (SR 48968) on citric acid-induced cough in guinea pigs (48). Under similar conditions, FK 888 and SR 48968 had small additive effects (50). Such potentiation or additive effects were also observed with these compounds in other experimental models including bronchoconstriction induced by intravenous SP, NKA, capsaicin, or resiniferatoxin, as well as by allergen challenge in guinea pigs (64,65).

The antitussive effects of tachykinin NK_3 receptor antagonists were first demonstrated with SR 142801 on acid-induced cough in unanesthetized guinea pigs. The compound was able to inhibit cough at doses selective for NK_3 receptors (56). This property of NK_3 receptor antagonists was recently confirmed using SSR 146977 (57) and SB 235375 (58).

Drugs with combined tachykinin receptor antagonist activities such as MDL 105212A (NK_1+NK_2) (66), S 16474 (NK_1+NK_2) (67), and SCH 206272 ($NK_1+NK_2+NK_3$) (68) have also been reported to possess antitussive effects in preclinical studies.

Finally, similar to the results obtained with tachykinin receptor antagonists, a wide range of agents inhibiting tachykinin release, such as opioid receptor agonists (26,35) and nociceptin (see Chapter 7 in this book), have been shown to inhibit cough in humans and in animal models.

Level of Action of Tachykinin Receptor Antagonists: Peripheral or Central?

It is difficult to be certain whether the antitussive activity of tachykinin receptor antagonists is related to a central or a peripheral action. Arguments for a peripheral effect are drawn from (i) the ability of some tachykinin receptor antagonists (FK 224, SR 48968) to inhibit cough when given by inhalation (48,51,69–71) and (ii) the ability of tachykinin receptor antagonists to inhibit cough despite low CNS penetration and an inability to cross the blood–brain barrier, as shown by pharmacological methods or pharmacokinetic studies. Indeed, the NK_1 receptor antagonist FK 888 inhibited cough induced by tobacco smoke, phosphoramidon, SP, or citric acid but, even at high doses, did not inhibit foot tapping induced by central administration of SP in gerbils (50). Similarly, the tachykinin NK_3 receptor antagonist SB 235375 inhibits cough induced by citric acid in guinea pigs, but has been shown to have no significant effect on i.c.v. senktide-induced behavioral effects in mice (58). Furthermore, even after administration of high doses, SB 235375 concentrations in the brain were below the limit of detection (58). However, it is possible that, albeit poor CNS penetrant compounds, these drugs may enter the brain in sufficient concentrations to exert inhibitory effects on pulmonary function but not on central responses. They may also exert an effect in areas not protected by the blood–brain barrier. In addition, species differences may explain the discrepancies between respiratory and CNS pharmacological responses and/or pharmacokinetic studies.

Evidence for a central site of action for tachykinin receptor antagonists has been reported in guinea pigs and in cats. In guinea pigs, Bolser et al. (53) have shown that both CP-99,994 and SR 48412 (the racemate compound of SR 48968) inhibited capsaicin-induced cough after i.c.v. administration and the doses necessary to inhibit cough were much lower than the minimally active systemic doses. Similarly, Emonds-Alt et al. (49) have shown that the antitussive effect of the NK_1 receptor antagonist SSR 240600 may be related to its ability to penetrate into the brain. These authors (49) suggest that there is some parallelism between antitussive activity and other centrally mediated activities of the tachykinin NK_1 receptor antagonists. SR 140333 was shown to have several activities in the rat CNS (72), but it was also reported to be devoid of activity in other models, namely, models for emesis, in which brain penetration of the compound is essential (73,74). In contrast, CP-99,994 showed potent antiemetic activity as well as other typical centrally mediated effects (73). Moreover, a potent antidepressant-like activity of SSR 240600 in guinea pigs was clearly demonstrated (75) as for other centrally active tachykinin NK_1 receptor antagonists (76).

In the cat, Bolser et al. (53) have shown that both CP-99,994 and SR 48968 were able to inhibit cough induced by mechanical stimulation of the intrathoracic trachea when given intravenously but also when they were delivered directly to the brainstem circulation via the vertebral artery. The effective dose ratio for i.v. to i.a. potencies was considerably higher than expected for a drug considered as centrally active (80 vs. 20). Furthermore, cough elicited by mechanical stimuli involves RARs and likely does not elicit the peripheral release of tachykinins from pulmonary or bronchial C-fibers. These results are consistent with recent studies showing the important role of tachykinins in the CNS, especially in the NTS (17,18). Furthermore, recent data on the role of NK_3 receptors in the cNTS (46) may explain a central effect of the antitussive actions of the CNS penetrant tachykinin NK_3 receptor antagonists SR 142801 and SSR 146977 (56,57).

Conclusion

Recent advances in our knowledge of the role of tachykinins in cough result from (i) a better understanding of the properties and plasticity of sensory nerves in the periphery and in the CNS and (ii) analysis of the antitussive effects of tachykinin receptor antagonists. However, most of the data have been obtained in animal models. The clinical relevance of these results and the potential of tachykinin receptor antagonists in the treatment of cough in humans have not yet been elucidated. The lack of clinical results could be due to species differences, inasmuch as the role of neurogenic inflammation has not clearly been established in the human lung. However, on the basis of the data obtained on the effects of tachykinins in the NTS, the discovery and characterization of new tachykinin receptor antagonists with potent central activity will be of interest.

References

1. Lundberg JM. Pharmacology of cotransmission in the autonomic nervous system: integrative aspects on amines, neuropeptides, adenosine triphosphate, amino acids and nitric oxide. Pharmacol Rev 1996; 48:113–178.
2. Lundberg JM, Saria A. Polypeptide-containing neurons in airway smooth muscle. Ann Rev Physiol 1987; 49:557–572.
3. Ollerenshaw SL, Jarvis D, Sullivan CE, Woolcock AJ. Substance P immunoreactive nerves in airways from asthmatics and nonasthmatics. Eur Respir J 1991; 4:673–682.
4. Ellis JL, Undem BJ. Pharmacology of non-adrenergic, non-cholinergic nerves in airway smooth muscle. Pulm Pharmacol 1994; 7:205–223.
5. Baluk P, McDonald DM. Proinflammatory peptides in sensory nerves of the airways. In: Said SI, ed. Proinflammatory and Anti-Inflammatory Peptides. New York: Dekker, 1998:45–68.
6. Fischer A, McGregor GP, Saria A, Phillipin B, KummerW. Introduction of tachykinin gene and peptide expression in guinea-pig nodose primary afferent neurons by allergic airway inflammation. J Clin Invest 1996; 98:2284–2291.
7. Canning BJ. Interactions between vagal afferent nerve subtypes mediating cough. Pulm Pharmacol Ther 2002; 156:187–192.
8. Germonpré PR, Bullock GR, Lambrecht BN, Van de Velde V, Luyten WH, Joos GF, Pauwels RA. Presence of substance P and neurokinin 1 receptors in human sputum macrophages and U-937 cells. Eur Respir J 1999; 14: 776–782.
9. Lambrecht BN, Germonpré PR, Everaert EG, Carro-Muino I, De Veerman M, De Felipe C, Hunt SP, Thielemans K, Joos GF, Pauwels RA. Endogenously produced substance P contributes to lymphocyte proliferation induced by dendritic cells and direct TCR ligation. Eur J Immunol 1999; 29:3815–3825.
10. Braun A, Wieber P, Pfeufer A, Gessner R, Renz H. Differential modulation of immunoglobulin isotype production by the neuropeptides substance P, NKA and NKB. J Neuroimmunol 1999; 97:43–50.
11. Joos GF, De Swert KO, Pauwels RA. Airways inflammation and tachykinins: prospects for the development of tachykinin receptor antagonists. Eur J Pharmacol 2001; 429:239–250.

12. Advenier C, Lagente V, Boichot E. The role of tachykinin receptor antagonists in the prevention of bronchial hyperresponsiveness, airway inflammation and cough. Eur Respir J 1997; 10:1892–1906.
13. Spina D, Page CP, Morley J. Sensory neuropeptides and bronchial hyperresponsiveness. In: Said SI, ed. Proinflammatory and Anti-Inflammatory Peptides. New York: Dekker, 1998:45–68.
14. Regoli D, Bourdon A, Fauchère JL. Receptors and antagonists for substance P and related peptides. Pharmacol Rev 1994; 46:551–599.
15. Myers AC, Undem BJ. Electrophysiological effects of tachykinins and capsaicin on guinea-pig bronchial parasympathetic ganglion neurones. J Physiol 1993; 470:665–679.
16. Canning BJ, Reynolds SM, Anukwu LU, Kajetar R, Myers AC. Endogenous neurokinins facilitate synaptic transmission in guinea-pig airway parasympathetic ganglia. Am J Physiol Regul Integr Comp Physiol 2002; 283:R320–R330.
17. Mazzone SB, Geraghty DP. Respiratory actions of tachykinins in the nucleus of the solitary tract: characterisation of receptors using selective agonists and antagonists. Br J Pharmacol 2000; 129:1121–1131.
18. Mazzone SB, Canning BJ. Synergistic interactions between airway afferent nerves subtypes mediating reflex bronchospasm in guinea-pigs. Am J Physiol Regul Integr Comp Physiol 2002; 283:R86–R98.
19. Lundberg JM, Saria A. Capsaicin-induced desensitization of airway mucosa to cigarette smoke, mechanical and chemical irritants. Nature 1983; 302:251–253.
20. Forsberg K, Karlsson JA, Theodorssont E, Lundberg JM, Persson CGA. Cough and bronchoconstriction mediated by capsaicin-sensitive sensory neurons in the guinea-pig. Pulm Pharmacol 1988; 1:33–39.
21. Lalloo UG, Fox AJ, Belvisi MG, Chung KF, Barnes PJ. Capsazepine inhibits cough induced by capsaicin and citric acid but not hypertonic saline in guinea-pig. J Appl Physiol 1995; 79:1082–1087.
22. Widdicombe JG. Neurophysiology of the cough reflex. Eur Respir J 1995; 8:1193–1202.
23. Undem BJ, Carr MJ, Kollarik M. Physiology and plasticity of putative cough fibres in the guinea-pig. Pulm Pharmacol Ther 2002; 15:193–198.
24. Laude EA, Higgins KS, Morice AH. A comparative study of the effects of citric acid, capsaicin and resiniferatoxin on the cough challenge in guinea-pig and man. Pulm Pharmacol 1993; 6:171–175.
25. Midgren B, Hansson L, Karlsson JA, Simonsson BG, Persson CGA. Capsaicin-induced cough in humans. Am Rev Resp Dis 1992; 146:347–351.
26. Widdicombe JG. Neuroregulation of cough: implications for drug therapy. Curr Opin Pharmacol 2002; 2:256–263.
27. Kohrogi H, Graf P, Sekizawa K, Borson D, Nadel J. Neutral endopeptidase inhibitors potentiate substance P and capsaicin-induced cough in awake guinea-pigs. J Clin Invest 1988; 82:2063–2068.
28. Takahama K, Fuchikama T, Isohama Y, Kai H, Miyata T. Neurokinin A but not neurokinin B and substance P induces codeine-resistant coughs in awaked guinea-pigs. Regul Pept 1993; 42:236–237.

29. Fox AJ, Bernareggi M, Lalloo UG, Chung KF, Barnes PJ, Belvisi MG. The effect of substance P on the cough reflex and airway sensory nerves in guinea-pigs. Am J Respir Crit Care Med 1996; 153:A161.
30. Moreaux B, Nemmar A, Vincke G, Halloy D, Beerens D, Advenier C, Gustin P. Role of substance P and tachykinin receptor antagonists in citric acid-induced cough in pigs. Eur J Pharmacol 2000; 408:305–312.
31. Joos GF, Pauwels RA, Van Der Straeten ME. Effect of inhaled substance P and neurokinin A on the airways of normal and asthmatic subjects. Thorax 1987; 42:779–783.
32. Katsumata U, Sekizawa H, Sasaki H, Takishima T. Inhibitory actions of procaterol, a $beta_2$-stimulant, on substance P-induced cough in normal subjects during upper respiratory tract infection. J Exp Med 1989; 158:105–106.
33. Prabhakar NR, Runold M, Yamamoto Y, Lagercrantz H, Cherniack NS, von Euler C. Role of the vagal afferents in substance P-induced respiratory responses in anaesthetized rabbits. Acta Physiol Scand 1987; 131:63–71.
34. Masumoto S, Takeda M, Saiki C, Takahashi T, Ojima K. Effects of tachykinins on rapidly adapting pulmonary stretch receptors and total lung resistance in anesthetized articicially ventilated rabbits. J Pharmacol Exp Ther 1997; 283:1026–1031.
35. Fox AJ. Modulation of cough and airway sensory fibres. Pulm Pharmacol 1996; 9:335–342.
36. Ho CY, Gu JL, Hong JL, Lee LY. Prostaglandin E_2 enhances chemical and mechanical sensitivities of pulmonary C-fibers. Am J Respir Crit Care Med 2000; 162:528–533.
37. Lee LY, Kwong K, Lin YS, Gu Q. Hypersensitivity of bronchopulmonary C-fibers induced by airway mucosal inflammation: cellular mechanisms. Pulm Pharmacol Ther 2002; 15:199–204.
38. Lee LY, Pisarry TE. Afferent properties and reflex functions of bronchopulmonary C-fibres. Respir Physiol 2001; 125:47–65.
39. Lee LY, Gu Q, Gleich GJ. Effect of human eosinophil granule-derived cationic proteins on C-fibre afferents in the rat lung. J Physiol 2001; 91:1318–1326.
40. Myers AC, Kajekar R, Undem BJ. Allergic inflammation-induced neuropeptide production in rapidly adapting afferent nerves in guinea-pig airways. Am J Physiol Lung Cell Mol Physiol 2002; 282:L775–L781.
41. Carr MJ, Hunter DD, Jacoby DB, Undem BJ. Expression of tachykinins in non-nociceptive vagal afferent neurons during respiratory tract viral infection in guinea-pigs. Am J Respir Crit Care Med 2002; 165:1071–1075.
42. Bergren DR. Sensory receptor activation by mediators of defence reflexes in guinea-pig lungs. Respir Physiol 1997; 108:195–204.
43. Joad JP, Kott KS, Bonham AC. Nitric oxide contributes to substance P-induced increases in lung rapidly adapting receptor activity in guinea-pigs. J Physiol 1997; 503:635–643.
44. Jordan D. Central nervous pathways and control of the airways. Respir Physiol 2001; 125:67–81.
45. Mutoh T, Bonham AC, Joad JP. Substance P in the nucleus of the solitary tract augments bronchopulmonary C-fiber reflex output. Am J Physiol 2000; 279:R1215–R1223.

46. Mazzone SB, Canning BJ. Central interactions between airway afferent nerve subtypes mediating cough. Am J Respir Crit Care Med 2003; 167:A146.

47. Mazzone SB, Geraghty DP. Respiratory action of capsaicin microinjected into the nucleus of the solitary tract: involvement of vanilloid and tachykinin receptors. Br J Pharmacol 1999; 127:473–481.

48. Girard V, Naline E, Vilain P, Emonds-Alt X, Advenier C. Effect of the two tachykinins antagonists, SR 48968 and SR 140333, on cough induced by citric acid in the unanaesthetized guinea-pig. Eur Respir J 1995; 8:1110–1114.

49. Emonds-Alt X, Proietto V, Steinberg R, Oury-Donat F, Vige X, Vilain P, Naline E, Daoui S, Advenier C, Le Fur G, Maffrand JP, Soubrié P, Pascal M. SR240600 [(R)-2-(1-[2-[4-[2-[3,5-bis(trifluoromethyl)phenyl]acetyl]-2-(3,4-dichlorophenyl)-2-morpholinyl]ethyl]-4-piperidinyl)-2-methylpropanamide], a centrally active nonpeptide antagonist of the tachykinin neurokinin-1 receptor: biochemical and pharmacological characterization. J Pharmacol Exp Ther 2002; 303:1171–1179.

50. Yasumitsu R, Hirayama Y, Imai T, Miyayasu K, Hiroi J. Effects of specific tachykinin receptor antagonists on citric acid-induced cough and bronchoconstriction in unanesthetized guinea-pigs. Eur J Pharmacol 1996; 300:215–219.

51. Ujiie Y, Sekizawa K, Aikawa T, Sasaki H. Evidence for substance P as an endogenous substance causing cough in guinea-pigs. Am Rev Respir Dis 1993; 148:1628–1632.

52. Advenier C, Girard V, Naline E, Vilain P, Emonds-Alt X. Antitussive effect of SR 48968, a non-peptide tachykinin NK_2 receptor antagonist. Eur J Pharmacol 1993; 250:169–171.

53. Bolser DC, De Genno FE, O'Reilly S, McLeod RL, Hay JA. Central antitussive activity of the tachykinin receptor antagonists CP 99994 and SR 48968 in the guinea pig and cat. Br J Pharmacol 1997; 121:165–170.

54. Emonds-Alt X, Advenier C, Cognon C, Croci C, Daoui S, Ducoux JP, Landi M, Naline E, Neliat G, Poncelet M, Proietto V, Van Broek D, Vilain P, Manara L, Soubrié P, Le Fur G, Maffrand JP, Brelière JC. Biochemical and pharmacological activities of SR 144190, a new potent non-peptide tachykinin NK2 receptor antagonist. Neuropeptides 1997; 31:449–458.

55. Lalloo UG, Fox AJ, Bernareggi M, Belvisi MG, Chung KF, Barnes PJ. Bradykinin sensitisation of airway sensory nerves: a mechanism for captopril-induced enhancement of the cough reflex. Am J Respir Crit Care Med 1996; 153:A162.

56. Daoui S, Cognon C, Naline E, Emonds-Alt X, Advenier C. Involvement of tachykinin NK_3 receptors in citric acid-induced cough and bronchial responses in guinea-pigs. Am J Respir Crit Care Med 1998; 158:42–48.

57. Emonds-Alt X, Proietto V, Steinberg R, Advenier C, Daoui S, Naline E, Gueudet C, Michaud JC, Oury-Donat F, Poncelet M, Vilain P, Le Fur G, Maffrand JP, Soubrié P, Pascal M. Biochemical and pharmacological activities of SSR 146977, a new potent nonpeptide tachykinin NK3 receptor antagonist. Can J Physiol Pharmacol 2002; 80:482–488.

58. Hay D, Giardina GA, Griswold DE, Underwood DC, Kotzer CJ, Bush B, Potts W, Sandhu P, Lundberg D, Foley JJ, Schmidt DB, Martin LD, Killian D, Legos JJ, Baronne FC, Luttmann MA, Grugni M, Raveglia LF, Sarau HM. Non

peptide tachykinin receptor antagonists. III SB 235375, a low central nervous system-penetrant, potent and selective neurokinin-3 receptor antagonist, inhibits citric acid-induced cough and airways hyper-reactivity in guinea-pigs. J Pharmacol Exp Ther 2002; 300:314–323.

59. Evangelista S, Ballati J, Perretti F. MEN 10,627, a new selective NK_2 receptor antagonist inhibits antigen-induced bronchoconstriction in sensitized guinea-pigs. Neuropeptides 1994; 26(suppl 1):39–40.

60. Megens AA, Ashton D, Vermeire JC, Vermote PC, Hens KA, Hillen LC, Fransen JF, Mahieu M, Heylen L, Leysen JE, Jurzak MR, Janssens F. Pharmacological profile of (2R-trans)-4-[1-[3,5-bis(trifluoromethyl)benzoyl]-2-(phenylmethyl-4-piperidinyl]-N-(2,6-dimethylphenyl)-1-acetamide(S)-hydroxy-butanedioate (R116301), an orally and centrally active neurokinin-1 receptor antagonist. J Pharmacol Exp Ther 2002; 302:696–709.

61. Fahy JV, Wong HH, Geppetti P, Nadel JA, Boushey HA. Effect of an NK_1 receptor antagonist (CP-99,994) on hypertonic saline-induced bronchocon-striction and cough in asthmatic subjects. Am J Respir Crit Care Med 1994; 149:A1057.

62. Ichinose M, Nakajima N, Takahashi T, Yamamuchi H, Inoue H, Takishima T. Protection against bradykinin-induced bronchoconstriction in asthmatic patients by neurokinin receptor antagonist. Lancet 1992; 340:1248–1251.

63. Robineau P, Petit C, Staczek J, Peglion JL, Brion JD, Canet E. NK_1 and NK_2 receptors involvement in capsaicin-induced cough in guinea-pigs. Am J Respir Crit Care Med 1994; 149:A186.

64. Foulon DM, Champion E, Masson P, Rodger IW, Jones TR. NK_1 and NK_2 receptors mediate tachykinin and resiniferatoxin-induced bronchospasm in guinea-pigs. Am Rev Respir Dis 1993; 148:915–921.

65. Bertrand C, Nadel JA, Graf PA, Geppetti P. Capsaicin increases airflow resis-tance in guinea-pigs *in vivo* by activating both NK_2 and NK_1 tachykinin recep-tors. Am Rev Respir Dis 1993; 148:909–914.

66. Kudlacz EM, Shatzer SA, Knippenberg RW, Logan DE, Poirot M, Van Giersbergen PLM, Burkholder TP. *In vitro* and *in vivo* characterization of MDL 105,212A, a nonpeptide NK-1/NK-2 tachykinin receptor antagonist. J Pharmacol Exp Ther 1996; 277:840–851.

67. Robineau P, Longchampt M, Kucharczyk N, Krause JE, Regoli D, Fauchere JL, Prost JF, Canet E. *In vitro* and *in vivo* pharmacology of S.16474, a novel dual tachykinin NK_1 and NK_2 receptor antagonist. Eur J Pharmacol 1995; 294:677–684.

68. Anthes JC, Chapman RW, Richard C, Eckel S, Corboz M, Hey JA, Fernandez X, Greefeder S, McLeod R, Sehring S, Rizzo C, Crawley Y, Shih NY, Piwinski J, Reichard G, Ting P, Carruthers N, Cuss FM, Billah M, Kreutner W, Egan RW. SCH 206272: a potent, orally active tachykinin NK(1), NK(2) and NK(3) recep-tors antagonist. Eur J Pharmacol 2002; 450:191–202.

69. Xiang A, Uchida Y, Nomura A, Lijima H, Dong F, Zhang MJ, Hasegawa S. Effects of airway inflammation on cough response in the guinea-pig. J Appl Physiol 1998; 85:1841–1854.

70. Ogawa H, Fujimura M, Saito M, Matsuda T, Akao N, Kondo D. The effect of the neurokinin antagonist FK-224 on the cough response to inhaled capsaicin

in a new model of guinea-pig eosinophilic bronchitis induced by intranasal polymixin B. Clin Auton Res 1994; 4:19–27.

71. Sekizawa K, Ebihara T, Sasaki H. Role of substance P in cough during bronchoconstriction in awake guinea-pigs. Am J Respir Crit Care Med 1995; 151:815–821.

72. Jung M, Calassi R, Maruani J, Barnouin MC, Souilhac J, Poncelet M, Gueudet C, Emonds-Alt X, Soubrié P, Brelière JC, Le Fur G. Neuropharmacological characterization of SR 140333, a non peptide antagonist of NK₁ receptors. Neuropharmacology 1994; 33:167–179.

73. Rupniak NMJ, Tattersall FD, Williams AR, Rycroft W, Carlson EJ, Cascieri MA, Sadowsi S, Ber E, Hale JJ, Mills SG, MacCoss M, Seward E, Huscroft I, Owen S, Swain CJ, Hill RG, Hargreaves RJ. *In vitro* and *in vivo* predictors of the anti-emetic activity of tachykinin NK₁ receptors antagonists. Eur J Pharmacol 1997; 326:201–209.

74. Diemunsch P, Grélot L. Potential of substance P antagonists as antiemetics. Drugs 2000; 60:533–546.

75. Steinberg R, Alonso R, Rouquier L, Desvignes C, Michaud JC, Cudennec A, Jung M, Simiand J, Griebel G, Emonds-Alt X, Le Fur G, Soubrie P. SSR240600 [(R)-2-(1-[2-[4-[2-[3,5-bis(trifluoromethyl)phenyl]acetyl]-2-(3,4-dichlorophenyl)-2-morpholinyl]ethyl]-4-piperidinyl)-2-methylpropanamide], a centrally active nonpeptide antagonist of the tachykinin neurokinin 1 receptor: II. Neurochemical and behavioral characterization. J Pharmacol Exp Ther 2002; 303:1180–1188.

76. Rupniak NM, Kramer MS. Discovery of the antidepressant and anti-emetic efficacy of substance P receptor (NK₁) receptors antagonist. Trends Pharmacol Sci 1999; 12:485–490.

5

ACE Inhibitor-Induced Cough: Lessons from Animal Models

YUKO MORISHIMA and
KIYOHISA SEKIZAWA

Department of Pulmonary Medicine,
 Institute of Clinical Medicine,
 University of Tsukuba,
Tsukuba, Japan

TAKASHI OHRUI and
HIDETADA SASAKI

Department of Geriatric and Respiratory
 Medicine, Tohoku University
 School of Medicine,
Sendai, Japan

Introduction

Since captopril was first introduced in the late 1970s (1), angiotensin-converting enzyme (ACE) inhibitors have become well established as useful antihypertensive drugs, along with diuretics, beta-blockers, and calcium antagonists. ACE inhibitors may lower blood pressure by blocking the conversion of angiotensin I to angiotensin II and by causing the accumulation of kinins. Hypertension is now a worldwide problem from which approximately one billion people suffer (2), and ACE inhibitors are currently administered to millions of patients. ACE inhibitors are recommended especially for those hypertensive patients who have associated high-risk conditions such as diabetes, chronic renal disease, cerebrovascular disease, ischemic heart disease, and heart failure (2). Numerous studies have demonstrated satisfactory outcomes resulting from the administration of these agents (3–6).

Few fatal side effects have been associated with the use of ACE inhibitors. However, cough has been observed in a variable percentage of hypertensive patients (0.2–33%) as an adverse effect during ACE inhibitor therapy (7). Moreover, the cough associated with ACE inhibitor treatment is a major concern of physicians when treating hypertensive patients, as it can degrade a patients' quality of life and is closely correlated with variations in compliance with treatment (8). Conversely, chronic cough was estimated to be due to ACE inhibitors 2% of the time in a prospective descriptive study (9), such that ACE inhibitor-induced cough is among the important differential diagnoses when physicians assess patients complaining of a persistent cough (10).

Although several mechanisms have been proposed since ACE inhibitor-related cough was first reported in the early 1980s (11–13), it remains uncertain how ACE inhibitors produce cough. In this chapter, we will focus on the findings from several animal studies that have characterized the mechanism of ACE inhibitor-induced cough. The purpose of this chapter is to demonstrate how animal studies can impact our understanding and management of ACE inhibitor-induced cough.

Clinical Aspects of ACE Inhibitor-Induced Cough

Dry cough is the most frequent and troublesome adverse effect seen during ACE inhibitor therapy (14), and it is also a major limitation to continuing treatment with these medications (8). Although the incidence of ACE inhibitor-induced cough varies widely among the numerous published reports, the average may be as high as 10% (7).

This type of cough seems to occur much more frequently in women and in nonsmokers (14–19), but the reasons for these higher rates have not yet been elucidated. One explanation might be that females have a lower threshold for coughing than males, regardless of ACE inhibitor use (20–22). In addition, smokers are typically used to having a cough, and they may therefore not complain of this symptom. ACE inhibitor-induced coughing is a class effect, and some studies report no significant differences with regard to dosage (23) or particular type of ACE inhibitor (24). However, contrary data have also been reported, e.g., that coughing is more commonly observed with a specific type of ACE inhibitor (25,26) and at a high dosage (19). It has also been reported that there were no significant differences in terms of sex (27) and smoking habits (8,15,23).

ACE inhibitor-induced cough can appear within several weeks sometimes may take months to develop after starting treatment (21,28). Postviral respiratory infection occasionally becomes a trigger for the onset of the symptom (21). The cough is chronic and nonproductive, and the symptoms resemble those of patients with cough-variant asthma. Patients complain of the sensation of a tickle in the throat, and of choking easily when they laugh, shout, or inhale smoke or cold air. Although in most cases the symptom is not particularly serious, there are reports of ACE inhibitor-induced cough associated with sleep disturbance, vomiting, voice changes, sore throat, and feelings of being fatigued and depressed (19,29). The cough usually disappears within several days after withdrawal of the ACE inhibitor but sometimes can require as long as 4 weeks to resolve (14). A randomized double-blind controlled trial revealed that, among patients who had previously experienced ACE inhibitor-related cough, the cough recurred in 71.7% within 19 days (range 17–20 days) during a period of rechallenge. In addition, it was reported that this type of cough took 26 days (range 24–27.5) to subside during a placebo washout period (17).

Since there is no specific laboratory test for ACE inhibitor-induced cough, the resolution of coughing after discontinuation of ACE inhibitor therapy may be the only reliable means to diagnose the condition. Physicians should always consider the possibility of an ACE inhibitor as the cause of a cough whenever they treat patients who are taking ACE inhibitors as antihypertensive drugs.

Enzymatic Modulation of ACE and ACE Inhibitors

First isolated in 1956 as a hypertensin-converting enzyme, ACE (EC 3.4.15.1) is a peptidyldipeptide hydrolase which converts angiotensin I to the vasopressor angiotensin II by hydrolysis of the C-terminal dipeptide, His-Leu (30). Kininase II is also considered to be an ACE; kininase II is known to degrade bradykinin, a vasodilator, by the hydrolysis of the C-terminal dipeptide, Phe-Arg (31). Substance P and other biologically active peptides such as luteinizing hormone-releasing hormone are also substrates for ACE (32–34).

ACE exists in two distinct forms: a somatic form of high molecular weight found on the plasma membrane in many tissues, and a germinal low molecular weight form found in the testes. Somatic ACE contains two homologous domains, a C-terminal active site and an N-terminal active site (35), each of which has independent catalytic activity (36), whereas germinal ACE contains only a single active site (37). Although the two domains of somatic ACE appear to hydrolyze all substrates, the enzymatic properties of the active sites in these two domains may differ (38). Both active sites have a much higher affinity for bradykinin than for angiotensin I (38). The C-terminal active site is more sensitive to chloride activation which enhances the hydrolysis of angiotensin I and substance P, whereas the N-terminal active site preferentially hydrolyzes luteinizing-hormone releasing hormone (38). Each domain of ACE contains a zinc-binding site at which ACE carries out enzymatic interactions with the substrate, converting the substrate via these catalytic interactions. Due to this zinc-related mechanism, the activity of ACE can be inhibited by Zn chelating agents. A soluble form of ACE also exists, which circulates within the plasma, and which is derived from cleavage of tissue-bound ACE (39). However, the tissue-bound form of ACE has been demonstrated to be functionally important for locally degrading peptides located near the target receptor (40). ACE is distributed throughout the body, but is particularly abundant on the surface of endothelial cells of the lung and on the brush-border epithelial linings of the kidney, small intestine, and placenta (41–44). Although its activity has been reported to be predominant in the lung vascular endothelium, it is also present in the tissue of the airways (45,46). Therefore, ACE can regulate the degradation of kinins at both vascular and epithelial sites.

Studies of ACE inhibitors progressed rapidly after the isolation of an ACE inhibitory factor from snake venom in the early 1970s (47–50). Based on these early snake venom studies, Ondetti et al. (1) first discovered an orally active ACE inhibitor, captopril, which enabled the general therapeutic use of ACE inhibitors. Subsequently, many synthetic ACE inhibitors have been introduced. These compounds are structurally divided into three classes: the sulfhydryl-containing inhibitors such as captopril and alacepril; the carboxyalkyldipeptides such as enalapril, ramipril, and lisinopril; and phosphorus-containing inhibitors such as fosinopril and ceranapril, some of which are prodrug esters that require activation in vivo. When considering the relationship between ACE inhibitors and cough, one must be aware of the differences between the enzymatic properties of these inhibitory compounds. Although no obvious differences among ACE inhibitors have been reported as regards their inhibitory effects on the degradation of angiotensin I and bradykinin (51), further experiments may be required to clarify the specificities of these inhibitory functions. The structural potency and tissue distribution (52,53), as well as the affinity for each active site, may differ among ACE inhibitors.

Pathogenesis of ACE Inhibitor-Induced Cough

Cough can be caused by several pathophysiological conditions of the airways, including changes in the reflex itself, airway smooth muscle contraction, excessive mucus production, release of inflammatory mediators, epithelial sloughing, and enhanced epithelial permeability (54–56). Cough is a complex reflex, with an afferent pathway contained within the vagus nerve (57,58) and an efferent component within the somatic nervous system. Although cough and bronchoconstriction are believed to have separate afferent neural pathways, they often occur simultaneously and are thought to be closely related (56). With regard to cough and bronchoconstriction, many neurotransmitters and neural mechanisms have been identified, as described in previous chapters. Peptides such as bradykinin and substance P have been extensively studied during the past several decades, and are known to play a key role in stimulating the cough reflex and are recognized as important mediators in various inflammatory diseases of the airways such as asthma (59,60).

Recently, type 1 angiotensin II receptor antagonists, a new class of antihypertensive agents, have been reported to be associated with a low incidence of dry cough (21). This suggests that ACE inhibitor-induced cough is not due to alterations in the renin–angiotensin system but rather to an inhibition of kininase II-related factors. Because ACE is an enzyme that degrades bradykinin (47,49,61) and substance P (32,33,62), inhibiting ACE will not only decrease the production of angiotensin II but also potentiate kinins, an effect which may stimulate unmyelinated afferent sensory C-fibers and consequently alter cough sensitivity (24,63). The role of C-fibers in the development of cough is controversial. Some investigators have argued that stimulation of C-fibers inhibits cough through the modulation of a central gating mechanism (64,65) whereas other researchers have emphasized the excitatory effects of C-fiber activation (66–68). Although a conclusion has not been reached, it is known that sensitized C-fibers release more substance P in response to tussive stimuli via axon reflex mechanisms (69). In addition, both bradykinin and substance P can stimulate phospholipase A_2 to cause activation of the arachidonic acid cascade. This in turn generates prostanoids, among which prostaglandin E_2 (24,70–72) and thromboxane A_2 (73) are important proinflammatory peptides and exert an influence on the cough reflex. Finally, the accumulation of kinins may promote nitric oxide generation (74,75) and histamine release from mast cells (14), both of which may contribute to the development of cough. Thus, many proinflammatory peptides may be involved intricately in the pathogenesis of ACE inhibitor-induced cough.

Bradykinin

Bradykinin is a 9-amino-acid peptide derived from the enzymatic activation of the kallikrein–kinin system. Bradykinin usually acts locally by binding to specific receptors, i.e., bradykinin B_1 and B_2 receptors, located on smooth-muscle cells, epithelium, endothelium, and sensory nerves (76–78). This peptide is known to be an important inflammatory mediator, and it has pharmacological activity that leads to plasma extravasation, mucous gland secretion, pain, and vasodilatation. Most of these functions are mediated by the B_2 receptor (76–78). Therefore, in the pathogenesis of bronchoconstriction and cough, bradykinin may be an important mediator (59,70). Bradykinin is considered to stimulate C-fibers via type J receptors and thus to evoke a cough reflex (68). As mentioned previously, ACE inhibitors have inhibitory effects on the degradation of bradykinin, which will prolong its half-life (79,80). Furthermore, ACE inhibitors are considered to have a stimulatory effect on the bradykinin receptor that is distinct from its enzymatic inactivation (81,82). Therefore, bradykinin is one of the crucial candidate mediators in cough induced by ACE inhibitor treatment.

Dusser et al. (46) demonstrated that the neutral endopeptidase (NEP) inhibitors leucine-thiorphan and phophoramidon and the ACE inhibitor captopril potentiated bradykinin-induced contraction of ferret trachea in a dose-dependent fashion. The combination of phophoramidon and captopril resulted in an additive potentiation of the contraction. However, a substance P antagonist did not modify the potentiation of bradykinin-induced contraction. In that study, it was also shown that bradykinin[(8–9)] and bradykinin[(1–7)], the major fragments generated by hydrolysis of bradykinin by NEP or ACE, had only a very weak effect or no effect on tracheal contraction. Therefore, the cleavage of bradykinin by ACE inactivates its contractile activity, whereas inhibition of the enzyme may elevate the concentration of the peptide to increase the contractile response. Fox et al. (66) have shown that treatment of guinea pigs with captopril for 2 weeks led to an increased cough response to aerosols of citric acid, and this increase was prevented by concomitant treatment with the bradykinin receptor antagonist Hoe140 (icatibant). They have also shown that the responses of single vagal C-fibers to capsaicin increased after perfusion with bradykinin in vitro. Because ACE degrades bradykinin, it is possible that increases in the local concentration of bradykinin produced by ACE inhibition may stimulate C-fibers and release substance P, thereby provoking cough. In support of this concept, a human study demonstrated that in asthmatic patients, bradykinin-induced bronchoconstriction and cough were inhibited by a tachykinin receptor antagonist (83). Thus, bradykinin and tachykinins are closely connected, and together, they modulate the cough response.

Substance P

Substance P, an 11-amino acid molecule, is a member of the tachykinin family of peptides which share a common sequence (Phe-X-Gly-Leu-Met-NH_2) at their C-terminal end (84). In the lower respiratory tract of various species, substance P is localized in the sensory nerve terminals innervating the airway epithelium, smooth muscle, and blood vessels (85). Although substance P has a weak affinity for neurokinin (NK) -2 and NK-3 receptors, it primarily activates NK-1 receptors. It has potent proinflammatory effects, including increased vascular permeability (85), neutrophil adhesion (86), vasodilatation (87), exocytosis in some mast cells (88), submucosal gland secretion (89), ion transport (90), smooth muscle contraction (91), cholinergic neurotransmission (92), and cough (93,94). In the airways, substance P is released from activated C-fibers in response to antidromic electrical stimulation of the vagus nerves and to stimulation of the nerves by capsaicin, cigarette smoke, acetylcholine, bradykinin, histamine, and other mediators released by antigen exposure (95–98). Substance P is degraded by a variety of enzymes, including NEP (32,99), serine proteases (100), mast cell kinase (101), and ACE (32,33,62). Although substance P is a circulating mediator, it is also a paracrine mediator. ACE inhibitors may inhibit the local degradation of substance P and as a result potentiate the ability of substance P to trigger the cough reflex (33).

To evaluate the role of endogenous substance P and ACE in the cough reflex, the cough response to capsaicin and citric acid was examined in guinea pigs treated orally with the ACE inhibitor cilazapril (102). Cilazapril caused the dose–response curves of capsaicin and citric acid to shift to the left, an effect that was inhibited by pretreatment with FK 888 aerosols (Fig. 1). FK 888 is a selective NK_1 receptor antagonist (103), suggesting that substance P is responsible for the hypersensitivity of the cough reflex enhanced by ACE inhibitors. Likewise, in humans, the concentration of substance P in induced sputum was reported to be increased in patients suffering from dry cough due to the use of ACE inhibitors (104). Subsequent studies have been conducted in pigs to distinguish the contributions of substance P and bradykinin to ACE inhibitor-induced cough (105). The citric acid-induced cough response was increased with intravenous enalapril but decreased with the combination of enalapril and antagonists of the three tachykinin receptors NK_1, NK_2, and NK_3. In contrast, citric acid-induced cough was decreased by the bradykinin B_2 receptor antagonist Hoe140 but increased when Hoe140 was administered simultaneously with enalapril. Therefore, ACE inhibitor-induced enhancement of the cough reflex may have been due primarily to substance P in that model.

ACE inhibitor-induced cough may also involve inflammatory responses in the airways (106). One such mechanism has been confirmed in a study in mice (107). Intravenous captopril and enalapril were shown to increase plasma extravasation in the whole body including the trachea, and this effect was inhibited by pretreatment with the NK_1 receptor antagonist SR140333 as well as with the bradykinin B_2 receptor antagonist Hoe140. These results support the hypothesis that bradykinin may activate afferent C-fibers to release substance P(108). Substance P is also suggested to sensitize the rapidly adapting receptors, thereby causing a cough by increasing microvascular leakage (109).

These findings provide evidence that substance P released from sensory nerves may be one factor leading to ACE inhibitor-related cough, with additional contributions from other mediators including bradykinin and prostaglandins.

Prostanoids

Prostaglandins and thromboxanes are additional candidate mediators in ACE inhibitor-induced cough. The accumulation of bradykinin and

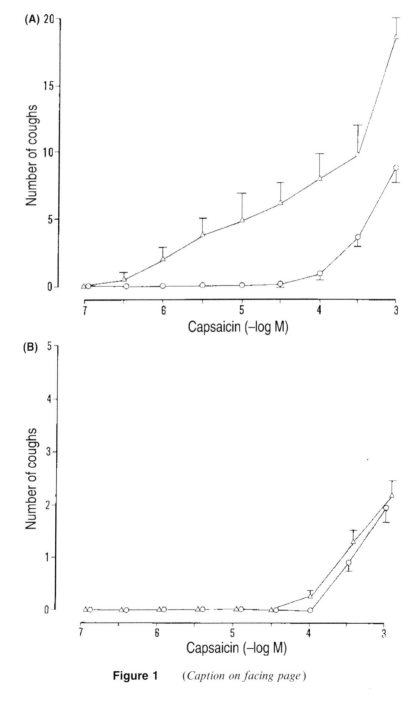

Figure 1   (*Caption on facing page*)

substance P may lead to the release of arachidonic acid and thereby evoke the synthesis of prostanoids such as prostaglandin E_2 and thromboxane B_2 via the stimulation of phospholipase A_2 (24,70–72). This cascade of events can contribute to the development of cough (58). In support of this, intravenous administration of captopril potentiated bradykinin-induced bronchoconstriction and enhanced the release of a prostaglandin-like substance from guinea pig lungs (70). Moreover, these actions were antagonized by the prostaglandin synthetase inhibitor indomethacin, suggesting that prostaglandins may be involved in the cough response induced by ACE inhibitors. Similarly, the number of citric acid-induced coughs was significantly enhanced by treatment with lisinopril and enalaprilat and this enhancement was diminished by pretreatment with indomethacin in guinea pigs (110).

Although the results have varied among published reports, some human studies have suggested that nonsteroidal anti-inflammatory agents (111–113) and thromboxane A_2 antagonists (114,115) can reduce cough induced by ACE inhibitors. However, the study groups were not large enough for reliable evaluation and thus there remains some controversy in this regard. Nevertheless, it is possible that at least some of the effects of bradykinin and substance P are mediated by prostanoids.

Other Factors

Recently, nitric oxide has been proposed as a possible cause of ACE inhibitor-induced cough (116). Nitric oxide, a vasorelaxant, has been shown to play a key role in the regulation of inflammation and has been implicated in the pathophysiology of various respiratory diseases including asthma, chronic obstructive pulmonary disease, and viral infections (117–119). Nitric oxide generation is altered by ACE inhibitors via the potentiation of kinins such as bradykinin leading to the induction of nitric oxide synthase (74,75,120,121). Based on this evidence, iron supplementation, which may decrease the activity of that synthetic enzyme, has been attempted to reduce the incidence of ACE inhibitor-induced cough in humans (116).

Many investigators have confirmed that ACE inhibitor-induced cough occurs more frequently in perimenopausal and postmenopausal women, but the reasons for this increased incidence remain unclear (14–16). In one study, danazol was administered to female guinea pigs to create a model

---

Figure 1   (*Facing page*) (**A**) Concentration–response curves showing the response to aerosols of capsaicin in guinea pigs treated with cilazapril (*open triangles*) and without the drug (*open circles*). (**B**) Effects of FK888, a selective NK_1 receptor antagonist, on the number of coughs induced by aerosols of capsaicin in guinea pigs treated with cilazapril (*open triangles*) and without the drug (*open circles*). Results are shown as mean $\pm$ SEM for seven animals. (Data taken from Ref. 102.).

of the perimenopausal and postmenopausal state (102). Danazol alone increased the sensitivity of the cough reflex to capsaicin and citric acid. Moreover, the combined administration of danazol and the ACE inhibitor cilazapril caused a further increase in the number of coughs compared with the administration of cilazapril alone. These effects were diminished by FK888, a selective substance P antagonist. Because danazol decreases the levels of circulating estrogen and progesterone (122,123), low plasma levels of these hormones may interfere with the release of substance P from C-fiber terminals, thereby increasing cough reflex sensitivity.

In human studies, genetic background has also been reported to influence the incidence of ACE-induced cough. ACE exists as three genetic variants—II, ID, and DD—and the relative order of enzymatic activity is II < ID < DD (124,125). One polymorphism, the I allele, has been reported to be associated with a high incidence of ACE inhibitor-induced cough in normal volunteers. Moreover, the frequencies of ACE inhibitor-induced cough and of the homozygous genotype (II) were found both to be approximately 15% (124,126). Such findings suggest that the enzymatic activity of ACE contributes to cough reflex hypersensitivity induced by ACE inhibitors (127–129). However, there remains much controversy about the interpretation of these findings (130,131). Further investigation will therefore be necessary to reach any definitive conclusion regarding the effects of such factors.

Hypersensitivity of the Cough Reflex Due to ACE Inhibitors

In animal studies, it is difficult to monitor spontaneous cough. The effects of ACE inhibitors are therefore usually examined by evoking the cough reflex or by measuring smooth muscle contractions associated with the application of physical and chemical stimuli such as distilled water, citric acid, capsaicin, and bradykinin. In other words, evaluation of the effects of ACE inhibitors in animals is conducted by means of airway hypersensitivity testing. In humans, however, ACE inhibitor-induced cough occurs spontaneously and studies of changes in cough reflex sensitivity due to ACE inhibitors have been inconclusive.

Morice et al. (63) demonstrated that oral administration of captopril potentiated the sensitivity of the cough response to capsaicin aerosols in normal subjects. Substance P released from sensory C-fibers might, in that case, have been responsible for ACE inhibitor-induced cough. Other investigators have also reported that cough reflex sensitivity is increased in patients with ACE inhibitor-induced cough (132–134) and returns to normal after ACE inhibitors are withdrawn (132). However, other studies have found that such hypersensitivity may be persistent, suggesting that individuals who develop ACE inhibitor-induced cough may have had pre-existing hypersensitivity (135).

Some reports have suggested that asthmatic patients are liable to develop cough when treated with ACE inhibitors, and that ACE inhibitor-induced cough has a tendency to be prolonged in individuals who are hyperreactive to methacholine (136,137). Moreover, ACE inhibitors may alter bronchial sensitivity in patients with asthma. Case reports have discussed similar events: for example, the condition of an asthmatic patient with symptoms such as dyspnea and wheezing worsened (138), and de novo asthma has been demonstrated (139,140) following antihypertensive therapy with ACE inhibitors. However, other studies have found that the incidence of ACE inhibitor-induced cough was not related to chronic respiratory disease such as asthma (19). It should be noted in this context that ACE inhibitors have been shown not to alter lung function or airway hypersensitivity in normal hypertensive patients (141). Similar results have also been obtained in patients with asthma and bronchial hyperreactivity (142–145). Considering these findings together, asthmatics do not appear to be at particular risk of ACE inhibitor-induced cough and can safely use ACE inhibitors as antihypertensive drugs.

Further well-designed comprehensive studies will be required to achieve a better understanding of the relationship between ACE inhibitors and hypersensitivity of the cough reflex.

Clinical Management of ACE Inhibitor-Induced Cough

Because ACE inhibitors are effective antihypertensive drugs and as they do not normally lead to irreversible respiratory dysfunction, treatment with ACE inhibitors can be continued provided that cough is not too bothersome. Although spontaneous remission of ACE inhibitor-induced cough has been reported (146), this type of cough does not typically diminish over time in most cases. Discontinuation of ACE inhibitor treatment may therefore be the only means to achieving a cessation of the symptom.

In specific circumstances that necessitate the continuation of an ACE inhibitor in spite of this type of cough, several medications can be safely considered. Nifedipine (a dihydropyridine calcium antagonist) (113) and nonsteroidal anti-inflammatory drugs such as indomethacin (113), an intermediate dose of aspirin (147), and sulindac (112) are all known to inhibit prostaglandin synthesis, and have been reported to be of some benefit in patients with ACE inhibitor-induced cough. Sodium cromoglycate may suppress tachykinin-induced activation of C-fibers and thereby ameliorate the cough (148,149). Furthermore, the thromboxane antagonists picotamide (115) and ozagrel (114), and a tachykinin receptor antagonist (83) are now available for clinical use, and these may also be effective in such cases.

Some investigators remain opposed to the use of these medications due to a lack of evidence as to their effectiveness, as well as the possibility of interference with the vasodepressor effect of the ACE inhibitor (150–152). Some studies have suggested switching to the ACE inhibitor imidapril, which has a weak inhibitory effect against the active portion of kininase, in such cases (25,26,153). However, ACE inhibitor-induced cough is a class effect, and therefore substituting one ACE inhibitor for another may not be effective (7,10,51). Recently, novel orally active nonpeptide inhibitors of the renin–angiotensin system, i.e., angiotensin II receptor antagonists, have become available as organoprotective antihypertensive agents (2,154–157). This new class of agents has the advantage of not producing cough as an adverse effect (2,17). Angiotensin II receptor antagonists can therefore be substituted for ACE inhibitors in cases in which it is necessary to eliminate ACE inhibitor-induced cough (158).

It should also be mentioned that ACE inhibitors may be of benefit for patients whose activities of daily living have deteriorated and whose cough reflex has decreased. For example, the risk of pneumonia was reduced by about one-third in hypertensive patients with a history of stroke when they were treated with an ACE inhibitor (159). Therefore, ACE inhibitors may have beneficial effects in the prevention of pneumonia in such patients.

Summary

This chapter has briefly reviewed some of the major contributions made by animal studies to the understanding of ACE inhibitor-induced cough. The genetic background of patients, patient management, and the potential paradoxical benefit for patients at risk for aspiration pneumonia were also addressed. Although many factors can influence the development of cough, ACE inhibitors are of particular interest because this is the only situation in which a systemically active drug is known to produce cough in humans. Understanding ACE inhibitor-induced cough may be of pivotal importance in advancing our understanding of the biochemical and physiologic mechanisms of the cough reflex. Although the mechanisms by which ACE inhibitors induce cough are not yet fully understood, animal studies have provided important clues in this regard. In contrast to human studies, animal studies lack confounding environmental and clinical variables. Furthermore, tissue analysis and testing procedures can be performed in animal studies that are not possible in human studies. Keeping species differences in mind, we can nonetheless attempt to extrapolate the experimental results to humans. Use of animal models may provide suggestions for future research, which may in turn provide much needed information for the benefit of hypertensive patients.

Two key substances, bradykinin and substance P, are known to be involved in the etiology of ACE inhibitor-induced cough. Inhibiting the enzymatic degradation of both bradykinin and substance P may cause the potentiation of these peptides, and subsequently might upregulate the synthesis of arachidonic acid metabolism-derived products such as prostaglandins (24,70–72) and thromboxane A_2 (73). These latter products may also play key roles in triggering the cough reflex. In addition, it is known that nitric oxide generation (74,75) and histamine release (14) are increased by the modulatory effect of kinins, and such events have been considered as additional candidates for inducing ACE inhibitor-induced cough. Several receptor antagonists and synthase inhibitors of the proinflammatory mediators are already currently available. The use of highly selective inhibitors of each candidate factor in future clinical studies will help elucidate the nature of ACE inhibitor-induced cough.

References

1. Ondetti MA, Rubin B, Cushman DW. Design of specific inhibitors of angiotensin-converting enzyme: new class of orally active antihypertensive agents. Science 1977; 196:441–444.
2. Chobanian AV, Bakris GL, Black HR, Cushman WC, Green LA, Izzo JL Jr, Jones DW, Materson BJ, Oparil S, Wright JT Jr, Roccella EJ. The Seventh Report of the Joint National Committee on Prevention, Detection, Evaluation, and Treatment of High Blood Pressure: the JNC 7 Report. JAMA 2003; 289:2560–2572.
3. The Heart Outcomes Prevention Evaluation Study Investigators. Effects of an angiotensin-converting-enzyme inhibitor, ramipril, on cardiovascular events in high risk patients. N Engl J Med 2000; 342:145–153.
4. Heart Outcomes Prevention Evaluation Study Investigators. Effects of ramipril on cardiovascular and microvascular outcomes in people with diabetes mellitus: results of the HOPE study and MICRO-HOPE substudy. Lancet 2000; 355:253–259.
5. PROGRESS Collaborative Group. Randomised trial of a perindopril-based blood-pressure-lowering regimen among 6105 individuals with previous stroke or transient ischaemic attack. Lancet 2001; 358:1033–1041.
6. The CAPRICORN Investigators. Effect of carvedilol on outcome after myocardial infarction in patients with left-ventricular dysfunction: the CAPRICORN randomised trial. Lancet 2001; 357:1385–1390.
7. Irwin RS, Boulet LP, Cloutier MM, Fuller R, Gold PM, Hoffstein V, Ing AJ, McCool FD, O'Byrne P, Poe RH, Prakash UBS, Pratter MR, Rubin BK. Managing cough as a defense mechanism and as a symptom. A consensus panel report of the American College of Chest Physicians. Chest 1998; 114: 133S–181S.
8. Yeo WW, Ramsay LE. Persistent dry cough with enalapril: incidence depends on method used. J Hum Hypertens 1990; 4:517–520.

9. Irwin RS, Curely FJ, Fench CL. Chronic Cough. The spectrum and frequency of causes, key components of the diagnostic evaluation and outcome of specific therapy. Am Rev Respir Dis 1990; 141:640–647.
10. Irwin RS, Madison JM. The persistently troublesome cough. Am J Respir Crit Care Med 2002; 165:1469–1474.
11. Havelka J, Boerlin HJ, Studer A, Greminger P, Tenschert W, Lüscher T, Siegenthaler W, Vetter W, Walger P, Vetter H. Long-term experience with captopril in severe hypertension. Br J Clin Pharmacol 1982; 14(suppl 2):71S–76S.
12. Havelka J, Vetter H, Studer A, Greminger P, Lüscher T, Wollnik S, Siegenthaler W, Vetter W. Acute and chronic effects of the angiotensin-converting enzyme inhibitor captopril in severe hypertension. Am J Cardiol 1982; 49: 1467–1474.
13. Sesoko S, Kaneko Y. Cough associated with the use of captopril. Arch Intern Med 1985; 145:1524.
14. Israili ZH, Hall WD. Cough and angioneurotic edema associated with angiotensin-converting enzyme inhibitor therapy. A review of the literature and pathophysiology. Ann Intern Med 1992; 117:234–242.
15. Os I, Bratland B, Dahlöf B, Gisholt K, Syvertsen JO, Tretli S. Female sex as an important determinant of lisinopril-induced cough. Lancet 1992; 339:372.
16. Chalmers D, Whitehead A, Lawson DH. Postmarketing surveillance of captopril for hypertension. Br J Clin Pharmacol 1992; 34:215–223.
17. Lacourcière Y, Brunner H, Irwin R, Karlberg BE, Ramsay LE, Snavely DB, Dobbins TW, Faison EP, Nelson EB, the Losartan Cough Study Group. Effects of modulators of the renin–angiotensin–aldosterone system on cough. J Hypertens 1994; 12:1387–1393.
18. Berkin KE. Respiratory effects of angiotensin converting enzyme inhibition. Eur Respir J 1989; 2:198–201.
19. Yeo WW, Foster G, Ramsay LE. Prevalence of persistent cough during long-term enalapril treatment: controlled study versus nifedipine. Q J Med 1991; 80:763–770.
20. Fujimura M, Sakamoto S, Kamio Y, Matsuda T. Sex difference in the inhaled tartaric acid cough threshold in non-atopic healthy subjects. Thorax 1990; 45: 633–634.
21. Lacourcière Y, Lefebvre J, Nakhle G, Faison EP, Snavely DB, Nelson EB. Association between cough and angiotensin converting enzyme inhibitors versus angiotensin II antagonists: the design of a prospective, controlled study. J Hypertens 1994; 12(suppl 2):S49–S53.
22. Kastelik JA, Thompson RH, Aziz I, Ojoo JC, Redington AE, Morice AH. Sex-related differences in cough reflex sensitivity in patients with chronic cough. Am J Respir Crit Care Med 2002; 166:961–964.
23. Gibson GR. Enalapril-induced cough. Arch Intern Med 1989; 149: 2701–2703.
24. Just PM. The positive association of cough with angiotensin-converting enzyme inhibitors. Pharmacotherapy 1989; 9:82–87.
25. Saruta T, Arakawa K, Iimura O, Abe K, Matsuoka H, Nakano T, Nakagawa M, Ogihara T, Kajiyama G, Hiwada K, Fujishima M, Nakajima M. Difference in the incidence of cough induced by angiotensin converting enzyme inhibi-

tors: a comparative study using imidapril hydrochloride and enalapril maleate. Hypertens Res 1999; 22:197–202.

26. Zweiker R, Stoschitzky K, Maier R, Klein W. Efficacy and safety of the ACE-inhibitor imidapril in patients with essential hypertension. Acta Med Austriaca 2002; 29:72–76.

27. Visser LE, Stricker BHCh, van der Velden J, Paes AHP, Bakker A. Angiotensin converting enzyme inhibitor associated cough: a population-based case-control study. J Clin Epidemiol 1995; 48:851–857.

28. Inman WHW, Rawson NSB, Wilton LV, Pearce GL, Speirs CJ. Postmarketing surveillance of enalapril. I: Results of prescription-event monitoring. B M J 1988; 297:826–829.

29. Fletcher AE, Palmer AJ, Bulpitt CJ. Cough with angiotensin converting enzyme inhibitors: how much of a problem? J Hypertens 1994; 12(suppl 2):S43–S47.

30. Skeggs LT Jr, Kahn JR, Shumway NP. The preparation and function of the hypertensin-converting enzyme. J Exp Med 1956; 103:295–299.

31. Yang HYT, Erdös EG. Second kininase in human blood plasma. Nature 1967; 215:1402–1403.

32. Skidgel RA, Engelbrecht S, Johnson AR, Erdös EG. Hydrolysis of substance P and neurotensin by converting enzyme and neutral endopeptidase. Peptides 1984; 5:769–776.

33. Cascieri MA, Bull HG, Mumford RA, Patchett AA, Thornberry NA, Liang T. Carboxyl-terminal tripeptidyl hydrolysis of substance P by purified rabbit lung angiotensin-converting enzyme and the potentiation of substance P activity *in vivo* by captopril and MK-422. Mol Pharmacol 1984; 25:287–293.

34. Skidgel RA, Erdös EG. Novel activity of human angiotensin I converting enzyme: release of the NH_2- and COOH-terminal tripeptides from the luteinizing hormone-releasing hormone. Proc Natl Acad Sci USA 1985; 82:1025–1029.

35. Soubrier F, Alhenc-Gelas F, Hubert C, Allegrini J, John M, Tregear G, Corvol P. Two putative active centers in human angiotensin I-converting enzyme revealed by molecular cloning.

36. Wei L, Alhenc-Gelas F, Corvol P, Clauser E. The two homologous domains of human angiotensin I-converting enzyme are both catalytically active. J Biol Chem 1991; 266:9002–9008Proc Natl Acad Sci USA 1988; 85:9386–9390.

37. Ehlers MRW, Fox EA, Strydom DJ, Riordan JF. Molecular cloning of human testicular angiotensin-converting enzyme: the testis isozyme is identical to the C-terminal half of endothelial angiotensin-converting enzyme. Proc Natl Acad Sci USA 1989; 86:7741–7745.

38. Jaspard E, Wei L, Alhenc-Gelas F. Differences in the properties and enzymatic specificities of the two active sites of angiotensin I-converting enzyme (kininase II). Studies with bradykinin and other natural peptides. J Biol Chem 1993; 268:9496–9503.

39. Beldent V, Michaud A, Wei L, Chauvet MT, Corvol P. Proteolytic release of human angiotensin-converting enzyme. Localization of the cleavage site. J Biol Chem 1993; 268:26428–26434.

40. Esther CR Jr, Marino EM, Howard TE, Machaud A, Corvol P, Capecchi MR, Bernstein KE. The critical role of tissue angiotensin-converting enzyme as revealed by gene targeting in mice. J Clin Invest 1997; 99:2375–2385.

41. Ng KKF, Vane JR. Conversion of angiotensin I to angiotensin II. Nature 1967; 216:762–766.
42. Ward PE, Erdös EG, Gedney CD, Dowben RM, Reynolds RC. Isolation of membrane-bound renal enzymes that metabolize kinins and angiotensins. Biochem J 1976; 157:643–650.
43. Lieberman J, Sastre A. Angiotensin-converting enzyme activity in postmortem human tissues. Lab Invest 1983; 48:711–717.
44. Johnson AR, Skidgel RA, Gafford JT, Erdös EG. Enzymes in placental microvilli: angiotensin I converting enzyme, angiotensinase A, carboxypeptidase, and neutral endopeptidase ("enkephalinase"). Peptides 1984; 5: 789–796.
45. Johnson AR, Ashton J, Schulz WW, Erdös EG. Neutral metalloendopeptidase in human lung tissue and cultured cells. Am Rev Respir Dis 1985; 132: 564–568.
46. Dusser DJ, Nadel JA, Sekizawa K, Graf PD, Borson DB. Neutral endopeptidase and angiotensin converting enzyme inhibitors potentiate kinin-induced contraction of ferret trachea. J Pharmacol Exp Ther 1988; 244:531–536.
47. Ferreira SH, Greene LJ, Alabaster VA, Bakhle YS, Vane JR. Activity of various fractions of bradykinin potentiating factor against angiotensin I converting enzyme. Nature 1970; 225:379–380.
48. Ondetti MA, Williams NJ, Sabo EF, Pluščec J, Weaver ER, Kocy O. Angiotensin-converting enzyme inhibitors from the venom of *Bothrops jararaca*. Isolation, elucidation of structure, and synthesis. Biochemistry 1971; 19:4033–4039.
49. Ferreira SH, Bartelt DC, Greene LJ. Isolation of bradykinin-potentiating peptides from *Bothrops jararaca* venom. Biochemistry 1970; 9:2583–2593.
50. Cheung HS, Cushman DW. Inhibition of homogeneous angiotensin-converting enzyme of rabbit lung by synthetic venom peptides of *Bothrops jararaca*. Biochim Biophys Acta 1973; 293:451–463.
51. Shionoiri H, Takasaki I, Minamisawa K, Ueda S, Kihara M, Shindo K, Hiroto S, Sugimoto K, Himeno H, Naruse M, Nagamochi I, Yasuda G. Cough-challenge trial with a new angiotensin-converting enzyme inhibitor, imidapril. J Clin Pharmacol 1998; 38:442–446.
52. Cushman DW, Wang FL, Fung WC, Grover GJ, Harvey CM, Scalese RJ, Mitch SL, DeForrest JM. Comparisons *in vitro, ex vivo*, and *in vivo* of the actions of seven structurally diverse inhibitors of angiotensin converting enzyme (ACE). Br J Clin Pharmacol 1989; 28(suppl 2):115S–131S.
53. Ondetti MA. Structural relationships of angiotensin converting-enzyme inhibitors to pharmacologic activity. Circulation 1988; 77(suppl I): I74–I78.
54. Salem H, Aviado DM. Antitussive drugs with special reference to a new theory for the initiation of the cough reflex and the influence of bronchodilators. Am J Med Sci 1964; 247:585–600.
55. Widdicombe JG. Respiratory reflexes and defence. In: Brain JD, Proctor DF, Reid LM, eds. Respiratory Defence Mechanisms. New York: Mercel Dekker, 1977:593–630.

56. Karlsson JA, Sant'Ambrogio G, Widdicombe J. Afferent neural pathways in cough and reflex bronchoconstriction. J Appl Physiol 1988; 65:1007–1023.
57. Widdicombe JG. Receptors in the trachea and bronchi of the cat. J Physiol 1954; 123:71–104.
58. Coleridge HM, Coleridge JCG, Ginzel KH, Baker DG, Banzett RB, Morrison MA. Stimulation of "irritant" receptors and afferent C-fibres in the lungs by prostaglandins. Nature 1976; 264:451–453.
59. Barnes PJ. Bradykinin and asthma. Thorax 1992; 47:979–983.
60. Sekizawa K, Jia YX, Ebihara T, Hirose Y, Hirayama Y, Sasaki H. Role of substance P in cough. Pulm Pharmacol 1996; 9:323–328.
61. Erdös EG. Kininases. In: Erdös EG, ed. Bradykinin, Kallidin and Kallikrein: Handbook of Experimental Pharmacology. Supplement to Vol. XXV. Heidelberg: Springer-Verlag, 1979:427–487.
62. Shore SA, Stimler-Gerard NP, Coats SR, Drazen JM. Substance P-induced bronchoconstriction in the guinea pig. Enhancement by inhibitors of neutral metalloendopeptidase and angiotensin-converting enzyme. Am Rev Respir Dis 1988; 137:331–336.
63. Morice AH, Lowry R, Brown MJ, Higenbottam T. Angiotensin-converting enzyme and the cough reflex. Lancet 1987; 2:1116–1118.
64. Tatar M, Webber SE, Widdicombe JG. Lung C-fibre receptor activation and defensive reflexes in anaesthetized cats. J Physiol 1988; 402:411–420.
65. Tatar M, Sant'Ambrogio G, Sant'Ambrogio FB. Laryngeal and tracheobronchial cough in anesthetized dogs. J Appl Physiol 1994; 76:2672–2679.
66. Fox AJ, Lalloo UG, Belvisi MG, Bernareggi M, Chung KF, Barnes PJ. Bradykinin-evoked sensitization of airway sensory nerves: a mechanism for ACE-inhibitor cough. Nat Med 1996; 2:814–817.
67. Fox AJ, Urban L, Barnes PJ, Dray A. Effects of capsazepine against capsaicin- and proton-evoked excitation of single airway C-fibres and vagus nerve from the guinea-pig. Neuroscience 1995; 67:741–752.
68. Kaufman MP, Coleridge HM, Coleridge JCG, Baker DG. Bradykinin stimulates afferent vagal C-fibers in intrapulmonary airways of dogs. J Appl Physiol 1980; 48:511–517.
69. Barnes PJ. Asthma as an axon reflex. Lancet 1986; 1:242–245.
70. Greenberg R, Osman GH Jr, O'Keefe EH, Antonaccio MJ. The effects of captopril (SQ 14,225) on bradykinin-induced bronchoconstriction in the anesthetized guinea pig. Eur J Pharmacol 1979; 57:287–294.
71. Swartz SL, Williams GH. Angiotensin-converting enzyme inhibition and prostaglandins. Am J Cardiol 1982; 49:1405–1409.
72. Hartung HP, Heininger K, Schäfer B, Toyka KV. Substance P and astrocytes: stimulation of the cyclooxygenase pathway of arachidonic acid metabolism. FASEB J 1988; 2:48–51.
73. Rossoni G, Omini C, Viganò T, Mandelli V, Folco GC, Berti F. Bronchoconstriction by histamine and bradykinin in guinea pigs: relationship to thromboxane A_2 generation and the effect of aspirin. Prostaglandins 1980; 20:547–557.
74. Linz W, Wohlfart P, Schölkens BA, Malinski T, Wiemer G. Interactions among ACE, kinins and NO. Cardiovasc Res 1999; 43:549–561.

75. Zhang X, Xie YW, Nasjletti A, Xu X, Wolin MS, Hintze TH. ACE inhibitors promote nitric oxide accumulation to modulate myocardial oxygen consumption. Circulation 1997; 95:176–182.

76. Hall JM. Bradykinin receptors: pharmacological properties and biological roles. Pharmacol Ther 1992; 56:131–190.

77. Regoli D, Barabé J. Pharmacology of bradykinin and related kinins. Pharmacol Rev 1980; 32:1–46.

78. Regoli D, Jukic D, Gobeil F, Rhaleb NE. Receptors for bradykinin and related kinins: a critical analysis. Can J Physiol Pharmacol 1993; 71:556–567.

79. Ferreira SH. A bradykinin-potentiating factor (BPF) present in the venom of *Bothrops jararaca*. Br J Pharmacol 1965; 24:163–169.

80. Erdös EG, Wohler JR. Inhibition *in vivo* of the enzymatic inactivation of bradykinin and kallidin. Biochem Pharmacol 1963; 12:1193–1199.

81. Marcic BM, Erdös EG. Protein kinase C and phosphatase inhibitors block the ability of angiotensin I-converting enzyme inhibitors to resensitize the receptor to bradykinin without altering the primary effects of bradykinin. J Pharmacol Exp Ther 2000; 294:605–612.

82. Benzing T, Fleming I, Blaukat A, Müller-Esterl W, Busse R. Angiotensin-converting enzyme inhibitor ramiprilat interferes with the sequestration of the B_2 kinin receptor within the plasma membrane of native endothelial cells. Circulation 1999; 99:2034–2040.

83. Ichinose M, Nakajima N, Takahashi T, Yamauchi H, Inoue H, Takishima T. Protection against bradykinin-induced bronchoconstriction in asthmatic patients by neurokinin receptor antagonist. Lancet 1992; 340:1248–1251.

84. Chang MM, Leeman SE, Niall HD. Amino-acid sequence of substance P. Nat New Biol 1971; 232:86–87.

85. McDonald DM, Mitchell RA, Gabella G, Haskell A. Neurogenic inflammation in the rat trachea. II. Identity and distribution of nerves mediating the increase in vascular permeability. J Neurocytol 1988; 17:605–628.

86. Umeno E, Nadel JA, Huang HT, McDonald DM. Inhibition of neutral endopeptidase potentiates neurogenic inflammation in the rat trachea. J Appl Physiol 1989; 66:2647–2652.

87. Pernow B. Role of tachykinins in neurogenic inflammation. J Immunol 1985; 135:812S–815S.

88. Piotrowski W, Foreman JC. On the actions of substance P, somatostatin, and vasoactive intestinal polypeptide on rat peritoneal mast cells and in human skin. Naunyn Schmiedebergs Arch Pharmacol 1985; 331:364–368.

89. Borson DB, Corrales R, Varsano S, Gold M, Viro N, Caughey G, Ramachandran J, Nadel JA. Enkephalinase inhibitors potentiate substance P-induced secretion of $^{35}SO_4$-macromolecules from ferret trachea. Exp Lung Res 1987; 12:21–36.

90. Al-Bazzaz FJ, Kelsey JG, Kaage WD. Substance P stimulation of chloride secretion by canine tracheal mucosa. Am Rev Respir Dis 1985; 131:86–89.

91. Lundberg JM, Martling CR, Saria A. Substance P and capsaicin-induced contraction of human bronchi. Acta Physiol Scand 1983; 119:49–53.

92. Tanaka DT, Grunstein MM. Mechanisms of substance P-induced contraction of rabbit airway smooth muscle. J Appl Physiol 1984; 57:1551–1557.

93. Kohrogi H, Graf PD, Sekizawa K, Borson DB, Nadel JA. Neutral endopeptidase inhibitors potentiate substance P- and capsaicin-induced cough in awake guinea pigs. J Clin Invest 1988; 82:2063–2068.
94. Ujiie Y, Sekizawa K, Aikawa T, Sasaki H. Evidence for substance P as an endogenous substance causing cough in guinea pigs. Am Rev Respir Dis 1993; 148:1628–1632.
95. Saria A, Theodorsson-Norheim E, Gamse R, Lundberg JM. Release of substance P- and substance K-like immunoreactivities from the isolated perfused guinea-pig lung. Eur J Pharmacol 1984; 106:207–208.
96. Lundberg JM, Saria A. Capsaicin-induced desensitization of airway mucosa to cigarette smoke, mechanical and chemical irritants. Nature 1983; 302: 251–253.
97. Saria A, Martling CR, Yan Z, Theodorsson-Norheim E, Gamse R, Lundberg JM. Release of multiple tachykinins from capsaicin-sensitive sensory nerves in the lung by bradykinin, histamine, dimethylphenyl piperazinium, and vagal nerve stimulation. Am Rev Respir Dis 1988; 137:1330–1335.
98. Kröll F, Karlsson JA, Lundberg JM, Persson CGA. Capsaicin-induced bronchoconstriction and neuropeptide release in guinea pig perfused lungs. J Appl Physiol 1990; 68:1679–1687.
99. Matsas R, Fulcher IS, Kenny AJ, Turner AJ. Substance P and [Leu]enkephalin are hydrolyzed by an enzyme in pig caudate synaptic membranes that is identical with the endopeptidase of kidney microvilli. Proc Natl Acad Sci USA 1983; 80:3111–3115.
100. Pernow B. Inactivation of substance P by proteolytic enzymes. Acta Physiol Scand 1955; 34:295–302.
101. Caughey GH, Leidig F, Viro NF, Nadel JA. Substance P and vasoactive intestinal peptide degradation by mast cell tryptase and chymase. J Pharmacol Exp Ther 1988; 244:133–137.
102. Ebihara T, Sekizawa K, Ohrui T, Nakazawa H, Sasaki H. Angiotensin-converting enzyme inhibitor and danazol increase sensitivity of cough reflex in female guinea pigs. Am J Respir Crit Care Med 1996; 153:812–819.
103. Wang ZY, Tung SR, Strichartz GR, Håkanson R. Investigation of the specificity of FK 888 as a tachykinin NK$_1$ receptor antagonist. Br J Pharmacol 1994; 111:1342–1346.
104. Tomaki M, Ichinose M, Miura M, Hirayama Y, Kageyama N, Yamauchi H, Shirato K. Angiotensin converting enzyme (ACE) inhibitor-induced cough and substance P. Thorax 1996; 51:199–201.
105. Moreaux B, Advenier C, Gustin P. Role of bradykinin and tachykinins in the potentiation by enalapril of coughing induced by citric acid in pigs. Fundam Clin Pharmacol 2001; 15:23–29.
106. Lindgren BR, Andersson RGG. Angiotensin-converting enzyme inhibitors and their influence on inflammation, bronchial reactivity and cough. A research review. Med Toxicol Adverse Drug Exp 1989; 4:369–380.
107. Emanueli C, Grady EF, Madeddu P, Figini M, Bunnett NW, Parisi D, Regoli D, Geppetti P. Acute ACE inhibition causes plasma extravasation in mice that is mediated by bradykinin and substance P. Hypertension 1998; 31:1299–1304.

108. Meeker DP, Wiedemann HP. Drug-induced bronchospasm. Clin Chest Med 1990; 11:163–175.
109. Bonham AC, Kott KS, Ravi K, Kappagoda CT, Joad JP. Substance P contributes to rapidly adapting receptor responses to pulmonary venous congestion in rabbits. J Physiol 1996; 493:229–238.
110. Ito K, Ito K, Sawada Y, Kamei J, Misawa M, Iga T. Toxicodynamic analysis of cough and inflammatory reactions by angiotensin-converting enzyme inhibitors in guinea pig. J Pharmacol Exp Ther 1995; 275:920–925.
111. Biour M, Le Jeunne C, Hugues FC, Cheymol G. Diclofenac and cough induced by converting enzyme inhibitors. Therapie 1988; 43:122–123.
112. McEwan JR, Choudry NB, Fuller RW. The effect of sulindac on the abnormal cough reflex associated with dry cough. J Pharmacol Exp Ther 1990; 255: 161–164.
113. Fogari R, Zoppi A, Tettamanti F, Malamani GD, Tinelli C, Salvetti A. Effects of nifedipine and indomethacin on cough induced by angiotensin-converting enzyme inhibitors: a double-blind, randomized, cross-over study. J Cardiovasc Pharmacol 1992; 19:670–673.
114. Umemura K, Nakashima M, Saruta T. Thromboxane A_2 synthetase inhibition suppresses cough induced by angiotensin converting enzyme inhibitors. Life Sci 1997; 60:1583–1588.
115. Malini PL, Strocchi E, Zanardi M, Milani M, Ambrosioni E. Thromboxane antagonism and cough induced by angiotensin-converting-enzyme inhibitor. Lancet 1997; 350:15–18.
116. Lee SC, Park SW, Kim DK, Lee SH, Hong KP. Iron supplementation inhibits cough associated with ACE inhibitors. Hypertension 2001; 38:166–170.
117. Kharitonov SA, Yates D, Robbins RA, Logan-Sinclair R, Shinebourne EA, Barnes PJ. Increased nitric oxide in exhaled air of asthmatic patients. Lancet 1994; 343:133–135.
118. Barnes PJ, Kharitonov SA. Exhaled nitric oxide: a new lung function test. Thorax 1996; 51:233–237.
119. Maziak W, Loukides S, Culpitt S, Sullivan P, Kharitonov SA, Barnes PJ. Exhaled nitric oxide in chronic obstructive pulmonary disease. Am J Respir Crit Care Med 1998; 157:998–1002.
120. Wiemer G, Popp R, Schölkens BA, Gögelein H. Enhancement of cytosolic calcium, prostacyclin and nitric oxide by bradykinin and the ACE inhibitor ramiprilat in porcine brain capillary endothelial cells. Brain Res 1994; 638:261–266.
121. Cannon RO III. Potential mechanisms for the effect of angiotensin-converting enzyme inhibitors on endothelial dysfunction: the role of nitric oxide. Am J Cardiol 1998; 82:8S–10S.
122. Donaldson VH. Danazol. Am J Med 1989; 87:49N–55N.
123. Barbieri RL, Ryan KJ. Danazol: endocrine pharmacology and therapeutic applications. Am J Obstet Gynecol 1981; 141:453–463.
124. Rigat B, Hubert C, Alhenc-Gelas F, Cambien F, Corvol P, Soubrier F. An insertion/deletion polymorphism in the angiotensin I-converting enzyme gene accounting for half the variance of serum enzyme levels. J Clin Invest 1990; 86:1343–1346.

125. Lee EJD. Population genetics of the angiotensin-converting enzyme in Chinese. Br J Clin Pharmacol 1994; 37:212–214.
126. Yeo WW, Ramsay LE, Morice AH. ACE inhibitor cough: a genetic link? Lancet 1991; 337:187.
127. Furuya K, Yamaguchi E, Hirabayashi T, Itoh A, Hizawa N, Ohnuma N, Kawakami Y. Angiotensin-I-converting enzyme gene polymorphism and susceptibility to cough. Lancet 1994; 343:354.
128. Morice AH, Turley AJ, Linton K. Human ACE gene polymorphism and distilled water induced cough. Thorax 1997; 52:111–113.
129. Takahashi T, Yamaguchi E, Furuya K, Kawakami Y. The ACE gene polymorphism and cough threshold for capsaicin after cilazapril usage. Respir Med 2001; 95:130–135.
130. Kreft-Jais C, Laforest L, Bonnardeaux A, Dumont C, Plouin PF, Jeunemaitre X. ACE inhibitors, cough, and genetics. Lancet 1994; 343:740.
131. Chadwick IG, Yeo WW, Higgins KS, Jackson PR, Ramsay LE, Morice AH. ACE inhibitors, cough, and genetics. Lancet 1994; 343:740–741.
132. Fuller RW, Choudry NB. Increased cough reflex associated with angiotensin converting enzyme inhibitor cough. Br Med J 1987; 295:1025–1026.
133. Hinojosa M, Quirce S, Puyana J, Codina J, Rull SG. Bronchial hyperreactivity and cough induced by angiotensin-converting enzyme-inhibitor therapy. J Allergy Clin Immunol 1990; 85:818–819.
134. McEwan JR, Choudry N, Street R, Fuller RW. Change in cough reflex after treatment with enalapril and ramipril. Br Med J 1989; 299:13–16.
135. Semple PF. Putative mechanisms of cough after treatment with angiotensin converting enzyme inhibitors. J Hypertens 1995; 13(suppl 3):S17–S21.
136. Bucknall CE, Neilly JB, Carter R, Stevenson RD, Semple PF. Bronchial hyperreactivity in patients who cough after receiving angiotensin converting enzyme inhibitors. Br Med J 1988; 296:86–88.
137. Kaufman J, Casanova JE, Riendl P, Schlueter DP. Bronchial hyperreactivity and cough due to angiotensin-converting enzyme inhibitors. Chest 1989; 95:544–548.
138. Semple PF, Herd GW. Cough and wheeze caused by inhibitors of angiotensin-converting enzyme. N Engl J Med 1986; 314:61.
139. Popa V. Captopril-related (and -induced?) asthma. Am Rev Respir Dis 1987; 136:999–1000.
140. Lipworth BJ, McMurray JJ, Clark RA, Struthers AD. Development of persistent late onset asthma following treatment with captopril. Eur Respir J 1989; 2:586–588.
141. Boulet LP, Milot J, Lampron N, Lacourcière Y. Pulmonary function and airway responsiveness during long-term therapy with captopril. JAMA 1989; 261:413–416.
142. Riska H, Stenius-Aarniala B, Sovijärvi ARA. Comparison of the effects of an angiotensin converting enzyme inhibitor and a calcium channel blocker on blood pressure and respiratory function in patients with hypertension and asthma. J Cardiovasc Pharmacol 1987; 10(suppl 10):S79–S81.
143. Sala H, Abad J, Juanmiquel L, Plans C, Ruiz J, Roig J, Morera J. Captopril and bronchial reactivity. Postgrad Med J 1986; 62(suppl 1):76–77.

144. Dixon CMS, Fuller RW, Barnes PJ. The effect of an angiotensin converting enzyme inhibitor, ramipril, on bronchial responses to inhaled histamine and bradykinin in asthmatic subjects. Br J Clin Pharmacol 1987; 23:91–93.
145. Kaufman J, Schmitt S, Barnard J, Busse W. Angiotensin-converting enzyme inhibitors in patients with bronchial responsiveness and asthma. Chest 1992; 101:922–925.
146. Reisin L, Schneeweiss A. Spontaneous disappearance of cough induced by angiotensin-converting enzyme inhibitors (captopril or enalapril). Am J Cardiol 1992; 70:398–399.
147. Tenenbaum A, Grossman E, Shemesh J, Fisman EZ, Nosrati I, Motro M. Intermediate but not low doses of aspirin can suppress angiotensin-converting enzyme inhibitor-induced cough. Am J Hypertens 2000; 13:776–782.
148. Dixon M, Jackson DM, Richards IM. The action of sodium cromoglycate on 'C' fibre endings in the dog lung. Br J Pharmacol 1980; 70:11–13.
149. Hargreaves MR, Benson MK. Inhaled sodium cromoglycate in angiotensin-converting enzyme inhibitor cough. Lancet 1995; 345:13–16.
150. Gilchrist NL, Richards AM, March R, Nicholls MG. Effect of sulindac on angiotensin converting enzyme inhibitor-induced cough: randomised placebo-controlled double-blind cross-over study. J Hum Hypertens 1989; 3:451–455.
151. Fujita T, Yamashita N, Yamashita K. Effect of indomethacin on antihypertensive action of captopril in hypertensive patients. Clin Exp Hypertens 1981; 3:939–952.
152. Koopmans PP, van Megen T, Thien T, Gribnau FWJ. The interaction between indomethacin and captopril or enalapril in healthy volunteers. J Intern Med 1989; 226:139–142.
153. Takahama K, Araki T, Fuchikami J, Kohjimoto Y, Miyata T. Studies on the magnitude and the mechanism of cough potentiation by angiotensin-converting enzyme inhibitors in guinea-pigs: involvement of bradykinin in the potentiation. J Pharm Pharmacol 1996; 48:1027–1033.
154. Lewis EJ, Hunsicker LG, Clarke WR, Berl T, Pohl MA, Lewis JB, Ritz E, Atkins RC, Rohde R, Raz I. Renoprotective effect of the angiotensin-receptor antagonist irbesartan in patients with nephropathy due to type 2 diabetes. N Engl J Med 2001; 345:851–860.
155. Brenner BM, Cooper ME, de Zeeuw D, Keane WF, Mitch WE, Parving HH, Remuzzi G, Snapinn SM, Zhang Z, Shahinfar S. Effects of losartan on renal and cardiovascular outcomes in patients with type 2 diabetes and nephropathy. N Engl J Med 2001; 345:861–869.
156. Dåhlof B, Devereux RB, Kjeldsen SE, Julius S, Beevers G, de Faire U, Fyhrquist F, Ibsen H, Kristiansson K, Lederballe-Pedersen O, Lindholm LH, Nieminen MS, Omvik P, Oparil S, Wedel H. Cardiovascular morbidity and mortality in the Losartan Intervention For Endpoint reduction in hypertension study (LIFE): a randomised trial against atenolol. Lancet 2002; 359:995–1003.
157. Lithell H, Hansson L, Skoog I, Elmfeldt D, Hofman A, Olofsson B, Trenkwalder P, Zanchetti A. The Study on Cognition and Prognosis in the Elderly

(SCOPE): principal results of a randomized double-blind intervention trial. J Hypertens 2003; 21:875–886.

158. Miyamoto H, Ito K, Ito K, Wakabayashi S, Suzaka H, Matsuo H, Iga T, Sawada Y. Comparative study of effects of angiotensin II receptor antagonist, KD3-671, and angiotensin converting enzyme inhibitor, enalaprilat, on cough reflex in guinea pig. Eur J Drug Metab Pharmacokinet 2001; 26:47–52.

159. Sekizawa K, Matsui T, Nakagawa T, Nakayama K, Sasaki H. ACE inhibitors and pneumonia. Lancet 1998; 352:1069.

6

Pharmacology of Putative Cough Receptors

**PIERANGELO GEPPETTI, MARCELLO TREVISANI, and
SELENA HARRISON**

Department of Critical Care Medicine and Surgery, Clinical Pharmacology Unit,
Medical School, University of Florence, Florence, Italy

Introduction

Cough is a protective reflex response that can be activated by a large variety
of stimuli of either physical or chemical origin. Acute cough affords protection against potentially harmful agents, either inhaled or produced within
the airways and lungs. Chronic cough may maintain this protective role,
but occasionally its persistence can cause severe discomfort to the patient.
Thus, both dry and productive chronic cough result in medical consultation
and a need for appropriate treatment. Unfortunately, apart from drugs to
treat the underlying diseases that cause the symptom, medicines directly
oriented to reduce or abolish cough are limited to narcotic or narcotic-like
drugs. The lack of availability of antitussive medication is due to many
causes, but mainly to the poor understanding of the molecular mechanisms
that underlie the cough response.

Central synapses in the brainstem express opiate receptors with an
inhibitory action on the cough response. These synapses represent anatomical sites where additional interesting therapeutic targets may exist. These
targets are usually receptors that may evoke either excitatory or inhibitory

responses, and include the metabotropic or ionotropic glutamate receptors, tachykinin receptors, gamma-aminobutyric acid (GABA) receptors, and many other receptors. Several factors have reduced the chances of discovery of new drugs in this field. The complexity of central connections underlying the cough response, the well-documented species variability between different mammals with regard to the roles of specific receptors, and the consequent difficulty in extrapolating from animal models to the human disease are among these problems.

A different strategy to develop antitussive drugs is to inhibit the cough pathway at a peripheral level. This strategy is based on an understanding of the mechanisms that initiate the cough response at the peripheral nerve endings of the subset of primary sensory neurons with the ability to encode cough signals to the central nervous system. This chapter will cover the molecular and pharmacological aspects of certain ion channels, particularly the capsaicin receptor, expressed on the plasma membrane of terminals of neurons that have a role in the initiation of the cough response.

Molecular Mechanisms Underlying the Cough Response in Primary Sensory Neurons

The precise anatomic, physiologic, and neurochemical characterization of the neurons that convey the cough response is still a matter for debate. However, there is consistent evidence that a subpopulation of neurons with thinly myelinated Aδ fibers is involved in the cough response and, thus, they have been classified as cough receptors. These neurons are defined as rapidly adapting receptors (RARs) and are stimulated by low-threshold mechanical stimuli. There is another neuronal population that conducts action potentials in the C-fiber range; however, these neurons are rarely activated by mechanical stimuli, although they are efficiently stimulated by chemical agents, including capsaicin, the hot principle component contained in plants of the genus *Capsicum*. Capsaicin is one of the most commonly used tussive agents. Thus, capsaicin-sensitive sensory neurons can be included in the subset of neurons involved in the cough response. However, it must be emphasized that, at the somatosensory level at least, a proportion of the Aδ fibers are also sensitive to capsaicin. The possibility that electrophysiologic characteristics of conduction velocity, sensitivity to capsaicin, and expression of specific molecular markers do not define a distinct subpopulation of neurons that initiate the cough response will emerge in the following sections of this chapter.

The Vanilloid Receptor (TRPV1)

Capsaicin is a powerful stimulus which causes cough in experimental animals and in man. There is a large amount of evidence that the excitatory effect of capsaicin on sensory neurons is due to its ability to increase the open probability of a channel previously defined as the "capsaicin receptor." This molecular entity has been cloned (1) and encodes a 426-amino acid protein, originally called vanilloid receptor-1 (VR1) and recognized as belonging to the transient receptor potential (TRP) family of ion channels. TRP channels can be subdivided into three main subclasses: TRPC, TRPM, and TRPV, the latter including the channel selectively stimulated by capsaicin and now termed TRPV1 (2). Additional and novel proposed subtypes of TRP channels are TRPP (PKD2-like channels; PKD2 is mutated in polycystic kidney disease), TRPML (mucolipidin-like channels; mucolipidin mutations are responsible for some lysosomal-like disorders), and TRPN (NOMPC-like channels; NOMPC is required for mechanosensory function in flies). More recently, ANKTM1, a TRP-like channel that responds to cold temperatures ($<15°C$) but not to menthol, has been cloned (3). ANKTM1 appears to be expressed in sensory neurons that also express TRPV1 but not in neurons that express the other putative cold receptor TRPM8 (3,4). TRPs do not seem to sense stimuli directly, but act downstream of various heterotrimeric G-protein-coupled receptors, most probably via the phospholipase C pathway (5).

TRPV1, like many other ion channels, possesses six putative transmembrane domains, with a proposed pore region between transmembrane domains 5 and 6. TRPs are thought to have cytoplasmic N- and C-termini. Once activated by vanilloid molecules, TRPV1 allows the influx of cations (Ca^{2+} and Na^+). In terminals of primary sensory neurons these ionic events result in nerve terminal depolarization and the subsequent generation of action potentials that, by orthodromic conduction, initiate reflex responses including cough. Ca^{2+} influx into the nerve endings triggers the local release of neuropeptides, including calcitonin gene-related peptide (CGRP) and the tachykinins, substance P (SP) and neurokinin A (NKA). Activation of CGRP receptors and tachykinin (NK_1, NK_2, and NK_3) receptors on effector cells, particularly at the vascular level, causes a series of inflammatory responses collectively referred to as neurogenic inflammation (6). TRPV1 is a thermosensor, activated by moderate noxious temperature between $42°C$ and $53°C$ (1). Previous indications that the capsaicin-receptor could be stimulated by low extracellular pH (6–8) have been confirmed in the recombinant TRPV1 channel (9). Additional stimuli of TRPV1 include elevated concentrations (in the μM range) of the endocannabinoid anandamide (10) and the lipoxygenase metabolites of arachidonic acid, leukotriene (LT)B_4, and 12-HPETE (11). More recently, *N*-arachidonoyl-dopamine has been also recognized as a TRPV1 stimulant, apparently more potent than anandamide (12).

Other Putative Cough Receptors

Other members of the TRPV family include a truncated form of TRPV1, which does not seem to be functionally active (13); TRPV2 (or VRL1), which is activated by temperatures above 52°C (14) but not by vanilloid molecules; TRPV4, which senses changes in osmolarity and temperature (15) and whose activity is regulated by cytochrome P450 metabolites of arachidonic acid (16); and, finally, TRPV5 and TRPV6, which are activated by ionic intracellular changes (17). Because TRPV1 is a heat sensor, the existence of additional channels that sense temperature is worth mentioning: TRPM3 ($\approx$20–40°C) (18) and TRPM8 (3,4), which are stimulated by moderately low temperatures (15–22°C) and by menthol, and ANKTM1, which is stimulated by temperatures <15°C (19). Both ANKTM1 and TRPM8 coexist with TRPV1, whereas TRPV2 and TRPV3 are expressed on different neurons. Some of these receptors may have a role in the initiation or inhibition of the cough response. For instance, the osmoreceptor TRPV4 could be involved in hypertonic saline-induced cough. In contrast, the clinical observation that menthol alleviates cough suggests that the low-temperature-sensing TRPM8 channel, activated by menthol, may have some inhibitory effect on initiation of the cough response. However, the fact that TRPM8 has an excitatory function and is coexpressed with TRPV1 on the same neurons makes it unclear how this same neuron could mediate two clearly different sensory modalities (heat and cold) and how its activation could possibly reduce (via activation of the menthol receptor) cough stimulated by TRPV1 agonists.

Exposure of human or guinea pig airways to low-pH solutions is an additional stimulus commonly used for cough provocation. In guinea pigs the pH threshold for activation of RARs by protons is 6.7, and this type of stimulation is rapidly inactivating and apparently insensitive to the TRPV1 antagonist capsazepine (20,21). In contrast, TRPV1-mediated and capsazepine-sensitive activation of sensory neurons is mediated by sustained exposure to low-pH solutions gradually decreasing from 7.4 to 5.3 (20). Acid-sensing ion channels (ASICs) are members of a large family of epithelial Na^+ channels and degenerins initially found in *Caenorhabidtes elegans* (22), with two putative transmembrane domains and several subunits forming the channel pore. At least five ASIC types have been cloned and sensory ganglia are enriched with mRNA of four of the five members (all but ASIC2a). The capsazepine-insensitive component of the response to protons has biophysical characteristics of certain ASICs and particularly of those expressed in nodose ganglion neurons, the type 3 ASICs (23). Unfortunately, these channels and their functions can be characterized only on the basis of their electrophysiological features, as antagonists including amiloride lack specificity. In agreement with in vivo data collected in guinea pig, rat, and human skin, pain responses to mild pH reduction seem to be due to ASIC-dependent mechanisms, whereas responses caused by lower-pH solutions are mediated by TRPV1 activation (24).

Modes of Activation and/or Sensitization of TRPV1

Activation

The ability of vanilloid molecules to cause robust activation of TRPV1, and thus cause the activation of neurogenic inflammatory and reflex responses, has already been mentioned. In the respiratory system the action of capsaicin, and the consequent TRPV1 activation, results in multiple and variable effects that are strongly dependent on the particular species of mammal. These effects include arteriolar vasodilatation (rodents), plasma protein extravasation, and leukocyte adhesion to the vascular endothelium of postcapillary venules (rodents), bronchoconstriction (guinea pig), bronchodilation (mouse), serous gland secretion (rodents, ferret), reflex bronchoconstriction and chest tightness (guinea pig and man), and cough (guinea pig and man). The preferred endogenous agonist of tachykinin NK_2 receptors, NKA, is a powerful bronchoconstrictor in human bronchi in vitro and in man in vivo. This observation and the responses described above in experimental animals suggest that pharmacological interventions to limit neurogenic inflammation could have beneficial effects in asthma and chronic obstructive pulmonary disease (COPD). Selective NK_1 and NK_2 receptor antagonists, however, have failed in this area of clinical investigation, whereas more wide-spectrum tachykinin receptor antagonists await clinical scrutiny. The negative results may be because the amounts of SP and NKA released from peripheral endings of primary sensory neurons in the airways, if any, do not reach sufficient levels to cause neurogenic inflammation or alternatively may mean that dual NK_1/NK_2 or triple $NK_1/NK_2/NK_3$ antagonists are required instead of selective antagonists. Regarding the failure of tachykinin antagonists to reduce cough (25), it should be emphasized that clinical studies where cough was the specific outcome have not been reported and that marked species variation has been noted in the tachykinin receptor subtypes involved in the cough reflex pathway, especially at the level of central synapses. This implies that the therapeutic potential of peptidergic receptor antagonists cannot easily be extrapolated from guinea pig studies to human pathophysiology. In contrast to tachykinin and tachykinin receptor distribution and function, the anatomic distribution and most of the biologic functions of TRPV1 appear to be conserved among species, thus indicating this receptor as a potential target in cough therapy.

A critical issue for the definition of the therapeutic potential of receptor antagonists is an understanding of whether endogenous agonists exist and under what circumstances receptors are activated by these agonists.

Accordingly, the search for endovanilloid molecules has been active for many years. There is no doubt that molecules with the ability to activate TRPV1 exist. So far, however, requirements to define these molecules as endovanilloids are still lacking. Specifically, it has not been proven that putative agonists, such as N-arachidonoyl-dopamine, anandamide, 12-HTEPE, and LTB_4, can be released in the vicinity of the receptor in adequate quantities to activate the receptors. However, a number of examples suggest that TRPV1 undergoes remarkable regulation under a large variety of conditions. In particular, upregulation of TRPV1 is often produced by exposure to proinflammatory agents, thus suggesting the general hypothesis that under inflammatory circumstances a "sensitized" TRPV1 can be activated by agonist concentrations much lower than those tested under experimental conditions.

TRPV1 Sensitization and Upregulation

As with other TRP channels, there are indications that expression of TRPV1 can be upregulated and that its activity can be sensitized. One clear example of TRPV1 upregulation derives from the observation that TRPV1 protein expression in cell bodies of dorsal root ganglion (DRG) neurons is upregulated by inflammation occurring in their peripheral receptive areas. This upregulation is mediated by nerve growth factor (NGF) and p38 MAP kinase, and results in increased TRPV1 protein transportation to the peripheral endings of sensory neurons and a parallel increase in heat hypersensitivity (26). A larger body of evidence has accumulated on TRPV1 sensitization. Anandamide was shown to sensitize TRPV1 to other channel agonists. Anandamide also caused lowering of the threshold temperature for TRPV1 stimulation, an effect that was mediated by a protein kinase C (PKC)-ε-dependent pathway (27). More interestingly, activation of bradykinin B_2 receptors was found to result in TRPV1 sensitization by diverse intracellular mechanisms, including PKC-ε (27,28), displacement of phosphatidylinositol-4,5-bisphosphate (PtdIns(4,5)P2) from TRPV1 binding (29), and production of 12- and 5-lipoxygenase metabolites (30,31). PKC-dependent TRPV1 sensitization seems to be promiscuously used by different stimuli as, in addition to anandamide, heat and protons sensitize the channel by this enzymatic pathway (32). cAMP-dependent PK (PKA) also seems to be involved in TRPV1 sensitization (33), as capsaicin responses in sensory neurons exhibit a robust potentiation by PKA, and PKA reduces TRPV1 desensitization and directly phosphorylates TRPV1 (34). The observations that prostaglandins may induce cough (35) and, more relevantly, that one major adverse effect of angiotensin converting enzyme (ACE or kinase II) inhibitors is cough (36) suggest that exaggeration of the cough response is mediated by bradykinin accumulation (due to ACE blockade), which either directly, via a PKC-dependent pathway, or indirectly, through prostanoid release and a PKA-dependent pathway, results in TRPV1 sensitization.

It has recently been shown that ethanol (37) and other alcohols (M. Trevisani, S. Harrison, and P. Geppetti, unpublished observations) cause responses apparently mediated by TRPV1. Specifically, exposure to 0.3–3% ethanol concentrations causes intracellular Ca^{2+} mobilization in rat DRG neurons in culture, SP/CGRP release from slices of rat dorsal spinal cord, and plasma extravasation in the rat esophagus, all effects that are inhibited by the TRPV1 antagonist capsazepine. The observation that human embryonic kidney (HEK) cells did not respond to ethanol, but that transfection of these cells with human TRPV1 conferred the ability to respond to capsaicin and ethanol in a capsazepine-sensitive manner, confirmed that ethanol is a TRPV1 agonist. Patch clamp experiments in human TRPV1-transfected HEK cells showed that ethanol potentiated currents produced by the TRPV1 agonists anandamide (by about 10-fold) and protons (by about 50-fold). More importantly, it lowered the threshold temperature to stimulate TRPV1 by about 8°C. Thus, it may be concluded that TRPV1, usually activated at 43°C, may already be active at the physiologically relevant temperature of 37°C in the presence of ethanol (37). Although this observation provides a mechanistic explanation for the burning painful sensation that follows ethanol exposure to wounds and mucosal surfaces, it apparently contrasts with the anecdotal evidence that ethanol inhibits cough (38). The apparent discrepancy may be due to the central inhibitory effects of ethanol masking a moderate excitatory TRPV1-dependent action on peripheral nerve endings. Nevertheless, this study indicates that exogenous agents of dietary origin can cause dramatic regulation of TRPV1 activity.

Sensitization and Upregulation of Other Channels

TRPV1 is not unique in undergoing regulation by diverse mechanisms, and in particular by lipid derivatives of the arachidonic acid cascade. TRPV4, an osmoceptor that also exhibits sensitivity for heat, is markedly sensitized by the release of cyt-P450 metabolites (16). Whether this channel is involved in the cough response induced by non-iso-osmolar solutions, however, is not known. Expression of ASIC3 is increased by several factors including serotonin, bradykinin, NGF (39), and formamide (40). The observations that ASIC3 immunoreactivity coexists with CGRP in sensory neurons (41) and that ASIC3 knockout mice exhibit impaired nociception caused by chemical, thermal, and mechanical stimuli (42) suggest that this channel may also be important for enhanced signaling, and perhaps for initiating and perpetuating the cough reflex response during inflammation.

Cough Threshold to Capsaicin in Humans

Capsaicin is a commonly used agent in cough provocation studies. There is a large body of experimental evidence to indicate that the cough threshold to capsaicin is lowered in certain diseases such as asthma (43) including cough-variant asthma (44), COPD (43,45), and gastroesophageal reflux (46). In contrast with these findings, patients suffering from recurrent pneumonia exhibit an increased cough threshold to capsaicin (47). Variations in cough threshold to capsaicin have been described according to gender (48) and smoking habits (49,50). Drug interventions can also modify the cough threshold to capsaicin. In patients treated with ACE inhibitors the sensitivity to capsaicin was raised (51). Furthermore, ACE inhibitors significantly lowered the cough threshold to capsaicin in healthy subjects (52) and once treatment with ACE inhibitors was stopped the sensitivity to capsaicin decreased (53). Lowering of the cough threshold to capsaicin has also been noted with the use of local anesthetics such as lidocaine (54), nonsteroidal anti-inflammatory drugs (NSAIDs) such as sulindac (55), and GABA agonists such as baclofen (56,57). Surprisingly, opiates such as codeine (58) and morphine (59) had no effect on capsaicin-induced cough. Furthermore, medications typically used in airways disease such as sodium cromoglycate (60), nedocromil sodium (61), and β_2-adrenergic receptor agonists (62) failed to affect the threshold of capsaicin-induced cough. These clinical observations underscore the hypothesis that TRPV1 may be a useful target for the development of antitussive drugs.

Pharmacological Intervention in TRPV1-Mediated Cough

Inhibition of Sensitization of Cough Receptors

It has been recognized for many years that capsaicin has a dual action on sensory neurons (63). First, capsaicin excites sensory nerve terminals by gating TRPV1 and allowing the influx of cations into the nerve terminal. However, after prolonged exposure to high (greater than micromolar) concentrations of the drug, capsaicin causes desensitization of the receptor/nerve terminal, which undergoes concentration-dependent changes ranging from inability of the nerve terminal to be excited by adequate stimuli to neuronal cell death (64). These properties have been used empirically in a series of capsaicin-containing pharmaceutical preparations for topical use, which produce prolonged local analgesia after an initial excitatory effect. Such treatments have been successfully used in postmastectomy pain, postherpetic neuralgia, osteoarthritis, and other diseases (6). In the upper airways, local application of solutions or suspensions containing capsaicin have been used to treat perennial and allergic rhinitis (65–68). These treatments also reduced sneezing, which is a typical feature of these diseases. Although the use of local capsaicin administration to desensitize nerve terminals in the lower airways can be considered in principle and could potentially have useful effects on certain types of cough, discomfort and the hazards intrinsic to the administration of the drug to the trachea and bronchi have likely hampered the exploration of this approach in practical terms.

Antagonists of TRPV1

A large variety of channels (and in particular TRP channels) have been reported to be expressed on terminals of primary sensory neurons and presumably some of these channels may be expressed on RARs, but specific agonists and antagonists exist only for TRPV1. Agents such as amiloride can, for instance, block ASIC3 (24), but this action is far from selective. Knowledge of selective exogenous TRPV1 agonists, including vanilloid molecules such as capsaicin and the ultrapotent resiniferatoxin (RTX), preceded by decades the cloning of the channel. The availability of small molecules with selectivity and high affinity for TRPV1 has boosted the development of a large variety of TRPV1 antagonists (69–71) (Table 1). However, most of the current knowledge regarding TRPV1 antagonists derives from the use of capsazepine, which was first described more than 10 years ago (75,88).

Capsazepine is a competitive TRPV1 antagonist with reasonable selectivity but only moderate affinity for the channel. Thus, when the concentrations required to achieve complete TRPV1 blockade reach or exceed the micromolar range, depending on the experimental circumstances, its selectivity may be lost (78). Species differences in the ability of capsazepine to inhibit nociceptive responses in guinea pig vs. rat (89) may result from differences in affinity of antagonists underlying the possible existence of TRPV1 receptor subtypes particularly present in guinea pigs (78). More recently, additional antagonists have been produced with the aim of developing novel analgesics. Some of these antagonists exhibit affinities similar to or only slightly more potent than capsazepine (69,81,82), and their use as pharmacological tools or as potential drugs has been limited. However, other antagonists seem to be more promising, showing significantly higher affinities for TRPV1 than previously described antagonists (71,85). However, to date limited information is available regarding these novel antagonists and their ability to antagonize effectively TRPV1 in vivo.

Recently, it has been reported that iodination of the ultrapotent TRPV1 agonist RTX maintained the remarkable affinity for channel binding but changed the pharmacodynamic property of the drug from an agonist to an antagonist (71). I-RTX completely blocked capsaicin-induced currents in recombinant systems expressing rat TRPV1 ($IC_{50} = 3.9$ nM) and in other systems expressing the native channel (71). In vivo I-RTX was shown be about 40 times more potent than capsazepine (71). A subsequent

Table 1 Affinities of Novel TRPV1 Antagonists

	K_i (nM)	K_D (nM)	IC_{50} (nM)	pA_2	pK_B	ED_{50}
Ruthenium red: ammoniated ruthenium oxychloride			14^a (72)		8.09^a (72)	
Capsazepine: N-[2-(4-chlorophenylethyl)]-1,3,4,5-tetrahydro-7,8-dihydroxy-2H-2-benzaepine-2-carbothioamide						
	120–5000 (73) $580–3300^b$ (74)	107–220 (75)	0.1^b (69) 230–254 (76) 420 (75)	$7.0–6.6^a$ (69)	7.52^a (72)	
Iodo-resiniferatoxin: 6,7-Deepoxy-6,7-didehydro-5-deoxy-21-dephenyl-21-(phenylmethyl)-daphnetoxin, 20-4(-hydroxy-5-iodo-3-methoxybenzeneacetate						
	$1.7–6.7^b$ (77) 5.8^a (71)	4.3^a (71)	$0.07–5.4^b$ (77) 0.7^a (77) 3.9^c (71) 0.01–0.9 (69,78)	6.3 (78)	10.9–6.8 (78,79)	16 ng/ mouse (71) 0.41 μmol/ kg (78)
6-Iodo-nordihydrocapsaicin						
	$330–2910^b$ (69)		10^b (69) 638.6 (69)	7.2–5.6 (69)		

SB 366791: 4'-Chloro-3-methoxycinnamailide

7.6[b] (70)
6.8 (80)

L-R4W2: R_4W_2-NH_2

7.7[b] (70)

100 (81)
100 (82)

Arg-Arg-Arg-Trp-Trp-NH_2

4-(2-Pyridyl)piperazine-1-carboxamdes

32 69[b] (69)

N-[2-(3,4-dimethylbenzyl)-3-pivaloyloxypropyl]-N'-[3-fluoro-4-(methylsulfonylamino)benzyl] thiourea

4.8–58 nM[a] (83)

JYL1421: [N-(4-tert-butylbenzyl)-N'-[3-fluoro-4-(methylsulfonylamino)benzyl] thiourea]

7.8[d] (84)

53.5[d] (85)

BCTC: N-(4-tertiarybutylphenyl)-4-(3-chloropyridin-2-yl)tetrahydropyrazine-1(2H)-carbox-amide

9.2[d] (85)

6–35[a] (86,87)

[a] Rat TRPV1 HEK293 cell line.
[b] Human TRPV1 HEK293 cell line.
[c] VRI *X. laevis* oocytes.
[d] r-VRI CHO cells.

study found I-RTX more potent than capsazepine in inhibiting neurogenic inflammatory paradigms in vitro and in vivo by about 1000 and 20 times, respectively (78). However, it should be emphasized that I-RTX may retain some agonist properties, as unmasked in studies in vivo where local application occasionally caused writhing responses in mice (78) and paw flinching in rats (77).

Antagonists of TRPV1 in Cough Studies

The identification of relatively selective TRPV1 antagonists has been instrumental in defining the mechanism by which various agents provoke cough. Thus, the observation that anandamide-induced cough is blocked by capsazepine (90) suggests that, as in other experimental settings (10), this lipid derivative produces its excitatory effects by TRPV1 gating. However, regarding anandamide, its property as a cannabinoid receptor agonist, and that cannabinoid receptor activation inhibits sensory neuron stimulation (91) as well as cough responses (92), should be underlined. Two modes of sensory activation by protons have been defined using extracellular recordings from single jugular or nodose vagal ganglion neurons that project their sensory fibers into the airways: a slowly inactivating mechanism, present in C-fibers but not in RAR-like fibers, that appears to be mediated by TRPV1 and a rapidly inactivating mechanism, independent of TRPV1, with characteristics similar to ASICs and present in both C-fibers and RAR-like fibers (20). From these studies it might be concluded that acid-induced cough should be largely resistant to TRPV1 antagonists. In contrast to this hypothesis, two independent studies (93,94) have shown that capsazepine almost abolished both citric acid-induced and capsaicin-induced cough in guinea pigs. The ability of protons to cause cough via TRPV1 activation is supported by the additional finding that I-RTX given by intraperitoneal administration or by aerosol reduced citric acid-induced cough in guinea pigs (94). Neither capsazepine nor I-RTX affected hypertonic saline-induced cough (94), thus indicating their selectivity.

Conclusions

Chronic cough is a condition sustained by a variety of mechanisms. Pharmacological intervention in the central nervous system to limit cough has been successful, but currently available drugs acting at this level are not without adverse effects. It is not difficult to predict that these problems will also occur with future similar drugs. Drugs acting peripherally may have a more advantageous safety profile, but targeting a specific receptor or pathway at the peripheral level may not be an effective strategy given the complex and pleiotropic stimuli that initiate the tussive response. TRPV1 appears promising as a target of different and clinically relevant cough stimuli. However, only clinical studies will answer the question of whether TRPV1 antagonists are effective drugs to treat chronic cough in conditions such as postnasal drip, gastroesophageal reflux, asthma, COPD, and other diseases.

Acknowledgment

This work was supported in part ARCA (Associazione per lo Ricerca sull'Asma), Padua, Italy.

References

1. Caterina MJ, Schumacher MA, Tominaga M, Rosen TA, Levine JD, Julius D. The capsaicin receptor: a heat-activated ion channel in the pain pathway. Nature 1997; 389:816–824.
2. Montell C, Birnbaumer L, Flockerzi V, Bindels RJ, Bruford EA, Caterina MJ, Clapham DE, Harteneck C, Heller S, Julius D, Kojima I, Mori Y, Penner R, Prawitt D, Scharenberg AM, Schultz G, Shimizu N, Zhu MX. A unified nomenclature for the superfamily of TRP cation channels. Mol Cell 2002; 9:229–231.
3. Peier AM, Moqrich A, Hergarden AC, Reeve AJ, Andersson DA, Story GM, Earley TJ, Dragoni I, McIntyre P, Bevan S, Patapoutian A. A TRP channel that senses cold stimuli and menthol. Cell 2002; 108:705–715.
4. McKemy DD, Neuhausser WM, Julius D. Identification of a cold receptor reveals a general role for TRP channels in thermosensation. Nature 2002; 416:52–58.
5. Montell C. New light on TRP and TRPL. Mol Pharmacol 1997; 52:755–763.
6. Geppetti P, Holzer P. Neurogenic Inflammation. Boca Raton: CRC Press, 1996.
7. Geppetti P, Del Bianco E, Patacchini R, Santicioli P, Maggi CA, Tramontana M. Low pH-induced release of calcitonin gene-related peptide from capsaicin-sensitive sensory nerves: mechanism of action and biological response. Neuroscience 1991; 41:295–301.
8. Bevan S, Geppetti P. Protons: small stimulants of capsaicin-sensitive sensory nerves. Trends Neurosci 1994; 17:509–512.
9. Tominaga M, Caterina MJ, Malmberg AB, Rosen TA, Gilbert H, Skinner K, Raumann BE, Basbaum AI, Julius D. The cloned capsaicin receptor integrates multiple pain-producing stimuli. Neuron 1998; 21:531–543.
10. Zygmunt PM, Petersson J, Andersson DA, Chuang H, Sorgard M, Di Marzo V, Julius D, Hogestatt ED. Vanilloid receptors on sensory nerves mediate the vasodilator action of anandamide. Nature 1999; 400:452–457.
11. Hwang SW, Cho H, Kwak J, Lee SY, Kang CJ, Jung J, Cho S, Min KH, Suh YG, Kim D, Oh U. Direct activation of capsaicin receptors by products of lipoxygenases: endogenous capsaicin-like substances. Proc Natl Acad Sci USA 2000; 97:6155–6160.

12. Harrison S, De Petrocellis L, Trevisani M, Benvenuti F, Bifulco M, Geppetti P, Di Marzo V. Capsaicin-like effects of N-arachidonoyl-dopamine in the isolated guinea pig bronchi and urinary bladder. Eur J Pharmacol 2003; 475:107–114.

13. Schumacher MA, Moff I, Sudanagunta SP, Levine JD. Molecular cloning of an N-terminal splice variant of the capsaicin receptor. Loss of N-terminal domain suggests functional divergence among capsaicin receptor subtypes. J Biol Chem 2000; 275:2756–2762.

14. Caterina MJ, Rosen TA, Tominaga M, Brake AJ, Julius D. A capsaicin-receptor homologue with a high threshold for noxious heat. Nature 1999; 398: 436–441.

15. Guler AD, Lee H, Iida T, Shimizu I, Tominaga M, Caterina M. Heat-evoked activation of the ion channel, TRPV4. J Neurosci 2002; 22:6408–6414.

16. Watanabe H, Vriens J, Prenen J, Droogmans G, Voets T, Nilius B. Anandamide and arachidonic acid use epoxyeicosatrienoic acids to activate TRPV4 channels. Nature 2003; 424:434–438.

17. Hoenderop JG, Voets T, Hoefs S, Weidema F, Prenen J, Nilius B, Bindels RJ. Homo- and heterotetrameric architecture of the epithelial Ca^{2+} channels TRPV5 and TRPV6. EMBO J 2003; 22:776–785.

18. Grimm C, Kraft R, Sauerbruch S, Schultz G, Harteneck C. Molecular and functional characterization of the melastatin-related cation channel TRPM3. J Biol Chem 2003; 278:21493–21501.

19. Story GM, Peier AM, Reeve AJ, Eid SR, Mosbacher J, Hricik TR, Earley TJ, Hergarden AC, Andersson DA, Hwang SW, McIntyre P, Jegla T, Bevan S, Patapoutian A. ANKTM1, a TRP-like channel expressed in nociceptive neurons, is activated by cold temperatures. Cell 2003; 112:819–829.

20. Kollarik M, Undem BJ. Mechanisms of acid-induced activation of airway afferent nerve fibres in guinea-pig. J Physiol 2002; 543:591–600.

21. Carr MJ, Undem BJ. Pharmacology of vagal afferent nerve activity in guinea pig airways. Pulm Pharmacol Ther 2003; 16:45–52.

22. Waldmann R, Champigny G, Bassilana F, Heurteaux C, Lazdunski M. A proton-gated cation channel involved in acid-sensing. Nature 1997; 386:173–177.

23. Sutherland SP, Benson CJ, Adelman JP, McCleskey EW. Acid-sensing ion channel 3 matches the acid-gated current in cardiac ischemia-sensing neurons. Proc Natl Acad Sci USA 2001; 98:711–716.

24. Ugawa S, Ueda T, Ishida Y, Nishigaki M, Shibata Y, Shimada S. Amiloride-blockable acid-sensing ion channels are leading acid sensors expressed in human nociceptors. J Clin Invest 2002; 110:1185–1190.

25. Fahy JV, Wong HH, Geppetti P, Reis JM, Harris SC, Maclean DB, Nadel JA, Boushey HA. Effect of an NK1 receptor antagonist (CP-99,994) on hypertonic saline-induced bronchoconstriction and cough in male asthmatic subjects. Am J Respir Crit Care Med 1995; 152:879–884.

26. Ji RR, Samad TA, Jin SX, Schmoll R, Woolf CJ. p38 MAPK activation by NGF in primary sensory neurons after inflammation increases TRPV1 levels maintains heat hyperalgesia. Neuron 2002; 36:57–68.

27. Premkumar LS, Ahern GP. Induction of vanilloid receptor channel activity by protein kinase C. Nature 2000; 408:985–990.

28. Sugiura T, Tominaga M, Katsuya H, Mizumura K. Bradykinin lowers the threshold temperature for heat activation of vanilloid receptor 1. J Neurophysiol 2002; 88:544–548.
29. Chuang HH, Prescott ED, Kong H, Shields S, Jordt SE, Basbaum AI, Chao MV, Julius D. Bradykinin and nerve growth factor release the capsaicin receptor from PtdIns(4,5)P2-mediated inhibition. Nature 2001; 411:957–962.
30. Carr MJ, Kollarik M, Meeker SN, Undem BJ. A role for TRPV1 in bradykinin-induced excitation of vagal airway afferent nerve terminals. J Pharmacol Exp Ther 2003; 304:1275–1279.
31. Shin J, Cho H, Hwang SW, Jung J, Shin CY, Lee SY, Kim SH, Lee MG, Choi YH, Kim J, Haber NA, Reichling DB, Khasar S, Levine JD, Oh U. Bradykinin-12-lipoxygenase-VR1 signaling pathway for inflammatory hyperalgesia. Proc Natl Acad Sci USA 2002; 99:10150–10155.
32. Vellani V, Mapplebeck S, Moriondo A, Davis JB, McNaughton PA. Protein kinase C activation potentiates gating of the vanilloid receptor VR1 by capsaicin, protons, heat and anandamide. J Physiol 2001; 534:813–825.
33. De Petrocellis L, Harrison S, Bisogno T, Tognetto M, Brandi I, Smith GD, Creminon C, Davis JB, Geppetti P, Di Marzo V. The vanilloid receptor (VR1)-mediated effects of anandamide are potently enhanced by the cAMP-dependent protein kinase. J Neurochem 2001; 77:1660–1663.
34. Bhave G, Zhu W, Wang H, Brasier DJ, Oxford GS, Gereau RWT. cAMP-dependent protein kinase regulates desensitization of the capsaicin receptor (VR1) by direct phosphorylation. Neuron 2002; 35:721–731.
35. Costello JF, Dunlop LS, Gardiner PJ. Characteristics of prostaglandin induced cough in man. Br J Clin Pharmacol 1985; 20:355–359.
36. Israili ZH, Hall WD. Cough and angioneurotic edema associated with angiotensin-converting enzyme inhibitor therapy. Ann Intern Med 1992; 117:234–242.
37. Trevisani M, Smart D, Gunthorpe MJ, Tognetto M, Barbieri M, Campi B, Amadesi S, Gray J, Jerman JC, Brough SJ, Owen D, Smith GD, Randall AD, Harrison S, Bianchi A, Davis JB, Geppetti P. Ethanol elicits and potentiates nociceptor responses via the vanilloid receptor-1. Nat Neurosci 2002; 5:546–551.
38. Calesnick B, Vernick H. Antitussive activity of ethanol. Q J Stud Alcohol 1971; 32:434–441.
39. Mamet J, Baron A, Lazdunski M, Voilley N. Proinflammatory mediators, stimulators of sensory neuron excitability via the expression of acid-sensing ion channels. J Neurosci 2002; 22:10662–10670.
40. Xie J, Price MP, Wemmie JA, Askwith CC, Welsh MJ. ASIC3 and ASIC1 mediate FMRFamide-related peptide enhancement of H^+-gated currents in cultured dorsal root ganglion neurons. J Neurophysiol 2003; 89:2459–2465.
41. Ichikawa H, Sugimoto T. The co-expression of ASIC3 with calcitonin gene-related peptide and parvalbumin in the rat trigeminal ganglion. Brain Res 2002; 943(2):287–291.
42. Chen CC, Zimmer A, Sun WH, Hall J, Brownstein MJ. A role for ASIC3 in the modulation of high-intensity pain stimuli. Proc Natl Acad Sci USA 2002; 99:8992–8997.

43. Barber CM, Curran AD, Fishwick D. Impaired cough reflex in patients with recurrent pneumonia. Thorax 2003; 58:645–646.

44. Cho YS, Lee CK, Yoo B, Moon HB. Cough sensitivity and extrathoracic airway responsiveness to inhaled capsaicin in chronic cough patients. J Korean Med Sci 2002; 17:616–620.

45. Higenbottam T. Chronic cough and the cough reflex in common lung diseases. Pulm Pharmacol Ther 2002; 15:241–247.

46. Nieto L, de Diego A, Perpina M, Compte L, Garrigues V, Martinez E, Ponce J. Cough reflex testing with inhaled capsaicin in the study of chronic cough. Respir Med 2003; 97:393–400.

47. Niimi A, Matsumoto H, Ueda T, Takemura M, Suzuki K, Tanaka E, Chin K, Mishima M, Amitani R. Impaired cough reflex in patients with recurrent pneumonia. Thorax 2003; 58:152–153.

48. Kastelik JA, Thompson RH, Aziz I, Ojoo JC, Redington AE, Morice AH. Sex-related differences in cough reflex sensitivity in patients with chronic cough. Am J Respir Crit Care Med 2002; 166:961–964.

49. Dicpinigaitis PV. Cough reflex sensitivity in cigarette smokers. Chest 2003; 123:685–688.

50. Millqvist E, Bende M. Capsaicin cough sensitivity is decreased in smokers. Respir Med 2001; 95:19–21.

51. Fuller RW, Warren JB, McCusker M, Dollery CT. Effect of enalapril on the skin response to bradykinin in man. Br J Clin Pharmacol 1987; 23:88–90.

52. Morice AH, Lowry R, Brown MJ, Higenbottam T. Angiotensin-converting enzyme and the cough reflex. Lancet 1987; 2:1116–1118.

53. Yeo WW, Chadwick IG, Kraskiewicz M, Jackson PR, Ramsay LE. Resolution of ACE inhibitor cough: changes in subjective cough and responses to inhaled capsaicin, intradermal bradykinin and substance-P. Br J Clin Pharmacol 1995; 40:423–429.

54. Millqvist E. Cough provocation with capsaicin is an objective way to test sensory hyperreactivity in patients with asthma-like symptoms. Allergy 2000; 55:546–550.

55. Foster G, Yeo WW, Ramsay LE. Effect of sulindac on the cough reflex of healthy subjects. Br J Clin Pharmacol 1991; 31:207–208.

56. Dicpinigaitis PV, Dobkin JB. Antitussive effect of the GABA-agonist baclofen. Chest 1997; 111:996–999.

57. Dicpinigaitis PV, Dobkin JB, Rauf K, Aldrich TK. Inhibition of capsaicin-induced cough by the gamma-aminobutyric acid agonist baclofen. J Clin Pharmacol 1998; 38:364–367.

58. Hutchings HA, Eccles R. The opioid agonist codeine and antagonist naltrexone do not affect voluntary suppression of capsaicin induced cough in healthy subjects. Eur Respir J 1994; 7:715–719.

59. Fuller RW, Karlsson JA, Choudry NB, Pride NB. Effect of inhaled and systemic opiates on responses to inhaled capsaicin in humans. J Appl Physiol 1988; 65:1125–1130.

60. Collier JG, Fuller RW. Capsaicin inhalation in man and the effects of sodium cromoglycate. Br J Pharmacol 1984; 81:113–117.

61. Hansson L, Choudry NB, Fuller RW, Pride NB. Effect of nedocromil sodium on the airway response to inhaled capsaicin in normal subjects. Thorax 1988; 43:935–936.
62. Fujimura M, Sakamoto S, Kamio Y, Bando T, Kurashima K, Matsuda T. Effect of inhaled procaterol on cough receptor sensitivity to capsaicin in patients with asthma or chronic bronchitis and in normal subjects. Thorax 1993; 48:615–618.
63. Szolcsanyi J. Tetrodotoxin-resistant non-cholinergic neurogenic contraction evoked by capsaicinoids and piperine on the guinea-pig trachea. Neurosci Lett 1983; 42:83–88.
64. Szolcsanyi J. A pharmacological approach to elucidation of the role of different nerve fibres and receptor endings in mediation of pain. J Physiol (Paris) 1977; 73:251–259.
65. Marabini S, Ciabatti PG, Polli G, Fusco BM, Geppetti P. Beneficial effects of intranasal applications of capsaicin in patients with vasomotor rhinitis. Eur Arch Otorhinolaryngol 1991; 248:191–194.
66. Blom HM, Van Rijswijk JB, Garrelds IM, Mulder PG, Timmermans T, Gerth van Wijk R. Intranasal capsaicin is efficacious in non-allergic, non-infectious perennial rhinitis. A placebo-controlled study. Clin Exp Allergy 1997; 27:796–801.
67. Blom HM, Severijnen LA, Van Rijswijk JB, Mulder PG, Van Wijk RG, Fokkens WJ. The long-term effects of capsaicin aqueous spray on the nasal mucosa. Clin Exp Allergy 1998; 28:1351–1358.
68. Stjarne P, Rinder J, Heden-Blomquist E, Cardell LO, Lundberg J, Zetterstrom O, Anggard A. Capsaicin desensitization of the nasal mucosa reduces symptoms upon allergen challenge in patients with allergic rhinitis. Acta Otolaryngol 1998; 118:235–239.
69. Appendino G, Harrison S, De Petrocellis L, Daddario N, Bianchi F, Schiano Moriello A, Trevisani M, Benvenuti F, Geppetti P, Di Marzo V. Halogenation of a capsaicin analogue leads to novel vanilloid TRPV1 receptor antagonists. Br J Pharmacol 2003; 139:1417–1424.
70. Davis JB, Gunthorpe MJ, Jerman JC, Gray J, Smith GD, Davies CH, Randall AD, Smart D, Rami HK, Wyman PA. Identification of a potent and selective antagonist of vanilloid receptor-1, SB366791 (abstract). Soc Neurosci 2001; 27:910.5.
71. Wahl P, Foged C, Tullin S, Thomsen C. Iodo-resiniferatoxin, a new potent vanilloid receptor antagonist. Mol Pharmacol 2001; 59:9–15.
72. Jerman JC, Brough SJ, Prinjha R, Harries MH, Davis JB, Smart D. Characterization using FLIPR of rat vanilloid receptor (rVR1) pharmacology. Br J Pharmacol 2000; 130:916–922.
73. Szallasi A, Goso C, Blumberg PM, Manzini S. Competitive inhibition by capsazepine of [3H]resiniferatoxin binding to central (spinal cord and dorsal root ganglia) and peripheral (urinary bladder and airways) vanilloid (capsaicin) receptors in the rat. J Pharmacol Exp Ther 1993; 267:728–733.
74. Lee J, Szabo T, Gonzalez AF, Welter JD, Blumberg PM. N-(3-acyloxy-2-benzylpropyl)-N′-dihydroxytetrahydrobenzazepine and tetrahydroisoquinoline

thiourea analogues as vanilloid receptor ligands. Bioorg Med Chem 2001; 9:1713–1720.

75. Bevan S, Hothi S, Hughes G, James IF, Rang HP, Shah K, Walpole CS, Yeats JC. Capsazepine: a competitive antagonist of the sensory neurone excitant capsaicin. Br J Pharmacol 1992; 107:544–552.

76. Dickenson AH, Dray A. Selective antagonism of capsaicin by capsazepine: evidence for a spinal receptor site in capsaicin-induced antinociception. Br J Pharmacol 1991; 104:1045–1049.

77. Seabrook GR, Sutton KG, Jarolimek W, Hollingworth GJ, Teague S, Webb J, Clark N, Boyce S, Kerby J, Ali Z, Chou M, Middleton R, Kaczorowski G, Jones AB. Functional properties of the high-affinity TRPV1 (VR1) vanilloid receptor antagonist (4-hydroxy-5-iodo-3-methoxyphenylacetate ester) iodo-resiniferatoxin. J Pharmacol Exp Ther 2002; 303:1052–1060.

78. Rigoni M, Trevisani M, Gazzieri D, Nadaletto R, Tognetto M, Creminon C, Davis JB, Campi B, Amadesi S, Geppetti P, Harrison S. Neurogenic responses mediated by vanilloid receptor-1 (TRPV1) are blocked by the high affinity antagonist, iodo-resiniferatoxin. Br J Pharmacol 2003; 138:977–985.

79. Undem BJ, Kollarik M. Characterization of the vanilloid receptor 1 antagonist iodo-resiniferatoxin on the afferent and efferent function of vagal sensory C-fibers. J Pharmacol Exp Ther 2002; 303:716–722.

80. Fowler CJ, Jonsson KO, Andersson A, Juntunen J, Jarvinen T, Vandevoorde S, Lambert DM, Jerman JC, Smart D. Inhibition of C6 glioma cell proliferation by anandamide, 1-arachidonoylglycerol, and by a water soluble phosphate ester of anandamide: variability in response and involvement of arachidonic acid. Biochem Pharmacol 2003; 66:757–767.

81. Himmel HM, Kiss T, Borvendeg SJ, Gillen C, Illes P. The arginine-rich hexapeptide R4W2 is a stereoselective antagonist at the vanilloid receptor 1: a Ca^{2+} imaging study in adult rat dorsal root ganglion neurons. J Pharmacol Exp Ther 2002; 301:981–986.

82. Planells-Cases R, Aracil A, Merino JM, Gallar J, Perez-Paya E, Belmonte C, Gonzalez-Ros JM, Ferrer-Montiel AV. Arginine-rich peptides are blockers of VR-1 channels with analgesic activity. FEBS Lett 2000; 481:131–136.

83. Sun Q, Tafesse L, Islam K, Zhou X, Victory SF, Zhang C, Hachicha M, Schmid LA, Patel A, Rotshteyn Y, Valenzano KJ, Kyle DJ. 4-(2-pyridyl)piperazine-1-carboxamides: potent vanilloid receptor 1 antagonists. Bioorg Med Chem Lett 2003; 13:3611–3616.

84. Lee J, Kang M, Shin M, Kim JM, Kang SU, Lim JO, Choi HK, Suh YG, Park HG, Oh U, Kim HD, Park YH, Ha HJ, Kim YH, Toth A, Wang Y, Tran R, Pearce LV, Lundberg DJ, Blumberg PM. N-(3-acyloxy-2-benzylpropyl)-N'-(4-(methylsulfonylamino)benzyl)thiourea analogues: novel potent and high affinity antagonists and partial antagonists of the vanilloid receptor. J Med Chem 2003; 46:3116–3126.

85. Wang Y, Szabo T, Welter JD, Toth A, Tran R, Lee J, Kang SU, Suh YG, Blumberg PM. High affinity antagonists of the vanilloid receptor. Mol Pharmacol 2002; 62:947–956.

86. Valenzano KJ, Grant ER, Wu G, Hachicha M, Schmid L, Tafesse L, Sun Q, Rotshteyn Y, Francis J, Limberis J, Malik S, Whittemore ER, Hodges D.

N-(4-tertiarybutylphenyl)-4-(3-chloropyridin-2-yl)tetrahydropyrazine -1(2H)-carbox-amide (BCTC), a novel, orally effective vanilloid receptor 1 antagonist with analgesic properties: I. in vitro characterization and pharmacokinetic properties. J Pharmacol Exp Ther 2003; 306:377–386.
87. Pomonis JD, Harrison JE, Mark L, Bristol DR, Valenzano KJ, Walker K. N-(4-tertiarybutylphenyl)-4-(3-cholorphyridin-2-yl)tetrahydropyrazine-1(2H)-carbox-amide (BCTC), a novel, orally effective vanilloid receptor 1 antagonist with analgesic properties: II. In vivo characterization in rat models of inflammatory and neuropathic pain. J Pharmacol Exp Ther 2003; 306:387–393.
88. Walpole CS, Bevan S, Bovermann G, Boelsterli JJ, Breckenridge R, Davies JW, Hughes GA, James I, Oberer L, Winter J, et al. The discovery of capsazepine, the first competitive antagonist of the sensory neuron excitants capsaicin and resiniferatoxin. J Med Chem 1994; 37:1942–1954.
89. Walker KM, Urban L, Medhurst SJ, Patel S, Panesar M, Fox AJ, McIntyre P. The VR1 antagonist capsazepine reverses mechanical hyperalgesia in models of inflammatory and neuropathic pain. J Pharmacol Exp Ther 2003; 304: 56–62.
90. Jia Y, McLeod RL, Wang X, Parra LE, Egan RW, Hey JA. Anandamide induces cough in conscious guinea-pigs through VR1 receptors. Br J Pharmacol 2002; 137:831–836.
91. Tognetto M, Amadesi S, Harrison S, Creminon C, Trevisani M, Carreras M, Matera M, Geppetti P, Bianchi A. Anandamide excites central terminals of dorsal root ganglion neurons via vanilloid receptor-1 (VR-1) activation. J Neurosci 2000; 21:1104–1109.
92. Patel HJ, Birrell MA, Crispino N, Hele DJ, Venkatesan P, Barnes PJ, Yacoub MH, Belvisi MG. Inhibition of guinea-pig and human sensory nerve activity and the cough reflex in guinea-pigs by cannabinoid (CB2) receptor activation. Br J Pharmacol 2003; 140:261–268.
93. Lalloo UG, Fox AJ, Belvisi MG, Chung KF, Barnes PJ. Capsazepine inhibits cough induced by capsaicin and citric acid but not by hypertonic saline in guinea pigs. J Appl Physiol 1995; 79:1082–1087.
94. Trevisani M, Milan A, Gatti R, Zanasi A, Harrison S, Fontana G, Morice AH, Geppetti P. Iodo-resiniferatoxin is a potent antitussive drug in guinea pigs. Thorax. In press.

7

Pharmacological Modulation of the Cough Reflex and Development of New Antitussives

K. F. CHUNG

National Heart & Lung Institute, Imperial College and
   Royal Brompton & Harefield NHS Trust,
London, U.K.

The Normal and Abnormal Cough Reflex

The cough reflex is subserved by vagal primary afferent nerves such as bronchopulmonary rapidly adapting receptors (RARs) which can be stimulated by mechanical stimulation and deformation of the airway epithelium, such as by particulate matter or mucus, and by airway smooth muscle contraction induced by constrictor agents (1,2). These are predominantly present in the larynx, trachea, and carina. Activation of bronchopulmonary C-fibers by chemicals such as bradykinin and capsaicin can also evoke cough (3,4), although these may also activate the RARs. Peptide neurotransmitters are often associated with capsaicin-sensitive afferent C-fibers in the airways. In rodents, stimulation of C-fibers initiates local axonal reflexes mediated by the release of neuropeptides such as neurokinin A and substance P which may also induce cough indirectly by causing edema, mucus secretion, and airway smooth muscle contraction. These in turn can stimulate RARs. Pulmonary C-fibers may also inhibit RAR fiber activity.

C-fibers and RARs project to different subnuclei in the nucleus tractus solitarius in the brain stem, considered to be a cough center. Second-order neurones project to other nuclei associated with the regulation of breathing. Integration of the various inputs occurs centrally. For example, slow-adapting receptor afferent input may have a facilitatory effect on the genesis of cough (5). Interaction of RAR with C-fiber activity in the brain stem may be needed to initiate cough, as supported by the overlap of C-fiber and RAR termination sites in the nucleus tractus solitarius (6).

The network of neurones in the brain stem mediating cough is closely associated with that of breathing, with distinct anatomical connections (7). The excitability of this network of anatomical connections during coughing has been postulated to be controlled by a "gating" mechanism that could be sensitive to antitussive drugs (8). Some of these elements participate in the excitation of expiratory premotor neurones during cough. Centrally acting antitussives have effects at the level of the nucleus tractus solitarius by modifying neuronal activity and neurotransmitter actions. Other parts of the brain may interact with the "cough" nuclei and cortical control is important since cough can be suppressed by volitional control (9).

The afferent pathways for cough include actions on laryngeal and skeletal respiratory muscles, and on airway smooth muscle and mucus glands in the airways. These produce the rapid changes in airflow, in cough sound production, together with the bronchoconstriction and mucus production that accompanies the act of coughing. Most antitussive therapies focus on blocking aspects of the afferent pathways.

The Enhanced Cough Reflex

The cough response is enhanced in patients with persistent cough, as demonstrated by the increased tussive response of these patients to inhaled irritants such as capsaicin (10). Although capsaicin is being used to test the cough reflex in disease, it may not test cough sensitivity initiated by other stimuli such as by mechanical stimulation.

This process of "sensitization" may invoke both "peripheral" and/or "central" mechanisms. Central sensitization may occur by integration of signals from various sensory nerve subtypes in the central nervous system to initiate exaggerated reflexes and sensation (11). Substance P has been implicated as an important central mechanism for sensitization of the cough reflex, and its persistence. In a model of allergic inflammation, neuroplastic changes in the response of vagal primary afferent neurons are present, such that $A\delta$ mechanosensor rapidly adapting fibers release substance P when, under normal conditions, they do not (12). Substance P in the nucleus tractus solitarius can increase bronchopulmonary C-fiber reflex activity (13). Peripheral mechanisms of heightened cough reflex may occur through the release of inflammatory mediators such as prostaglandins or bradykinin that could enhance the response of the cough receptor. The cough receptor itself may respond abnormally with increased transduction of the stimulatory signals.

Thus, many mechanisms may lead to the increase in the cough reflex found in patients with persistent cough. Such mechanisms include enhanced excitability of the afferent nerve terminals, augmentation of neurotransmitters in the brain stem with increased synaptic transmission, and even changes in the efficiency of the transduction of mechanical stimuli in afferent nerves. In addition, different types of cough receptors may be involved, with different mechanisms of enhancement. This means that effective antitussives may need to possess both peripheral and central inhibitory effects (14) (Fig. 1), and may need to target several mechanisms simultaneously, making the development of effective inhibitors very difficult. In this chapter, I will review the pharmacological properties of several classes of potential antitussives.

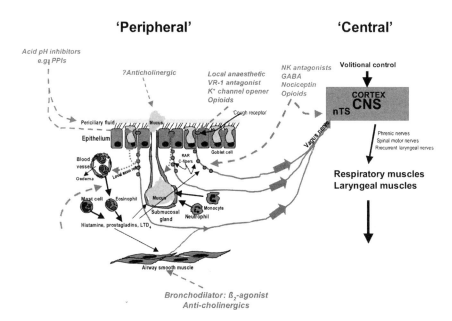

Figure 1   Pharmacology of inhibition of cough reflex pathway. Antitussives could act at the level of the cough receptor, centrally, or at both sites. *Abbreviations*: RAR, rapidly adapting receptor; NK, neurokinin; LTD$_4$, leukotriene D$_4$; VR1, vanilloid receptor; PPI, proton pump inhibitor; GABA, γ-aminobutyric acid; NTS, nucleus tractus solitarius.

Current Cough Treatments

The first task of the physician is to reach a diagnosis as to the cause of the cough and apply appropriate treatment to the disease. In terms of current cough treatments, the major unmet need is the lack of effective direct anticough medicines, irrespective of the cause of the cough. However, the treatment of the cause is often successful in suppressing the cough, and therefore, trying to determine the cause of cough first is a very reasonable approach. In conditions such as asthma, cough-variant asthma, or eosinophilic bronchitis, inhaled corticosteroid therapy is usually successful, or in rhinosinusitis, topical corticosteroids sometimes with a nasal decongestant, antibiotics, or antihistamines, or in gastroesophageal reflux, proton pump inhibitors or histamine H2-receptor antagonists. However, often cough may not respond to treatment of the cause, or the associated disease may not be treatable, e.g., lung cancer or there is no obvious cause of the cough. Under these circumstances, treatment aimed at targets involved in the cough reflex either at the central or peripheral level would be considered as direct anticough medicines.

There is some controversy as to whether the cough in conditions usually associated with the production of mucus such as chronic obstructive pulmonary disease (COPD) or bronchiectasis should be suppressed since it is envisaged that such suppression may lead to mucus accumulation in the lungs with an increased risk of lung infections. However, in COPD an enhanced cough reflex has been demonstrated, and therefore cough may not be caused only by excessive secretions. In such conditions, changing the composition and quality of the secretions may improve clearance and possibly the work of coughing has been approached although expectorants and mucolytic medications such as acetylcysteine are not very effective.

Potential Novel Classes of Antitussives (Table 1)

Opioid Receptor Agonists (μ, κ, and δ)

Opioid receptor agonists are classified by their activities at the opioid receptors μ, κ, and δ. The current compounds, morphine and codeine, are mostly μ-receptor agonists. While these drugs are classically thought of as acting centrally, they may also possess peripheral actions. The antitussive effect of codeine is antagonized by systemic administration of the quartenary opioid receptor antagonist N-methylnalorphine (15), indicating a peripheral action. BW443C, a μ-opioid receptor agonist and a pentapeptide polar agonist, by aerosol acts on μ-receptors on sensory receptors in the lung and has peripheral antitussive activity in the lungs (15). This compound inhibits

Table 1 Potential New Antitussives

Opioids: μ-, κ-, and δ-receptor agonists
Nociceptin (orphanin)
Neurokinin receptor antagonists (NK_1, NK_2, and NK_3)
Bradykinin B_2 receptor antagonists
Vanilloid receptor-1 antagonists
γ-Aminobutyric acid receptor B ($GABA_B$) agonists
Large conductance Ca^{2+}-dependent K^+ channel (BK_{Ca}) openers
ATP-dependent K^+ channels openers
5-Hydroxytryptamine receptor ($5\text{-}HT_{A1}$)
Furosemide and other diuretics
Local anesthetics (voltage-dependent sodium channel blockers)
ATP receptor antagonists
Dopamine receptor agonists
Eicosanoid inhibitors or antagonists

---

activity of airway sensory nerves from RARs and C-fiber receptors. In humans, BW443C did not have any antitussive activity (16).

Opioids may also act on κ-opioid receptors for their antitussive effects (17). A δ-selective receptor agonist (SB221122) was shown to inhibit citric acid-induced cough in the guinea pig (18), an effect prevented by a δ-receptor antagonist (SB244525). However, another δ-receptor antagonist, naltrindole, had dose-dependent anti-tussive activity in mice and rats (19), an action attributed to both δ-receptor antagonism and activation of κ-opioid receptors. Whether these conflicting data regarding δ-opioid receptor involvement in tussive or antitussive activity are due to species differences or to other effects of naltrindole such as agonist effects at μ and κ receptors is not entirely resolved. Nevertheless, an oral selective opioid δ-receptor antagonist, TRK-851, with 100–250 times greater potency in inhibiting cough in rat and guinea pig than codeine, is being developed as a potential antitussive (20).

The development of other opioid agonists such as κ- and δ-agonists may help towards a more acceptable opioid antitussive in terms of side effects. μ-Opioid agonists, such as codeine, cause respiratory depression, nausea, constipation, and physical dependence, while δ-agonists cause diuresis and sedation. δ-Opioid agonists are less prone to these side effects.

Levodropropizine, a nonopioid antitussive and derivative of phenylpiperazino-propane, inhibits vagally induced cough in the guinea pig by activating a reflex mediated by capsaicin-sensitive afferents, and not by a central mechanism of action (21). It inhibits C-fiber activity induced by chemical stimuli (22). Compared with dextromethorphan, it has a more favorable benefit/risk profile in patients with nonproductive cough (23).

Nociceptin

Nociceptin/orphanin is the endogenous peptide ligand for the orphan "opioid-like" NOP_1, which is a G-protein-coupled seven transmembrane receptor. Nociceptin does not stimulate opioid receptors. NOP_1 receptors are widely distributed in the central nervous system and are also present in airway nerves in the guinea pig (24), where nociceptin has been found to inhibit nonadrenergic noncholinergic responses (25). Capsaicin-induced bronchoconstriction is attenuated by nociceptin (26), an action possibly due to inhibition of tachykinin release from sensory C-fibers. Nociceptin diminishes the increase in intracellular calcium concentration in isolated nodose ganglia stimulated by capsaicin, with stimulation of an inward-recitifier K^+ channel (27).

Nociceptin administered intravenously or via the intracerebroven-tricular route suppresses capsaicin- and mechanically induced cough (28,29), effects blocked by an NOP_1 antagonist, J113397, but not by an opioid receptor antagonist. There are no data on humans.

Tachykinin Receptor Antagonists

Tachykinins are present in capsaicin-sensitive primary afferent nerves and their effects are mediated via 3 tachykinin receptor subtypes, NK1R, NK2R, NK3R, of the G-protein coupled, seven-transmembrane-spanning receptors (30). In rodents, capsaicin and other irritants can cause the release of tachy-kinins from peripheral nerve endings in the lungs via a local axon reflex. Tachy-kinins are potent bronchoconstrictors, increase microvascular permeability, and have various proinflammatory effects. These effects, together with a direct effect on myelinated Aδ-fibers, contribute to stimulation of cough. Tachy-kinins may enhance the responses of RARs and cough receptors. Tachykinins have been implicated in the central "sensitization" of cough.

In the guinea pig, an NK2 receptor antagonist, SR48968, inhibited citric acid-induced cough, while an NK1 receptor antagonist was ineffective (31,32). NK1 receptor antagonism may also prevent cough in the guinea pig (33). A study in asthmatic subjects found no effect of CP-99,994 against bronchoconstriction and cough induced by hypertonic saline (34). In the guinea pig, the antitussive effect of tachykinin NK1 and NK2 receptor antagonists may result from both a peripheral and central action, while in the cat, the suppressive effect is mostly central (35). A peripheral antitussive mechanism may involve prevention of tachykinin effects such as broncho-constriction, mucus production and airways edema, while a central effect may involve suppression of the neuroplasticity of cough reflex pathways.

There has been some interest in the role of NK3 receptors in cough. SR142801 is a selective, reversible, and competitive receptor antagonist for the NK3 receptor. It has been shown to inhibit citric acid-induced cough in guinea pigs (36). A nonpeptide NK3 receptor antagonist (SB235375), with low penetrance into the central nervous system, inhibited citric acid-induced cough and airways hyperreactivity in the guinea pig (37) but its development has been suspended.

Bradykinin B2 Receptor Antagonists

Bradykinin is a short peptide produced by the action of proteases, and activates B1 and B2 receptors. B2 receptors are found on a variety of cells such as airway and vascular smooth muscle cells, fibroblasts, epithelium, and also sensory nerves. Bradykinin can induce inflammation, and stimulate sensory nerve endings to induce the release of neuropeptides. In asthmatics, the bronchoconstrictor effect of bradykinin is inhibited by a mixed NK1/NK2 receptor antagonist (38). Bradykinin activates RAR activity, together with bronchoconstriction (39). It also activates airway C-fibers and can cause coughing in the guinea pig and in patients with asthma. A B2 receptor antagonist, HOE140, inhibited citric acid-induced cough in the guinea pig (40). In the guinea-pig, an inhibitor of angiotensin-converting enzyme caused sensitization of the cough reflex, and this was inhibited by a B2 receptor antagonist (HOE 140, icatibant) (41). There are a number of B2 receptor antagonists that have been developed (42) but B2 receptor antagonists have not been tried in humans.

Capsaicin Receptor Antagonists

Capsaicin, the pungent ingredient of chilli peppers, stimulates airway C- and Aδ-fibers, and also causes the release of neuropeptides in the airways of guinea pigs and rats, leading to airway smooth muscle constriction and plasma extravasation. These lead to an increase in the activity of RARs. Capsaicin activates vanilloid receptors on subpopulations of primary afferent neurons (43). Capsazepine is a receptor antagonist of the capsaicin receptor, the vanilloid receptor (VR)1, and blocks not only capsaicin-induced cough but also cough stimulated by citric acid in the guinea pig (44). The VR1 receptor is localized to small-diameter afferent neurons in dorsal root and vagal sensory ganglia (45). It is an ion channel that is stimulated by protons, the endogenous receptor agonist of VR1 and an endogenous eicosanoid, anandamide, and inflammatory mediators such as 12-HPETE and leukotriene B_4. Anandamide may stimulate sensory nerves in the guinea pig (46). VR1 channel activity is strongly modulated by the action of inflammatory mediators such as prostaglandins and bradykinin, through a protein kinase A- or C-mediated receptor phosphorylation (45,47).

Protons can increase the opening probability of VR1 ion channel, which can be inhibited by capsazepine or the more potent iodo-resiniferatoxin (48,49). Acid-induced cough as may occur with gastroesophageal reflux may be blocked by VR1 antagonists. Novel VR1 antagonist such as iodo-resiniferatoxin (i-RTX) are very potent blockers being 450-fold more potent that capsazepine. Noncompetitive VR1 antagonists consisting of tri- mers of *N*-alkylglycines are also effective in reducing capsaicin-induced neurogenic inflammation (50). An orally effective VR1 antagonist has been shown to possess analgesic properties but yet remains to be tested in cough models (51).

Ion Channel Modulators

Potassium Channels

Several potassium channels are located on vagal sensory neurons. A benzi- midazalone compound, NS1619, is an opener of a large conductance Ca^{2+}- activated K^+ channel (BK_{Ca}). It inhibits citric acid-induced cough and the generation of action potentials in guinea pig tracheal Aδ- and C-fibers sti- mulated by hyperosmolality (52). These effects were prevented by iberio- toxin, a BK_{Ca} channel selective blocker. An ATP-sensitive K^+ channel opener, pinacidil, also inhibits cough induced by capsaicin in the guinea- pig, an effect reversed by the ATP-sensitive K^+ channel blocker, glibencla- mide (53). Moguistine may work as an ATP-sensitive K^+ channel opener (53). Phase II studies have shown a reduction in cough frequency in chronic bronchitis.

Chloride Channels and Diuretics

Isotonic solutions of low chloride concentration can stimulate action poten- tial discharge of a subpopulation of Aδ- and C-fibers in guinea pigs (54), and activated afferent fibers in the dog (55). Low chloride solutions induce cough in man, and the diuretic furosemide inhibits cough induced by low chloride content solutions but not by capsaicin (56). Furosemide inhibits to some extent airway afferent action potential discharge, and sensitizes slow adapting receptors and desensitizes RARs in rat airways (57). The mechanism by which furosemide works is unknown (58). A preliminary study in patients with cough did not show any effect.

γ-Aminobutyric Acid Receptors (GABA$_B$)

γ-Aminobutyric acid is an inhibitory neurotransmitter present in the central and peripheral nervous system, and the development of selective GABA receptor agonists and antagonists has led to the discovery of potential anti- tussive effects of these compounds. GABA$_B$ receptors modulate cholinergic and tachykininergic nerves (59). Capsaicin-induced cough is inhibited in the conscious guinea pig by GABA$_B$ receptor agonists, baclofen, and the more potent 3–aminopropylphosphinic acid, an effect that was mediated through GABA$_B$, not GABA$_A$, receptors (60). This effect of baclofen was shown to result from central not peripheral stimulation of GABA$_B$ receptors (61). In the guinea pig, the dose of baclofen needed to cause respiratory depression was greater than that required for inhibition of cough (62). In human volunteers, there was an inhibitory effect of baclofen on capsaicin-induced cough (63), but only a small beneficial effect was shown in two patients with chronic cough (64).

Local Anesthetics

Afferent nerves need voltage-gated sodium channels for action potential conduction from the nerve terminals to the central nervous system. Local anesthetics such as lidocaine, benzonatate, bupivicaine, and mexilitine inhibit this action potential generation and transmission in afferent nerves. Lidocaine and bupivicaine are local anesthetics by virtue of their sodium channel blocking activity, and block the cough response when delivered to the upper and lower airways by aerosol (65). These agents also dampen upper airway protective reflexes, and may occasionally induce bronchoconstriction, and therefore need to be used with care. It is reported that lidocaine inhalation inhibits cough at doses that do not affect reflex bronchoconstriction (66). Their duration of action is only of the order of 15 min or less. Lidocaine topically applied to the mucosal surface of the upper airways is commonly used during fiberoptic bronchoscopies to suppress the cough caused by mechanical irritation caused by the bronchoscope. Delivery of local anesthetic by a metered dose inhaler delivery system to target the upper airways as well as the lower airways would represent progress. In addition, a local anesthetic with a duration of action of at least a few hours would be useful. At present, these are usually reserved for the most severe persistent coughers (67).

Mexilitine, an orally active local anesthetic, reduced histamine-induced reflex bronchoconstriction in subjects with mild asthma (68), and suppressed cough induced by tartaric acid but not by capsaicin in humans (69). The effects of mexilitine may be longer lasting than those of lidocaine.

Carcainium chloride (RSD931) is a quartenary ammonium compound that is structurally related to lidocaine and mexilitine, but its actions are not due to local anesthetic effects. It inhibits citric acid and capsaicin-induced cough in the guinea pig (70). In rabbits pretreated with ozone to increase cough sensitivity to citric acid, the drug was as effective as codeine in suppressing cough. Carcainium chloride inhibited histamine-induced discharge of RARs in the tracheobronchial tree of rabbits, but without affecting spontaneous and capsaicin-evoked discharges in pulmonary and bronchial C-fibers.

5-Hydroxytryptamine (5-HT)

5-Hydroxytryptamine or serotonin receptors are present in nodose ganglia and facilitate neural transmission in visceral C-fiber afferents. Activation of central 5-HT pathways mediates the antitussive activity of opiates in experiments performed in mice (71). Infusion of 5-HT and of 5-hydroxytryptophan reduced cough responses to chloride-deficient solutions, but had no effect on capsaicin responses (72). In guinea pigs, an agonist at the 5-HT_{1A} receptor, 8-OH-DPAT (8-hydroxy-2-(di-*n*-propylamino)-tetralin), showed both excitatory and inhibitory influences on the cough reflex to capsaicin, which may be initiated via postsynaptic stimulation of central serotoninergic neurons and/or coexisting peripheral sites (73).

Cromones

The prophylactic asthma drugs, disodium cromoglycate and nedocromil sodium, produce some antitussive effects by inhibiting sensory nerves, and activating of C-fiber activity by capsaicin (74,75). It appears that these drugs can induce a long-lasting chloride-dependent nerve depolarization and reduce the firing of action potentials following desensitization of the nerve (76). Nedocromil sodium delays the onset of cough to citric acid in dogs (77) and in some clinical studies, they have been shown to reduce the severity of cough in patients with asthma (78). Both sodium cromoglycate and nedocromil sodium abolished voltage-dependent Ca^{2+} currents while cromoglycate alone also reduced Ca^{2+}-dependent Cl^- currents in airway smooth muscle, but without effects on the contractile response (79). The effects on afferent nerves have not been studied.

Lipid Mediator Antagonists

Lipid mediators, particularly eicosanoids such as prostaglandins and leukotrienes, are released during allergic inflammation, and may potentiate cough responses through a process of peripheral sensitization. Prostaglandins are recognized to be able to activate or increase the excitability of afferent nerves. Excitatory effects of prostaglandins E_2, D_2, and I_2 have been demonstrated in studies of vagal afferent ganglion neuron cell bodies (80,81). Prostaglandins inhibit calcium-activated potassium currents involved in hyperpolarization, and may cause an increase in hyperpolarization activation cation currents (82). At nerve terminals, low concentrations of prostaglandins E_2 that did not cause action potential discharge in airway afferent nerves effectively sensitized pulmonary C-fiber afferents to capsaicin or mechanical stimulation during lung inflation (83,84). Thromboxane, and prostaglandins E_2, I_2, and $F_{2\alpha}$ increased the rate of baseline discharge in airway RARs and C-fibers (84–88). In vivo, prostaglandins $F_{2\alpha}$ and

E_2 can increase the sensitivity of the cough response in human volunteers (89–91).

Inhalation of leukotriene C_4 caused activation of RAR fibers in guinea pig airways, but this could have been secondary to the bronchoconstrictor effect (92). In vagal sensory ganglion neural cell bodies, cysteinyl-leukotrienes inhibited the after-spike hyperpolarization and caused membrane depolarization of neuron cell bodies isolated from vagal afferent ganglia (80,93).

Specific inhibitors of eicosanoids have not been systematically tried in chronic cough. There are no reports of prostaglandin synthesis inhibitors yet, although they could have a beneficial effect in "allergic-based" or "asthmatic" cough. There are anecdotal reports of cough-variant asthma not responsive to inhaled corticosteroid therapy that has been controlled with leukotriene receptor antagonists. However, an inhibitor of cyclooxygenase-2 and an antagonist of the Cys-LT1 receptor did not alter capsaicin cough responses in patients with asthma (94,95).

ATP Receptor Antagonists

ATP and related purines stimulate action potential discharge in pulmonary C-fibers, an effect inhibited by P2X receptor selective antagonists (96). There have been no studies on cough so far.

Dopamine Receptor Agonists

Agonists of dopamine receptors D_1–D_5 may modulate cough (97). Dopamine receptor activation inhibits the release of neuropeptides from peripheral airway nerves and the activation of RARs (98). Dopamine receptors are present on sensory nerves in the human vagus (99). A more recent investigation of a dual dopamine D_2 and β_2-adrenoceptor agonist, sibenadet, did not demonstrate significant effects on cough in patients with COPD (100).

Conclusion

There is a lack of effective antitussives available and the mechanisms of persistent cough remain unclear. It is unclear whether peripheral or central mechanisms of cough sensitization, or both, are important in the persistence of the cough. Despite this, research into the cough reflex has led to potential new targets. Opioids or opioid-like drugs may be improved and they are the most effective antitussives. Most of the novel targets have been studied in animals often only in in vitro systems, and they need to be tested in man particularly in cough associated with an enhanced cough reflex. It is the need for studying these novel drugs in pathological cough that is probably hampering the development of these potential antitussives. The most likely models for use are the postviral cough, which is usually transient, or the persistent chronic dry cough. In conditions of chronic persistent cough associated with known causes of cough, for example eosinophilia, asthma, gastroesophageal reflux, or rhinosinusitis, newer compounds to treat these conditions may provide as effective antitussive control.

References

1. Widdicombe JG. Neurophysiology of the cough reflex. Eur Respir J 1995; 8:1193–1202.
2. Karlsson J-A, Sant'Ambrogio G, Widdicombe J. Afferent neural pathways in cough and reflex bronchoconstriction. J Appl Physiol 1988; 65:1007–1023.
3. Karlsson JA. The role of capsaicin-sensitive C-fibre afferent nerves in the cough reflex. Pulm Pharmacol 1996; 9:315–321.
4. Fox AJ. Modulation of cough and airway sensory fibres. Pulm Pharmacol 1996; 9:335–342.
5. Hanacek J, Davies A, Widdicombe JG. Influence of lung stretch receptors on the cough reflex in rabbits. Respiration 1984; 45:161–168.
6. Jordan D. Central nervous pathways and control of the airways. Respir Physiol 2001; 125:67–81.
7. Shannon R, Baekey DM, Morris KF, Lindsey BG. Ventrolateral medullary respiratory network and a model of cough motor pattern generation. J Appl Physiol 1998; 84:2020–2035.
8. Bolser DC, Hey JA, Chapman RW. Influence of central antitussive drugs on the cough motor pattern. J Appl Physiol 1999; 86:1017–1024.
9. Hutchings HA, Morris S, Eccles R, Jawad MSM. Voluntary suppression of cough induced by inhalation of capsaicin in healthy volunteers. Respir Med 1993; 87:379–382.
10. Choudry NB, Fuller RW. Sensitivity of the cough reflex in patients with chronic cough. Eur Respir J 1992; 5:296–300.
11. Canning BJ. Interactions between vagal afferent nerve subtypes mediating cough. Pulm Pharmacol 2002; 15:187–192.
12. Myers AC, Kajekar R, Undem BJ. Allergic inflammation-induced neuropeptide production in rapidly adapting afferent nerves in guinea pig airways. Am J Physiol (Lung Cell Mol Physiol) 2002; 282:L775–L781.
13. Mutoh T, Bonham AC, Joad JP. Substance P in the nucleus of the solitary tract augments bronchopulmonary C fiber reflex output. Am J Physiol (Regul Integr Comp Physiol) 2000; 279:R1215–R1223.
14. Bolser DC. Mechanisms of action of central and peripheral antitussive drugs. Pulm Pharmacol 1996; 9:357–364.
15. Adcock JJ, Schneider C, Smith TW. Effects of codeine, morphine and a novel opioid pentapeptide BW443C on cough, nociception and ventilation in the unanaesthetized guinea-pig. Br J Pharmacol 1988; 93:93–100.
16. Choudry NB, Gray SJ, Posner J, Fuller RW. The effect of 443C81, a mu opioid receptor agonist, on the response to inhaled capsaicin in healthy volunteers. Br J Clin Pharmacol 1991; 32:633–636.

17. Kamei J, Tanihara H, Kasuya Y. Antitussive effects of two specific κ-opioid agonists, U-50, 448H and U-62, 066E, in rats. Eur J Pharmacol 1990; 199: 281–286.
18. Kotzer CJ, Hay DW, Dondio G, Giardina G, Petrillo P, Underwood DC. The antitussive activity of delta-opioid receptor stimulation in guinea pigs. J Pharmacol Exp Ther 2000; 292:803–809.
19. Kamei J, Iwamoto Y, Suzuki T, Misawa M, Nagase H, Kasuya Y. Antitussive effects of naltrindole, a selective delta-opioid receptor antagonist, in mice and rats. Eur J Pharmacol 1993; 249:161–165.
20. Ueno S, Saitoh A, Kawai K, Natsume K, Sakami S, Maeda M et al. The rational drug design and antitussive effects of a novel opioid delta receptor antagonist TRK-851. Jpn J Pharmacol 2001; 85:S32–S34.
21. Lavezzo A, Melillo G, Clavenna G, Omini C. Peripheral site of action of levodropropizine in experimentally-induced cough: role of sensory neuropeptides. Pulm Pharmacol 1992; 5:143–147.
22. Shams H, Daffonchio L, Scheid P. Effects of levodropropizine on vagal afferent C-fibres in the cat. Br J Pharmacol 1996; 117:853–858.
23. Catena E, Daffonchio L. Efficacy and tolerability of levodropropizine in adult patients with non-productive cough. Comparison with dextromethorphan. Pulm Pharmacol Ther 1997; 10:89–96.
24. Fischer A, Forssmann WG, Undem BJ. Nociceptin-induced inhibition of tachykinergic neurotransmission in guinea pig bronchus. J Pharmacol Exp Ther 1998; 285:902–907.
25. Shah S, Page CP, Spina D. Nociceptin inhibits non-adrenergic non-cholinergic contraction in guinea-pig airway. Br J Pharmacol 1998; 125:510–516.
26. Corboz MR, Rivelli MA, Egan RW, Tulshian D, Matasi J, Fawzi AB et al. Nociceptin inhibits capsaicin-induced bronchoconstriction in isolated guinea pig lung. Eur J Pharmacol 2000; 402:171–179.
27. Jia Y, Wang X, Aponte SI, Rivelli MA, Yang R, Rizzo CA et al. Nociceptin/orphanin FQ inhibits capsaicin-induced guinea-pig airway contraction through an inward-rectifier potassium channel. Br J Pharmacol 2002; 135: 764–770.
28. McLeod RL, Parra LE, Mutter JC, Erickson CH, Carey GJ, Tulshian DB et al. Nociceptin inhibits cough in the guinea-pig by activation of ORL(1) receptors. Br J Pharmacol 2001; 132:1175–1178.
29. Bolser DC, McLeod RL, Tulshian DB, Hey JA. Antitussive action of nociceptin in the cat. Eur J Pharmacol 2001; 430:107–111.
30. Geppetti P, Tognetto M, Trevisani M, Amadesi S, Bertrand C. Tachykinins and kinins in airway allergy. Expert Opin Investig Drugs 1999; 8: 947–956.
31. Advenier C, Giraud V, Naline E, Villain P, Emonds-Alt X. Antitussive effect of SR 48968, a non-peptide tachykinin NK2 receptor antagonist. Eur J Pharmacol 1992; 250:169–173.
32. Girard V, Naline E, Vilain P, Emonds-Alt X, Advenier C. Effect of the two tachykinin antagonists, SR 48968 and SR 140333, on cough induced by citric acid in the unanaesthetized guinea pig. Eur Respir J 1995; 8:1110–1114.

33. Ujiie Y, Sekizawa K, Aikawa T, Sasaki H. Evidence for substance P as an endogenous substance causing cough in guinea pigs. Am Rev Respir Dis 1993; 148:1628–1632.
34. Fahy JV, Wong HH, Geppetti P, Reis JM, Harris SC, Maclean DB, et al. Effect of an NK1 antagonist (CP-99,994) on hypertonic saline-induced bronchoconstriction and cough in male asthmatic subjects. Am J Respir Crit Care Med 1995; 152:879–884.
35. Bolser DC, Degennaro FC, O'Reilly S, McLeod RL, Hey JA. Central antitussive activity of the NK1 and NK2 tachykinin receptor antagonists, CP-99,994 and SR 48968, in the guinea-pig and cat. Br J Pharmacol 1997; 121:165–170.
36. Daoui S, Cognon C, Naline E, Emonds-Alt X, Advenier C. Involvement of tachykinin NK3 receptors in citric acid-induced cough and bronchial responses in guinea pigs. Am J Respir Crit Care Med 1998; 158:42–48.
37. Hay DW, Giardina GA, Griswold DE, Underwood DC, Kotzer CJ, Bush B, et al. Nonpeptide tachykinin receptor antagonists. III. SB 235375, a low central nervous system-penetrant, potent and selective neurokinin-3 receptor antagonist, inhibits citric acid-induced cough and airways hyper-reactivity in guinea pigs. J Pharmacol Exp Ther 2002; 300:314–323.
38. Ichinose M, Nakajima N, Takahashi T, Yamauchi H, Inoue H, Takishima T. Protection against bradykinin-induced bronchoconstriction in asthmatic patients by neurokinin receptor antagonist. Lancet 1992; 340:1248–1251.
39. Bergren DR. Sensory receptor activation by mediators of defense reflexes in guinea-pig lungs. Respir Physiol 1997; 108:195–204.
40. Featherstone RL, Parry JE, Evans DM, Jones DM, Olsson H, Szelke M, et al. Mechanism of irritant-induced cough: studies with a kinin antagonist and a kallikrein inhibitor. Lung 1996; 174:269–275.
41. Fox AJ, Lalloo UG, Bernareggi M, Belvisi MG, Chung KF, Barnes PJ. Bradykinin and captopril-induced cough in guinea-pigs. Nat Med 1996; 2:814–817.
42. Bock MG, Longmore J. Bradykinin antagonists: new opportunities. Curr Opin Chem Biol 2000; 4:401–406.
43. Caterina MJ, Schumacher MA, Tominaga M, Rosen TA, Levine JD, Julius D. The capsaicin receptor: a heat-activated ion channel in the pain pathway. Nature 1997; 389:816–824.
44. Lalloo UG, Fox AJ, Belvisi MG, Chung KF, Barnes PJ. Inhibition by capsazepine of cough induced by capsaicin and citric acid, but not by hypertonic saline in awake guinea-pigs. J Appl Physiol 1995; 79:1082–1087.
45. Szallasi A, Blumberg PM. Vanilloid (capsaicin) receptors and mechanisms. Pharmacol Rev 1999; 51:159–212.
46. Tucker RC, Kagaya M, Page CP, Spina D. The endogenous cannabinoid agonist, anandamide stimulates sensory nerves in guinea-pig airways. Br J Pharmacol 2001; 132:1127–1135.
47. Premkumar LS, Ahern GP. Induction of vanilloid receptor channel activity by protein kinase C. Nature 2000; 408:985–990.
48. Kollarik M, Undem BJ. Mechanisms of acid-induced activation of airway afferent nerve fibres in guinea-pig. J Physiol 2002; 543:591–600.

49. Wahl P, Foged C, Tullin S, Thomsen C. Iodo-resiniferatoxin, a new potent vanilloid receptor antagonist. Mol Pharmacol 2001; 59:9–15.
50. Garcia-Martinez C, Humet M, Planells-Cases R, Gomis A, Caprini M, Viana F, et al. Attenuation of thermal nociception and hyperalgesia by VR1 blockers. Proc Natl Acad Sci USA 2002; 99:2374–2379.
51. Pomonis JD, Harrison JE, Mark L, Bristol DR, Valenzano KJ, Walker K. BCTC (N-(4-tertiarybutylphenyl)-4-(3-cholorphyridin-2-yl) tetrahydropryazine-1(2H)-carbox-amide), a novel, orally-effective vanilloid receptor 1 antagonist with analgesic properties: II. In vivo characterization in rat models of inflammatory and neuropathic pain. J Pharmacol Exp Ther 2003; 306: 387–393.
52. Fox AJ, Barnes PJ, Venkatesan P, Belvisi MG. Activation of large conductance potassium channels inhibits the afferent and efferent function of airway sensory nerves in the guinea pig. J Clin Invest 1997; 99:513–519.
53. Morita K, Kamei J. Involvement of ATP-sensitive K^+ channels in the antitussive effect of moguisteine. Eur J Pharmacol 2000; 395:161–164.
54. Fox AJ, Urban L, Barnes PJ, Dray A. Effects of capsazepine against capsaicin- and proton-evoked excitation of single airway C-fibres and vagus nerve from the guinea-pig. Neurosci Lett 1995; 67:741–752.
55. Sant'Ambrogio FB, Sant'Ambrogio G, Anderson JW. Effect of furosemide on the response of laryngeal receptors to low-chloride solutions. Eur Respir J 1993; 6:1151–1155.
56. Ventresca PG, Nichol GM, Barnes PJ, Chung KF. Inhaled furosemide inhibits cough induced by low chloride solutions but not by capsaicin. Am Rev Respir Dis 1990; 142:143–146.
57. Sudo T, Hayashi F, Nishino T. Responses of tracheobronchial receptors to inhaled furosemide in anesthetized rats. Am J Respir Crit Care Med 2000; 162:971–975.
58. Chung KF, Barnes PJ. Loop diuretics and asthma. Pulm Pharmacol 1992; 5:1–7.
59. Chapman RW, Hey JA, Rizzo CA, Bolser DC. GABA$_B$ receptors in the lung. Trends Pharmacol Sci 1993; 14:26–29.
60. Bolser DC, Aziz SM, Degennaro FC, Kreutner W, Egan RW, Siegel MI, et al. Antitussive effects of GABA$_B$ agonists in the cat and guinea-pig. Br J Pharmacol 1993; 110:491–495.
61. Bolser DC, Degennaro FC, O'Reilly S, Chapman RW, Kreutner W, Egan RW, et al. Peripheral and central sites of action of GABA-B agonists to inhibit the cough reflex in the cat and guinea pig. Br J Pharmacol 1994; 113:1344–1348.
62. Hey JA, Mingo G, Bolser DC, Kreutner W, Krobatsch D, Chapman RW. Respiratory effects of baclofen and 3-aminopropylphosphinic acid in guinea-pigs. Br J Pharmacol 1995; 114:735–738.
63. Dicpinigaitis PV, Dobkin JB, Rauf K, Aldrich TK. Inhibition of capsaicin-induced cough by the gamma-aminobutyric acid agonist baclofen. J Clin Pharmacol 1998; 38:364–367.
64. Dicpinigaitis PV, Dobkin JB. Antitussive effect of the GABA-agonist baclofen. Chest 1997; 111:996–999.

65. Hansson L, Midgren B, Karlsson JA. Effects of inhaled lignocaine and adrenaline on capsaicin-induced cough in humans. Thorax 1994; 49:1166–1168.
66. Choudry NB, Fuller RW, Anderson N, Karlsson J-A. Separation of cough and reflex bronchoconstriction by inhaled local anaesthetics. Eur Respir J 1990; 3:579–583.
67. Howard P, Cayton RM, Brennan SR, Anderson PB. Lignocaine aerosol and persistent cough. Br J Dis Chest 1977; 71:19–24.
68. Groeben H, Foster WM, Brown RH. Intravenous lidocaine and oral mexiletine block reflex bronchoconstriction in asthmatic subjects. Am J Respir Crit Care Med 1996; 154:885–888.
69. Fujimura M, Kamio Y, Myou S, Hashimoto T. Effect of oral mexiletine on the cough response to capsaicin and tartaric acid. Thorax 2000; 55:126–128.
70. Adcock JJ, Douglas GJ, Garabette M, Gascoigne M, Beatch G, Walker M, et al. RSD931, a novel anti-tussive agent acting on airway sensory nerves. Br J Pharmacol 2003; 138:407–416.
71. Kamei J, Hosokawa T, Yanaura S, Hukuhara T. Involvement of central serotonergic mechanisms in the cough reflex. Jpn J Pharmacol 1986; 42:531–538.
72. Stone RA, Worsdell YM, Fuller RW, Barnes PJ. Effects of 5-hydroxytryptamine and 5-hydroxytryptophan infusion on the human cough reflex. J Appl Physiol 1993; 74:396–401.
73. Stone RA, Barnes PJ, Chung KF. Effect of 5-HT$_{1A}$ receptor agonist, 8-OH-DPAT, on cough responses in the conscious guinea pig. Eur J Pharmacol 1997; 332:201–207.
74. Dixon M, Jackson DM, Richards IM. The action of sodium cromoglycate on C-fibre endings in the dog lung. Br J Pharmacol 1980; 70:11–13.
75. Dixon M, Jackson DM, Richards IM. A study of the afferent and efferent nerve distribution to the lungs of dogs. Respiration 1980; 39:144–149.
76. Jackson DM, Pollard CE, Roberts SM. The effect of nedocromil sodium on the isolated rabbit vagus nerve. Eur J Pharmacol 1992; 221:175–177.
77. Jackson DM, Norris AA, Eady RP. Nedocromil sodium and sensory nerves in the dog lung. Pulm Pharmacol 1989; 2:179–184.
78. Jones PW. Quality of life, symptoms and pulmonary function in asthma: long-term treatment with nedocromil sodium examined in a controlled multicentre trial. Nedocromil Sodium Quality of Life Study Group. Eur Respir J 1994; 7:55–62.
79. Janssen LJ, Wattie J, Betti PA. Effects of cromolyn and nedocromil on ion currents in canine tracheal smooth muscle. Eur Respir J 1998; 12:50–56.
80. Undem BJ, Weinreich D. Electrophysiological properties and chemosensitivity of guinea pig nodose ganglion neurons in vitro. J Auton Nerv Syst 1993; 44:17–33.
81. Weinreich D, Wonderlin WF. Inhibition of calcium-dependent spike after-hyperpolarization increases excitability of rabbit visceral sensory neurones. J Physiol 1987; 394:415–427.
82. Ingram SL, Williams JT. Modulation of the hyperpolarization-activated current (Ih) by cyclic nucleotides in guinea-pig primary afferent neurons. J Physiol 1996; 492:97–106.

83. Ho CY, Gu Q, Hong JL, Lee LY. Prostaglandin E_2 enhances chemical and mechanical sensitivities of pulmonary C fibers in the rat. Am J Respir Crit Care Med 2000; 162:528–533.

84. Coleridge HM, Coleridge JCG, Ginzel KH, Baker DG, Banzett RB, Morrison MA. Stimulation of 'irritant' receptors and afferent C-fibres in the lungs by prostaglandins. Nature 1976; 264:451–453.

85. Mohammed SP, Higenbottam TW, Adcock JJ. Effects of aerosol-applied capsaicin, histamine and prostaglandin E_2 on airway sensory receptors of anaesthetized cats. J Physiol 1993; 469:51–66.

86. Roberts AM, Schultz HD, Green JF, Armstrong DJ, Kaufman MP, Coleridge HM, et al. Reflex tracheal contraction evoked in dogs by bronchodilator prostaglandins E_2 and I_2. J Appl Physiol 1985; 5:1823–1831.

87. Bergren DR, Gustafson JM, Myers DL. Effect of prostaglandin F2 alpha on pulmonary rapidly-adapting-receptors in the guinea pig. Prostaglandins 1984; 27:391–405.

88. Karla W, Shams H, Orr JA, Scheid P. Effects of the thromboxane A2 mimetic, U46,619, on pulmonary vagal afferents in the cat. Respir Physiol 1992; 87:383–396.

89. Nichol GM, Nix A, Barnes PJ, Chung KF. Enhancement of capsaicin-induced cough by inhaled prostaglandin $F_{2\alpha}$: modulation by beta-adrenergic agonist and anticholinergic agent. Thorax 1990; 45:694–698.

90. Choudry NB, Fuller RW, Pride NB. Sensitivity of the human cough reflex: effect of inflammatory mediators prostaglandin E_2, bradykinin, and histamine. Am Rev Respir Dis 1989; 140:137–141.

91. Stone R, Barnes PJ, Fuller RW. Contrasting effects of prostaglandins E2 and F2 alpha on sensitivity of the human cough reflex. J Appl Physiol 1992; 73:649–653.

92. Bergren DR, Kincaid RJ. Rapidly-adapting receptor activity and intratracheal pressure in guinea pigs. II. Action of aspirin and salicylic acid in antagonizing mediators of allergic asthma. Prostaglandins Leukot Med 1984; 16:163–171.

93. McAlexander MA, Myers AC, Undem BJ. Inhibition of 5-lipoxygenase diminishes neurally evoked tachykinergic contraction of guinea pig isolated airway. J Pharmacol Exp Ther 1998; 285:602–607.

94. Dicpinigaitis PV. Effect of the cyclooxygenase-2 inhibitor celecoxib on bronchial responsiveness and cough reflex sensitivity in asthmatics. Pulm Pharmacol Ther 2001; 14:93–97.

95. Dicpinigaitis PV, Dobkin JB. Effect of zafirlukast on cough reflex sensitivity in asthmatics. J Asthma 1999; 36:265–270.

96. Pelleg A, Hurt CM. Mechanism of action of ATP on canine pulmonary vagal C fibre nerve terminals. J Physiol 1996; 490:265–275.

97. Schwartz JC, Diaz J, Bordet R, Griffon N, Perachon S, Pilon C, et al. Functional implications of multiple dopamine receptor subtypes: the D1/D3 receptor coexistence. Brain Res Brain Res Rev 1998; 26:236–242.

98. Jackson DM, Simpson WT. The effect of dopamine on the rapidly adapting receptors in the dog lung. Pulm Pharmacol Ther 2000; 13:39–42.

99. Birrell MA, Crispino N, Hele DJ, Patel HJ, Yacoub MH, Barnes PJ, et al. Effect of dopamine receptor agonists on sensory nerve activity: possible

therapeutic targets for the treatment of asthma and COPD. Br J Pharmacol 2002; 136:620–628.

100. Laursen LC, Lindqvist A, Hepburn T, Lloyd J, Perrett J, Sanders N, et al. The role of the novel D2/beta2-agonist, Viozan (sibenadet HCl), in the treatment of symptoms of chronic obstructive pulmonary disease: results of a large-scale clinical investigation. Respir Med 2003; 97(suppl A):S23–S33.

8

Analysis of the Cough Sound

JOHN EARIS

Aintree Chest Centre, University
   Hospital Aintree,
Liverpool, U.K.

JACLYN SMITH

Manchester Royal Infirmary,
Manchester, U.K.

Introduction

Cough is readily recognized by the human ear and can easily be distinguished from other upper airway sounds such as speech, laughing, throat clearing, and snoring. In addition, individuals can sometimes be recognized by the characteristics of their cough and specific cough qualities have been attributed to different chest conditions. Medical textbooks describe cough by a number of descriptors (e.g., dry, moist, productive, brassy, bovine, barking, rattling, hoarse, wheezy, loose, etc), which can be broadly divided into those coughs produced with and without the presence of sputum within the airways. A recent systematic study of cough descriptors using cluster analysis (1) has confirmed that commonly used terms do indeed divide cough into those associated with sputum (moist, productive, rattling, and loose) and those without sputum production (dry, brassy, barking, and hoarse). Moreover, although some practitioners can also recognize a wheezy quality to cough, there was a very limited ability to recognize individual chest diseases by their cough characteristics.

Analysis of speech, the commonest upper airway sound, provides an insight into possible methods of cough analysis. Two broad approaches have been used: first, the identification of interesting features either in the time or frequency domain and second, research directed toward understanding the mechanism of speech production and its relationship to the anatomy of the upper airway. From this research an acoustic/computer model of speech production has been developed based on a series of tubes of different and varying diameters. Speech can now be represented by the parameters of these digital models and this has enabled lower bit-rate transmission for telecommunications, and the development of speech recognition programs. Although there has been some attempt to understand the mechanism of cough production, so far little research has been directed toward computer modeling of the cough sound. However, the acoustic features of the cough sound are the result of its generation and modification by the physical dimensions and resonances of the larynx, vocal cords, and nasal and thoracic cavities. Thus, in time, research should lead to a more fundamental understanding of cough production and facilitate the development of cough recognition algorithms.

Cough Production Mechanism

The mechanical process producing a cough was first described in the early part of the 19th century from direct observation in animals and in humans with neck lacerations and later studied in more detail with the advent of laryngoscopy (2). Classically, four phases of a cough are described: inspiration, contraction of muscles of respiration against a closed glottis, sudden opening of the glottis with expulsion of air, and partial closure of the glottis (3–5). The relationships between the changes in airflow, subglottic pressure, and the sound of cough during these cough phases was first described in voluntary coughs from healthy volunteers (3). Significant correlations between the volume of inspired and expired air, maximum flow rate (which could reach 10 L/sec), and first peak pressure were found and two main patterns in subglottic pressure and flow were identified (Fig. 1). The first example (Fig. 1A) contains a second rise in pressure with an associated dip in flow. This was probably a consequence of the second partial closure of the glottis, while the second example (Fig. 1B) has only one pressure peak. These studies have demonstrated that the initial rapid increase in airflow and sudden glottic opening is associated with the main sound of cough. However, later work questioned the need for glottic closure and high flow rates to produce effective coughs. Young et al. (2) described voluntary and involuntary coughs in both healthy volunteers and patients with chronic obstructive pulmonary disease (COPD) and despite flow rates as low as 0.15 L/sec coughs were still associated with sputum expectoration. Moreover, in patients who cannot produce airway closure because they have undergone a laryngectomy,

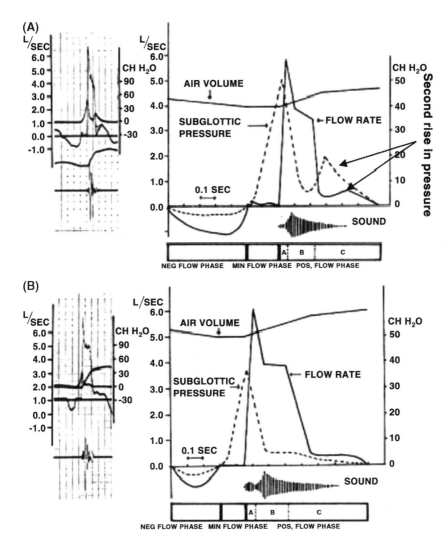

Figure 1   Flow rate, subglottic pressure, and sound production in a typical cough. (From Ref. 3.)

recognizable cough sounds are still possible, although they are markedly reduced when compared to those of age-matched healthy volunteers (6).

Recording and Analysis of the Cough Sound

Recording

Although cough sounds have traditionally been recorded onto analog tape there has been a change in recent years towards the use of digital media such as DAT tape, computer hard disks, or digital devices designed to record music. If the latter devices are used the recorded sound is often modified by the use of compression algorithms (e.g., MP3). This will remove data from the signal, which may affect subsequent acoustic analysis but has the advantage of facilitating monitoring over long periods of time. The advent of these digital storage systems now opens up the possibility of cough monitoring for 24 hr or more. Recording of the cough sound onto any of these media may be with a free-field microphone or by a contact sensor attached to the chest wall or neck. Free-field microphones provide the potential of a wide bandwidth (up to 18 kHz) so that the full acoustic features of cough sounds can be stored. In contrast, chest wall sensors, most commonly air coupled microphones or contact sensors, provide a much narrower bandwidth (with little power above 2 kHz). This is due in part to the high-pass filtering properties of tissue and secondly to the fact that sensors attached to the chest have limited ability to pick up higher frequencies.

Basic Features of the Cough Sound

The time domain waveform (i.e., relative amplitude plotted against time) of a typical cough recorded by a free-field microphone with the accompanying glottal activity is shown in Fig. 2. The term tussiphonogram is sometimes used for this representation and then derived measurements of intensity and duration are often included with a representation of the waveform. Typically, a cough amplitude plot may be divided into three phases (Fig. 2) (4,7,8). The first explosive phase (also termed the first cough sound) corresponds to glottic opening and is followed by an intermediate second phase that is usually much lower in amplitude and is associated with steady-state airflow through the open glottis. The division between the first and second phases is arbitrary as one merges into the other and thus it can be impossible to delineate them clearly. Typically, there is also a third "voiced" phase (the second cough sound) generated by the partial closing and, hence, vibration of the vocal cords. Unlike the chaotic and noise-like phases 1 and 2, this third phase consists of a regular (periodic) waveform similar to speech. The second cough sound (third phase) is not always present and its absence was once thought to be typical of psychogenic cough (9). However, several investigators have since described this type of cough in asthma and COPD (7,10) (Fig. 3).

Cough events may also occur in "peals" or "bursts" of cough sounds within a single inspiration, as seen in Fig. 4, and the phases then become much more difficult to define. In patients with COPD it has been observed that sputum expectoration more often follows peals than groups of single coughs (2). Similar cough morphologies have been recorded in response to inhaled capsaicin (11).

Position of Glottis

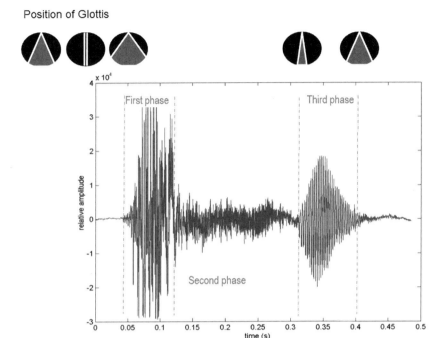

Figure 2 Typical three-phase cough sound with position of glottis shown. (Adapted from Ref. 4.)

A more detailed examination of the cough waveform is often undertaken by outlining its envelope, thus producing an amplitude profile of the wave. The raw signal is rectified and smoothed by low-pass filtering so that the overall shape of the signal amplitude can be easily appreciated (Fig. 5). Systematic investigation of the cough sound envelope in different diseases has demonstrated that only 50% of coughs have a second sound. Although there is considerable variability in the shape of the first sound both within and between patients, typically a rapid rise in power is followed by a rapid fall that then merges into the second intermediate cough phase.

The frequency content of cough sounds has been investigated using the Fourier transform, which is most commonly implemented using the fast Fourier transform (FFT). A Fourier spectrograph can be plotted which breaks down the cough signal into its constituent frequencies and this shows how these evolve over time. However, this technique has to be undertaken with care to prevent spurious results arising from problems such as aliasing or use of incorrect windowing. The output from an FFT may be presented graphically. First, a power spectrogram presents the relative power of all the frequencies within the measured range of the signal

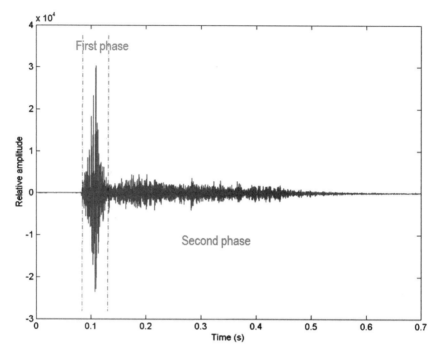

Figure 3 Two-phase cough sound.

(Fig. 6); this representation enables frequency peaks to be easily recognized. Second, a three-dimensional spectrograph can be drawn with time on the horizontal axis, frequency on the vertical, and the intensity represented by color (yellow indicating the highest and blue the lowest amplitudes). Figure 7 is a spectrograph of an asthmatic cough using a frequency range of 100–8000 Hz. The wide range of frequencies contained in the cough sounds is readily appreciated and the highly periodic final voiced sound can be clearly seen as a series of parallel frequency bands representing the harmonics of the sound. Many numeric ways of representing the frequency content of a signal such as cough can be obtained from the FFT, such as ratios between frequency bands, maximal frequency, median frequency (frequency below which half the power lies), and frequency quartiles (frequency at which 25% or 75% of the power lies).

Cough Studies in Healthy Volunteers

Because of the variability of spontaneous coughs occurring as part of a disease process, much of the work investigating the acoustic properties of cough sounds has been undertaken using voluntary coughs or those induced by the inhalation of chemical irritants such as capsaicin or citric acid. The

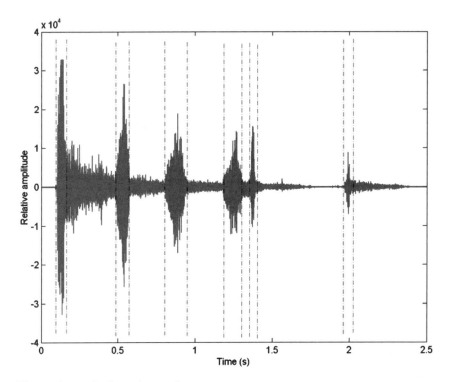

Figure 4 Peal of cough sounds.

recordings have usually been made with free-field microphones rather than those attached to the chest wall or throat and thus the resulting analysis uses a wide bandwidth. Little is known about the relationships between the acoustic properties of voluntary, spontaneous, and induced coughs.

Olia et al. (8) compared the acoustic parameters of cough sounds in 234 coughs from males and females ($n = 24$) and described the duration, intensity, dominant frequencies, and continuous frequencies within the coughs. Although most parameters had a high coefficient of variation between individuals they described a mean cough length (350 msec) similar to that in previous investigations. A final third "voiced" phase was present in 53.3% of coughs, with no gender difference. Frequencies were generally higher in females, probably due to anatomical differences in the upper airways between the sexes. The most consistent feature was the number of continuous frequencies in the second phase of cough; an example is seen as a horizontal stripe in the first cough in Fig. 7.

Capsaicin-induced cough sounds in 13 healthy volunteers were investigated by Doherty et al. (11). They examined the envelope of the cough signals (root mean square plots) and showed repeatable patterns both within

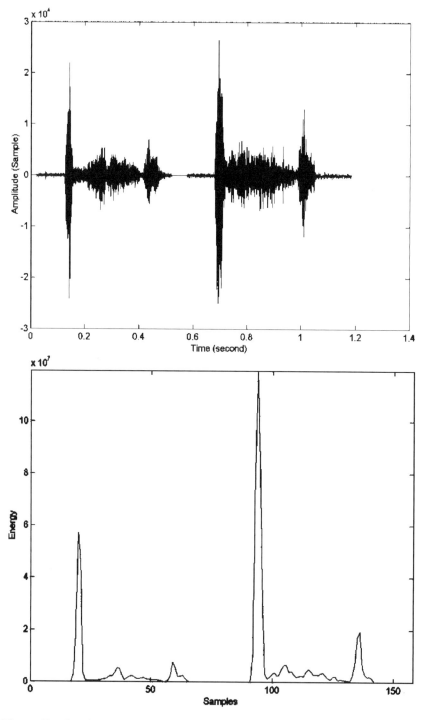

Figure 5 Cough sounds in time domain, raw signal (*top*), and signal envelope (*bottom*).

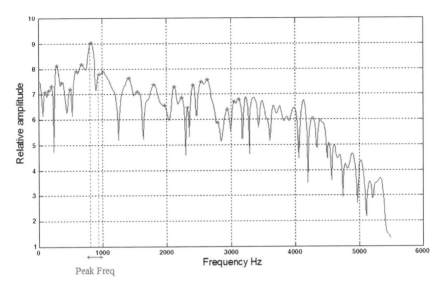

Figure 6 Power spectrograph of cough sound in COPD.

and between study days. Although there was some overall visual similarity in the spectrographs between individuals, the finer details of relative spectral energy distribution were more consistent within than between individuals. It was felt that these "cough signatures" were due to the coloration of the cough sound by individual anatomical variations responsible for resonances in the upper airway. Further evidence that voluntary cough sounds are affected by the anatomy of the upper airways was provided by Debreczeni et al. (12) who showed that the frequency content of cough sounds both in health and in disease was altered by the application of a nose clip.

Korpas et al. (13), comparing voluntary and citric acid-induced cough sounds in 36 healthy volunteers, found no significant differences in frequency content, duration, and intensity. Although they concluded that spontaneous and voluntary coughs were identical, their sound analysis was more limited than in some other studies, it was not clear which part of the cough sound was analyzed, and it was also assumed that chemically induced coughs are the same as spontaneous coughs.

Studies by Van Hirtum and Berckmans (14) of 48 coughs analyzed from free-field microphone recordings in a soundproof room compared spontaneous and voluntary cough in nine healthy volunteers and three pathological subjects, and arrived at a different conclusion. Principal components analysis was used to condense the sound parameters measured into just a few dimensions. Using a fuzzy logic approach, coughs could be correctly classified as voluntary or spontaneous 96% of the time, suggesting definite acoustic differences.

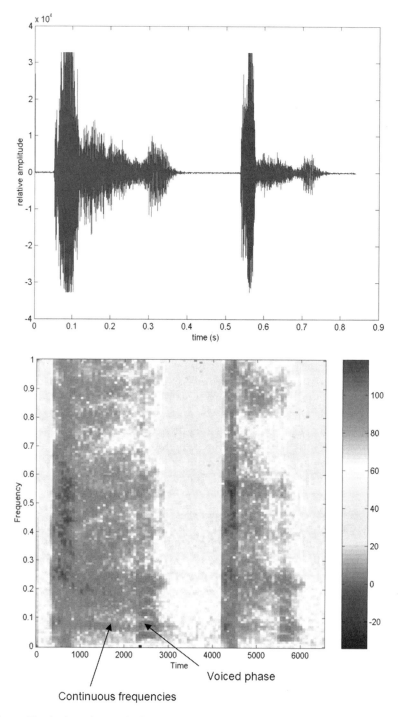

Figure 7   Asthmatic coughs in the time and frequency domains (spectrogram).

Cough Sounds Associated with Pulmonary Disease

Korpas and coworkers (4,13,15–17) have published extensively on their studies of the acoustic properties of voluntary coughs in different diseases using time amplitude plots, "tussiphonography." They describe different time domain tussiphonographic patterns of voluntary coughs in normal subjects and patients with mild bronchitis, laryngitis, tracheitis, and severe laryngotracheobronchitis (Fig. 8). After examining the morphology of over 15,000 cough recordings they claim that the tussiphonogram is useful in diagnosis and screening for effectiveness of treatment. From their observations of voluntary cough they hypothesize that the changes in the first cough sound reflect turbulent flow in the airways peripheral to the tracheal bifurcation and the second sound reflects laryngeal abnormalities. The intermediate sound reflects disease affecting the trachea. Although they have reported that voluntary and induced cough in normal individuals produce similar patterns, the differences with spontaneous cough in diseased states using tussiphonography have not been defined.

One research group to have investigated acoustic features and flow characteristics of spontaneous cough sounds under different conditions is Piirila and Sovijarvi (10). Cough sounds were recorded in an acoustic chamber using a condenser microphone attached to the sternum while subjects breathed and coughed into a mouthpiece. A mean of 12.4 ($\pm$6.2) coughs per patient were recorded from individuals suffering from asthma exacerbations ($n = 7$), pulmonary fibrosis ($n = 7$), tracheobronchial collapse syndrome ($n = 5$), and acute ($n = 5$) and chronic ($n = 7$) bronchitis. The duration of recording was not stated and thus whether all coughs under these conditions were truly spontaneous is difficult to ascertain; in other studies, long periods of recordings have been required to record these numbers of spontaneous coughs. The implied hypothesis is that the diagnostic groups are homogenous and that there are differences in the acoustic properties of cough between the diagnostic groups.

The parameters measured for each group were mean duration, upper frequency limit, dominant frequencies, and the presence of wheeze. The first sound was prolonged in the asthmatic group; however, the way the first sound was defined is unclear. Upper-frequency limits were all between 5 and 6 kHz, which is lower than previously reported (11,18). Wheezing sounds were heard in all patients but were greatest in the asthmatics. The maximal intensity of the cough sounds occurred at a frequency of 436 Hz with no difference between the groups; however, the standard deviation was large, at 544 Hz, with the majority of the variability being confined to the two bronchitis groups. Despite the small number of patients and coughs, this work provides interesting insights into cough in disease.

Voluntary cough sounds in asthmatic children have been analyzed by Thorpe and coworkers (7,19,20). The coughs were recorded from a micro-

Cough sound

Pattern   Intensity   Duration

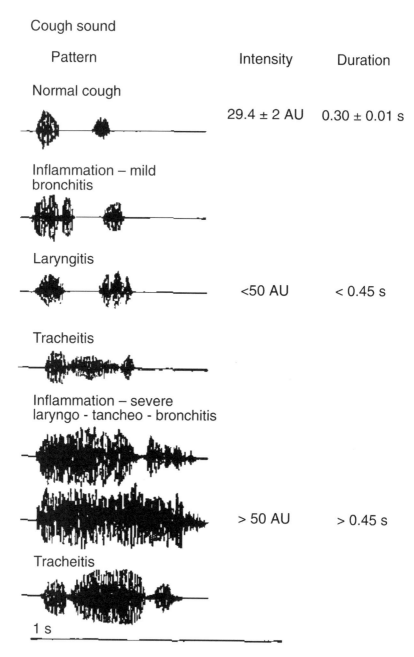

Figure 8   Tussiphonograms in different diseases. (From Ref. 5.)

phone positioned in the output of a pneumotachograph in 12 asthmatic children and 5 healthy volunteers before and after exercise. Temporal and spectral features were extracted from the first two phases of the cough sounds. Principal component analysis and multivariate discriminant analysis were performed to identify features that discriminated between the asthmatic and nonasthmatic cough sounds. Asthmatic cough sounds had a shorter first phase (first cough sound), more commonly contained a third phase (second cough sound), and had a decreased zero crossing rate when compared to healthy volunteers but the increased overall cough duration previously reported was not found. Possible explanations are that these coughs were in children not adults, that they were voluntary rather than spontaneous, and the relatively small numbers of subjects and coughs per subject.

Murata et al. (18) examined 10 voluntary productive and 10 nonproductive coughs in each of five patients with chronic bronchitis. Comparisons were made with healthy volunteer coughs. They found a significant increase in the length and sound pressure levels in the second phase of cough when the cough was productive of sputum, allowing acoustic discrimination between productive and nonproductive coughs. These findings were confirmed in another study by the same group (21), which looked at voluntary cough sounds in patients with productive and nonproductive chronic cough and the properties of sputum. Yield and ciliary transportability were found to correlate significantly with the energy and duration of the second phase.

A recent study performed acoustic analysis on 1393 spontaneous coughs from 35 patients with a range of respiratory diseases: asthma ($n = 9$), idiopathic pulmonary fibrosis ($n = 8$), cystic fibrosis ($n = 9$), and COPD ($n = 9$) (unpublished data). These coughs were extracted from overnight recordings performed in patients' homes, in all but the Cystic Fibrosis patients (who were recorded in individual hospital rooms). The duration, number of cough phases, and frequency content of a median of 46 (range 10–54) coughs per patient were measured. These cough parameters were not normally distributed, forcing the use of nonparametric statistics. Similar to other investigators the median length of cough sounds for all diagnoses was 322 msec (range 105–590). However, the variability of the duration of all phases was considerable. In this study the differences in cough parameters between individuals were more significant than the differences between the disease groups.

Cough Counting

When compared to the measurement and characterization of other biological signals such as ECG and EEG, little progress has been made in the measurement of cough. The severity of cough is usually assessed subjectively

from the patient's or a relative's perception of the symptom derived from
the clinical history, by the use of a structured questionnaire assessing effects
on quality of life (22,23), or by using a severity scale. Because of the inher-
ent variability of such subjective assessments, objective cough counting has
been suggested.

Objective cough counting has proved very difficult to achieve mainly
due to the intermittent nature of coughing necessitating prolonged monitoring times (ideally 24 hr), which makes manual cough counting impractical.
Second, the use of simple algorithms to count the coughs has so far met
with limited success because of the variability of the cough signal and difficulty in separating it from other upper airway sounds, particularly speech,
sneezing, and laughter.

An alternative approach is to measure other features of the cough
event such as the intercostal electromyograph (EMG) signal, sudden movement of the chest wall with a "movement" sensor (24), or by recording continuous chest wall movement with impedance devices devised to look at
flow and volume measurements (e.g., RespiTrace™, LifeShirt™). Attempts
to produce a cough monitor using such surrogates can only provide the
number and temporal distribution of cough events rather than any information about cough quality. Thus, a combination of acoustic features and
other signals has been employed to try and develop clinically useful cough
monitoring.

The initial attempt to count coughs from sound recordings was by
Woolf and Rosenberg in 1964 (25). They used a microphone positioned
above a patient's bed connected to an analog tape-recorder. A time base
was achieved by the use of a chiming clock and the coughs were counted
manually to quantify the effects of antitussive agents over a 4-day period.
A number of similar laboratory-based studies were performed in the late
1960s to quantify cough in pulmonary tuberculosis, chronic bronchitis,
and pneumonia (26,27) and to investigate the effect of codeine (28,29).
The main limitation of these systems was their nonambulatory nature,
and the measured cough rates of patients recorded under laboratory
conditions may be different from ambulatory recordings in the community.

With advances in electronics, two ambulatory monitors have been
reported in the last decade. Both systems identify cough from a combination of two signals, a contact microphone and EMG electrodes. The
Brompton Cough Monitor has been used in a number of studies to monitor
adults (30), children (31), infants (32), healthy volunteers, patients with
cough variant asthma, idiopathic chronic cough patients (30), and cystic
fibrosis (33). The coughs are recorded on triggering of the EMG signal
but must still be manually counted from a visual display of the signals.
Cough is quantified as "cough epochs," but the length of each epoch cannot be measured. Chang et al. have used an adapted Holter monitor to produce a similar system, which records continuously. This system has been

used to study children with recurrent cough (34–36), to investigate the effects of beclomethasone and salbutamol on cough (37), and to compare cough counts with cough challenge thresholds and subjective scores (38). Manual counting of coughs is again necessary.

Another system automatically analyzes cough sounds from a contact microphone or accelerometer attached to a radio transmitter (39), but again coughs must still be identified by a trained observer. Up to 24 hr recordings are made, via a receiver, onto the hard drive of a personal computer. Patients are confined to their own homes for the recording, as the range of the radio transmitter is limited. The system by design has been limited to analysis of acute cough. The published data describe a meta-analysis of six studies examining the effect of dextromethorphan on objective cough frequency, cough bouts, cough effort, and cough latency.

A number of groups have been working to develop automated cough recognition algorithms. Advanced digital signal processing techniques used in speech recognition have been used with some degree of success in identifying spontaneous cough in ambulatory sound recordings in different respiratory diseases (40,41) and in differentiating voluntary from involuntary cough sounds in laboratory recordings (14). Recently, a cough recognition algorithm has been reported for use in acute cough with an average sensitivity of 94% (42). Apart from achieving adequate sensitivity, the main challenges to making these algorithms useful are high specificity and repeatability. High specificity is needed to accurately quantify cough over long time periods where the amount of talking is substantially greater than the amount of coughing. Moreover, to accurately measure changes in cough frequency over time and the effects of treatment, the sensitivity of an algorithm must be consistent within an individual studied on different occasions.

Another important aspect in cough recording and recognition is the method for quantifying cough sounds. The most obvious technique is to count the number of explosive cough phases. However, in long bursts of coughing the phases become difficult to differentiate and most studies have not used this measure. Some groups have measured cough epochs, which are defined as a close succession of coughs (<2 sec between each individual cough) (33,43). An alternative approach described recently is to measure the amount of time that an individual spends coughing, defined as "cough seconds" per unit time (i.e., cough seconds per hour) (44). This improves algorithm accuracy while still taking into account the length of a peal of coughs.

Conclusions

The current situation with research into acoustic properties of the cough sound leaves many questions yet to be answered. Most studies have only investigated a small number of patients and have often used voluntary coughs rather than naturally occurring involuntary coughing. A major problem in investigating natural cough is its spasmodic nature, which sometimes necessitates many hours of recording to provide an adequate number of coughs for analysis. A number of the studies described have shown some differences in the acoustic properties of cough in different diseases but these are very difficult to compare with one another as the differences in sound acquisition sensors, microphone position, and quality of recording (sampling rates) vary enormously. Much larger studies with carefully defined diagnostic groups are needed to establish whether the acoustic properties of cough are specific to the underlying disease. The simple aim of producing a robust and accurate cough counter has proved elusive but current research may soon prove successful. In addition, research is also needed to define the mechanism of the neural stimulation that results in cough and the origins and pathophysiology of the sound of cough.

References

1. Ashurst L, Smith JA, Jack S, Woodcock AA, Earis JE. Subjective recognition of cough sounds by respiratory professionals (abstract). Eur Respir J 2003; 22(suppl 45):172s.
2. Young S, Abdul SN, Caric D. Glottic closure and high flows are not essential for productive cough. Bull Eur Physiopathol Respir 1987; 23(suppl 10): 11s–17s.
3. Yanagihara N, Von Leden H, Werner-Kukuk E. The physical parameters of cough: the larynx in a normal single cough. Acta Otolaryngol 1966; 61:495–510.
4. Korpas J, Sadlonova J, Salat D, Masarova E. The origin of cough sounds. Bull Eur Physiopathol Respir 1987; 23(suppl 10):47s–50s.
5. Korpas J, Sadlonova J, Vrabec M. Analysis of the cough sound: an overview. Pulm Pharmacol 1996; 9:261–268.
6. Fontana GA, Pantaleo T, Lavorini F, Mutolo D, Polli G, Pistolesi M. Coughing in laryngectomized patients. Am J Respir Crit Care Med 1999; 160:1578–1584.
7. Thorpe CW, Toop LJ, Dawson KP. Towards a quantitative description of asthmatic cough sounds. Eur Respir J 1992; 5:685–692.
8. Olia PM, Sestini P, Vagliasindi M. Acoustic parameters of voluntary cough in healthy non-smoking subjects. Respirology 2000; 5:271–275.
9. Korpas J, Salat D, Korpasova-Sadlonova J. Phonographic analysis of psychogenic cough. Bratisl Lek Listy 1982; 77:656–661.
10. Piirila P, Sovijarvi AR. Differences in acoustic and dynamic characteristics of spontaneous cough in pulmonary diseases. Chest 1989; 96:46–53.
11. Doherty MJ, Wang LJ, Donague S, Pearson MG, Downs P, Stoneman SA, et al. The acoustic properties of capsaicin-induced cough in healthy subjects. Eur Respir J 1997; 10:202–207.

12. Debreczeni LA, Korpas J, Salat D. Spectral analysis of cough sounds recorded with and without a nose clip. Bull Eur Physiopathol Respir 1987; 23(suppl 10):57s–61s.
13. Korpas J, Vrabec M, Sadlonova J. Comparison of voluntary and chemically induced cough sounds. Proceedings of 3rd High Tatras International Health Symposium, 1994:147–151.
14. Van Hirtum A, Berckmans D. Automated recognition of spontaneous versus voluntary cough. Med Eng Phys 2002; 24:541–545.
15. Korpas J, Sadlonova J, Salat D, Debreczeni LA. Tussiphonography: a new tool for the diagnosis of airways inflammation. Proceedings of 1st High Tatras International Health Symposium, 1992:252–257.
16. Sadlonova J, Korpas J, Salat D, Vrabec M. Possibilities to observe pathological conditions of the airways on the basis of tussiphonography. Proceedings of 1st High Tatras International Health Symposium, 1992:258–264.
17. Debreczeni LA, Korpas J, Vertes C, Sadlonova J, Radich K, Laszlo A. Role of spectral analysis of the voluntary cough sounds in screening. Proceedings of 1st High Tatras International Health Symposium, 2003:265–271.
18. Murata A, Taniguchi Y, Hashimoto Y, Kaneko Y, Takasaki Y, Kudoh S. Discrimination of productive and non-productive cough by sound analysis. Intern Med 1998; 37:732–735.
19. Thorpe CW, Fright WR, Toop LJ, Dawson KP. A microcomputer-based interactive cough sound analysis system. Comput Methods Programs Biomed 1991; 36:33–43.
20. Toop LJ, Dawson KP, Thorpe CW. A portable system for the spectral analysis of cough sounds in asthma. J Asthma 1990; 27:393–397.
21. Hashimoto Y, Murata A, Mikami M, Nakamura S, Yamanaka E, Kudoh S. Influence of the rheological properties of airway mucus on cough sound generation. Respirology 2003; 8:45–51.
22. French CT, Irwin RS, Fletcher KE, Adams TM. Evaluation of a cough-specific quality-of-life questionnaire. Chest 2002; 121:1123–1131.
23. Birring SS, Prudon B, Carr AJ, Singh SJ, Morgan MD, Pavord ID. Development of a symptom specific health status measure for patients with chronic cough: Leicester Cough Questionnaire (LCQ). Thorax 2003; 58:339–343.
24. Kohler D, Klauke M, Schonhofer B. A new portable cough recorder for long-term cough recording. Pneumologie 1997; 51:555–559.
25. Woolf CR, Rosenberg A. Objective assessment of cough suppressants under clinical conditions using a tape recorder system. Thorax 1964; 19:125–130.
26. Loudon RG, Brown LC. Cough frequency in patients with respiratory disease. Am Rev Respir Dis 1967; 96:1137–1143.
27. Loudon RG, Spohn SK. Cough frequency and infectivity in patients with pulmonary tuberculosis. Am Rev Respir Dis 1969; 99:109–111.
28. Sevelius H, Colmore JP. Objective assessment of antitussive agents in patients with chronic cough. J New Drugs 1966; 6:216–223.
29. Sevelius H, McCoy JF, Colmore JP. Dose response to codeine in patients with chronic cough. Clin Pharmacol Ther 1971; 12:449–455.

30. Hsu JY, Stone RA, Logan-Sinclair RB, Worsdell M, Busst CM, Chung KF. Coughing frequency in patients with persistent cough: assessment using a 24 hour ambulatory recorder. Eur Respir J 1994; 7:1246–1253.
31. Munyard P, Bush A. How much coughing is normal? Arch Dis Child 1996; 74:531–534.
32. Corrigan DL, Paton JY. Pilot study of objective cough monitoring in infants. Pediatr Pulmonol 2003; 35:350–357.
33. Hamutcu R, Francis J, Karakoc F, Bush A. Objective monitoring of cough in children with cystic fibrosis. Pediatr Pulmonol 2002; 34:331–335.
34. Chang AB, Newman RG, Phelan PD, Robertson CF. A new use for an old Holter monitor: an ambulatory cough meter. Eur Respir J 1997; 10:1637–1639.
35. Chang AB, Phelan PD, Robertson CF, Newman RG, Sawyer SM. Frequency and perception of cough severity. J Paediatr Child Health 2001; 37:142–145.
36. Chang AB, Newman RG, Carlin JB, Phelan PD, Robertson CF. Subjective scoring of cough in children: parent-completed vs. child-completed diary cards vs. an objective method. Eur Respir J 1998; 11:462–466.
37. Chang AB, Phelan PD, Carlin JB, Sawyer SM, Robertson CF. A randomised, placebo controlled trial of inhaled salbutamol and beclomethasone for recurrent cough. Arch Dis Child 1998; 79:6–11.
38. Chang AB, Phelan PD, Robertson CF, Roberts RG, Sawyer SM. Relation between measurements of cough severity. Arch Dis Child 2003; 88:57–60.
39. Pavesi L, Subburaj S, Porter-Shaw K. Application and validation of a computerized cough acquisition system for objective monitoring of acute cough: a meta-analysis. Chest 2001; 120:1121–1128.
40. Hiew YH, Smith JA, Cheetham BMG, Earis JE, Woodcock AA. Automatic cough detection using digital signal processing techniques—the Manchester cough algorithm (abstract). Am J Respir Crit Care Med 2002; 165(8):A832.
41. Hiew Y, Smith JA, Tait D, Cheetham BMG, Earis JE, Woodcock AA. Long-term objective cough recognition and quantification. IEE Med Appl Signal Process Lond 2002; 20:1–4.
42. Subburaj S, Van Hirtum A, Quanten S, Berkmans D. An algorithm to automatically identify cough sounds from clinical recordings (abstract). Eur Respir J 2003; 22(suppl 45):172s.
43. Power JT, Stewart IC, Connaughton JJ, Brash HM, Shapiro CM, Flenley DC, et al. Nocturnal cough in patients with chronic bronchitis and emphysema. Am Rev Respir Dis 1984; 130:999–1001.
44. Smith JA, Hiew YH, Cheetham BMG, Earis JE, Woodcock AA. Cough seconds—a new measure of cough (abstract). Am J Respir Crit Care Med 2002; 165(8):A832.

9

Capsaicin Inhalation Cough Challenge

PETER V. DICPINIGAITIS

Albert Einstein College of Medicine and Montefiore Medical Center,
Bronx, New York, U.S.A.

Capsaicin

Capsaicin, the pungent extract of hot pepper, is a compound of the vanilloid
class. Capsaicin induces cough in animals and man by stimulation of
sensory receptors within the airways. The specific role and relative contribution of the two types of afferent fibers relevant to cough, the bronchial
C-fibers and rapidly adapting pulmonary stretch receptors (RARs), remain
controversial (1,2). The recent discovery of the "capsaicin receptor," the
type 1 vanilloid receptor (VR1), will likely allow further elucidation of the
mechanism of action of capsaicin (3).

Cough Inhalation Challenge

Experimentally induced cough in humans was first described a half century
ago (4). The goal of the investigators, who developed a reproducible model
employing citric acid as the tussive agent, was to allow the evaluation of
potential antitussive medications using cough reflex sensitivity as an objective parameter. Subsequently, citric acid became a commonly used stimulus

in cough research. Other acid tussigenic agents, such as tartaric acid, have been described, but the experience with these compounds is limited. A modest but growing literature on the use of ultrasonically nebulized distilled water as a provocative agent is accumulating.

Capsaicin Inhalation Challenge

Background

The use of capsaicin to experimentally induce cough in humans was first described two decades ago (5). Capsaicin soon gained favor among investigators as a tussive agent because of its ability to induce cough in a dose-dependent and reproducible manner (6). It offered an advantage by not inducing a choking sensation or pharyngeal discomfort, as had been reported with the use of citric acid (6). Significant tachyphylaxis does not occur with capsaicin, especially if the interval between cough challenges is at least 4 hr (6–8). Furthermore, capsaicin does not induce clinically-significant bronchoconstriction in healthy volunteers or in asthmatics (5,9).

Methodology

Preparation and Storage of Capsaicin Solutions

The author prepares capsaicin solutions as previously described (10,11). Capsaicin (Sigma Chemical Co., St. Louis, Missouri, U.S.A.) 30.5 mg is dissolved in 1 mL pure ethanol and 1 mL polyoxyethylene sorbitan (Tween 80) and further dissolved in 8 ml physiological saline solution to yield a stock solution of 0.01 M. Without the detergent Tween 80, a cloudy rather than crystal-clear solution results. The solution is subsequently diluted with saline to make serial doubling concentrations ranging from 0.49 to 1000 µM. If healthy volunteers are to be tested, the lowest concentration prepared is 0.98 µM since, in the author's experience, induction of cough at this concentration is rare.

Fresh dilutions from stock solution are prepared on each day of testing. Stock solution is maintained at approximately −10°C. It is unclear how often fresh stock solution should be prepared. A recent study concluded that capsaicin solutions of 4 µM or higher concentration are stable for 1 year if stored at 4°C protected from light (12).

Administration of Capsaicin

The two main methods of capsaicin delivery during cough challenge testing are the single-dose and the dose–response methods (13). In the former method, a single concentration of capsaicin is employed. The dose–response method can involve either the administration of single, vital-capacity breaths of incremental concentrations of capsaicin via a dosimeter-controlled nebulizer, or the tidal-breath inhalation of incremental concentrations of tussive agent, each over a fixed time period, usually 15–60 sec (Table 1).

The author favors the single-breath dose–response method because of the accuracy and reproducibility of dose delivered and the ease with which a tussive response can be determined. With capsaicin inhalation occurring over a prolonged time period, variations in respiratory rate and tidal volume are likely to cause significant variations in the amount of aerosol delivered from subject to subject, as well as from one concentration to another in an individual subject. This would be of particular concern during administration of concentrations that induce significant coughing, thereby preventing the subject from inhaling the tussive agent for a significant portion of the fixed time period of aerosol delivery. Nevertheless, a recently published comparison of the tidal breathing and dosimeter methods of capsaicin inhalation challenge demonstrated both to be reproducible, with good agreement between the two methods (14).

Optimization of Reproducibility of Capsaicin Cough Challenges

Inspiratory Flow Rate

The rate of inspiratory flow will affect the pattern of deposition of aerosol within the airways. Variations in inspiratory flow rate have been demonstrated to affect the results of capsaicin cough challenge (15). Therefore, unless inspiratory flow rate is controlled, variable amounts of tussive agent will be delivered to different subjects, and even breath-to-breath variations may occur within the same study in a given subject. Such potential variability in aerosol delivery may affect the results of studies in which reproducibility of cough challenge is crucial, such as in pharmacological studies incorporating cough sensitivity measurement before and after drug therapy, and in epidemiological studies comparing different subject populations.

To control for inspiratory flow rate, the author uses a compressed air-driven nebulizer (model 646; DeVilbiss Health Care Inc., Somerset, Pennsylvania, U.S.A.) controlled by a dosimeter (KoKo DigiDoser; Pulmonary Data Service Instrumentation, Inc., Louisville, Colorado, U.S.A.) which is modified by the addition of an inspiratory flow regulator valve (RIFR, PDS Instrumentation, Inc.) (Fig. 1). The valve limits inspiratory flow rate

Table 1 Methods of Capsaicin Administration

Single-dose method
    Single concentration of capsaicin administered
Dose–response method: incremental concentrations administered
    Single (vital capacity) breath method
    Inhalation over fixed time period (usually 15–60 sec)

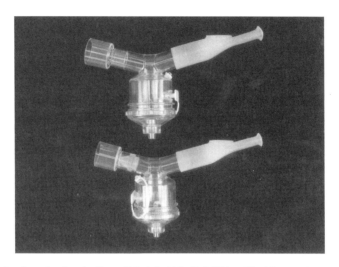

Figure 1   Standard nebulizer (Model 646; DeVilbiss Healthcare Inc., Somerset, Pennsylvania, U.S.A.) (*top*); and modified version containing inspiratory flow regulator valve (RIFR, PDS Instrumentation, Inc., Louisville, Colorado, U.S.A.), which limits inspiratory flow rate to 0.5 L/sec (*bottom*).

to 0.5 L/sec regardless of excessive inspiratory force, thereby guaranteeing a consistent and reproducible inspiratory effort with each breath. Thus, with appropriate instruction to inhale with sufficient force, all subjects achieve an identical inspiratory flow rate during each inhalation of aerosol.

Nebulizer Characteristics

Significant variation in the amount of aerosol delivered per inhalation may occur with a standard nebulizer, even in an individual subject who attempts to maintain a constant inspiratory flow rate. The importance of controlling for inspiratory flow rate is discussed above. The second major determinant of aerosol output is related to the structure of the nebulizer itself. For example, in the DeVilbiss 646 model, the straw and baffle assembly is a removable component of the nebulizer. When this structure is detached for washing and then reattached, variable distances result between the straw and baffle assembly and the source of pressurized air, the jet orifice (Fig. 2). The variation in distance, albeit minute, will result in variation in nebulizer output. Therefore, to optimize reproducibility, the author uses a nebulizer that is modified in two ways. First, an inspiratory flow regulator valve is installed, as described in the preceding text. Second, the straw and baffle assembly of the nebulizer is welded in place, thereby eliminating the variations in nebulizer output that may occur when these components are separated and then reattached with resulting variable distances between the jet orifice and straw. After these modifications are performed, the exact output

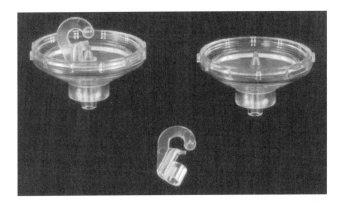

Figure 2 Standard nebulizer (Model 646; DeVilbiss Healthcare Inc., Somerset, Pennsylvania, U.S.A.) with straw and baffle assembly in place (*left*), and with straw and baffle (*bottom*) removed from the nebulizer (*right*). Jet orifice is located in the center of the nebulizer (*right*).

(mL/min) of the nebulizer is determined (characterized nebulizer, PDS Instrumentation, Inc.). When the exact output of a nebulizer is known, modulation of the duration of aerosol delivery will allow the determination of aerosol output per inhalation. For example, the author uses a nebulizer with an output of 1.007 mL/min, programmed to deliver aerosol for 1.2 sec, thereby providing 0.02 mL per breath.

Given the potential variations in nebulizer output, it is essential that research investigations utilize equipment tailored to optimize reproducibility, and that the same nebulizer, or one with identical output, is used in studies incorporating serial cough challenges in individual subjects, or studies comparing distinct subject populations. Given the reality that different types of equipment will continue to be used by cough researchers worldwide, perhaps one way to attempt standardization of cough challenge studies, to some degree, would be to control for nebulizer output per breath, as described previously.

Placebo Inhalations

To increase cough challenge blindness, inhalations of physiologic saline (placebo) should be randomly interspersed between incremental concentrations of capsaicin (13,16). This strategy may reduce the effects of voluntary suppression or conditioned responses in subjects who otherwise would be anticipating progressively higher concentrations of tussive agent.

Instructions to Subjects

Subjects undergoing cough challenge should be specifically instructed not to attempt to suppress any coughs, and not to talk immediately after inhalation of tussive agent, since this may potentially suppress cough. The author instructs subjects to "allow yourself to cough if you need to, and as much as you need to." Subjects should not be told that the induction of a specific number of coughs is the end point of the study (17) (see discussion of C_2 and C_5, end points of cough challenge testing, in the following text).

Determination of Tussive Response to Cough Challenge

When employing the single-breath method of capsaicin administration, the tussive response to each dose of aerosol is immediate and brief. Therefore, only coughs occurring within 15 sec of capsaicin delivery should be counted (13,18,19). Coughs that occur beyond this time period may not be capsaicin induced.

Interpretation of Cough Challenge Data

The most commonly used end points of cough challenge testing, especially with the dose–response method, are C_2 and C_5, the concentrations of capsaicin inducing two or more, and five or more coughs, respectively (Figs. 3 and 4). Differing opinions exist among investigators regarding which is the more highly reproducible measurement. Often, published studies will report both values but, not infrequently, only C_5 is reported. It is the author's opinion that

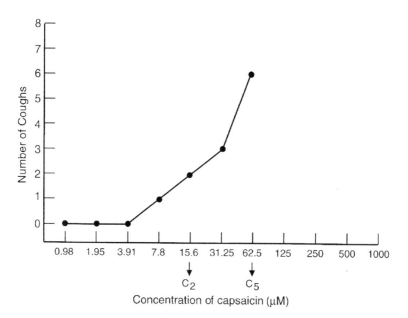

Figure 3 Dose–response curve of capsaicin cough challenge. In this study, C_2, the concentration of capsaicin inducing two or more coughs, is 15.6 μM and C_5, the concentration of capsaicin inducing five or more coughs, is 62.5 μM.

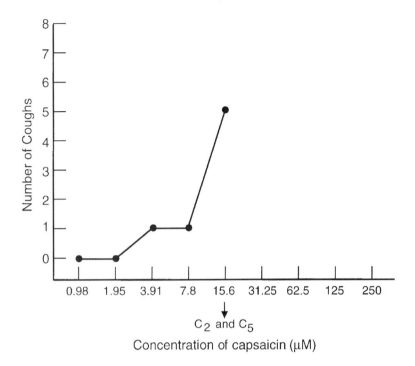

Figure 4 Dose–response curve of capsaicin cough challenge. In this study, C_2 and C_5 are identical, 15.6 μM (see definition of C_2 and C_5 in text).

C_5 is the clinically superior value (17), though other studies have found C_2 to be more reproducible (16).

A potential problem with the use of C_2 in serial cough challenges involves what the author has termed the "startle phenomenon." Occasionally, a subject undergoing an initial cough challenge will cough, usually one to three times, at a particular concentration of capsaicin, but then will not cough (or cough less) after the subsequent one or two incremental doubling concentrations. As the cough challenge study proceeds, a normal dose–response curve often results. Since the number of coughs associated with the "startle" of one's initial exposure to capsaicin is usually less than five, C_5 is much less likely to succumb to this potential pitfall.

Conversely, another potential issue relevant to cough challenge testing preferentially affects the measurement of C_5. In a small subgroup of individuals with relatively high cough thresholds, the inhalation of high concentrations of capsaicin (almost always greater than C_2) is precluded by a strong, burning sensation in the upper airway. As a result, the subject is unable to complete a full inhalation of capsaicin aerosol. If less than five coughs are induced by such a partial inhalation, an accurate determination of C_5 cannot be made. Such subjects would need to be excluded from clinical trials because a true C_5 cannot be discerned.

In some studies employing the fixed time period method of capsaicin administration, the total number of coughs occurring during the period of capsaicin inhalation (usually 15–60 sec) is counted.

An issue that has been raised by some investigators is whether the results of a subject's initial cough study should be excluded because of the observation that sometimes, the initial cough challenge yields lower cough thresholds than subsequent studies (20,21). This observation may to some extent be explained by the aforementioned "startle phenomenon." However, review of the results of serial cough challenges performed in the author's laboratory revealed no consistent trend in a subject's initial cough challenge relative to subsequent studies (17). Those data, therefore, do not support the contention that a subject's initial cough challenge is invalid and should be discarded.

Significance of Capsaicin Cough Sensitivity Measurements

It should be understood that an isolated measurement of capsaicin sensitivity (C_2 or C_5) has no intrinsic significance, due to the huge variation in cough reflex sensitivity among the population, and the lack of standardization in the methodology and equipment used by different investigators to measure this parameter. This stands in contrast to the assessment of bronchial responsiveness, where the PC_{20} (provocative concentration of methacholine inducing a 20% or greater decrement in FEV_1 from baseline) has a generally agreed-upon normal range, as well as standardized protocols for its measurement (22). Nevertheless, because cough reflex sensitivity to inhaled capsaicin is highly reproducible when performed by a individual investigator or laboratory using appropriate methodology (6,13,17), capsaicin cough challenge has established itself as an important tool in pharmacological studies incorporating serial cough challenges, as well as epidemiological studies comparing distinct populations.

Unfortunately, because of the lack of standardization of capsaicin cough challenge methodology, in terms of equipment, preparation of capsaicin solutions, method of capsaicin administration, nebulizer output, inspiratory flow rate, dose of aerosol per breath, etc. (see preceding text), comparisons of cough sensitivity data from different institutions are not valid.

Published Data: Reproducibility of Capsaicin Cough Challenge

The high degree of reproducibility of capsaicin cough challenge testing has been reported by numerous investigators employing the dose–response method, with both the single-breath technique (14,16,17) as well as with a fixed time period of capsaicin inhalation (5–7,14,23,24). However, these studies, performed mainly in healthy volunteers, evaluated short-term reproducibility of capsaicin-induced cough, with intervals between studies ranging from 20 min to 14 days. Two recently published studies, both employing the single-breath dose–response method, have confirmed the reproducibility of capsaicin cough challenge over longer periods of time: 3 months (25) and greater than 6 months (17). The latter study demonstrated good reproducibility of cough reflex sensitivity measurement in a group of 40 healthy volunteers in whom intervals between cough challenge studies were 16.7 ± 2.4 (SEM) months, with a range of 6–62 months (17).

Issues Relevant to Capsaicin Cough Challenge Testing in Specific Populations

Gender

Several studies have shown that healthy women have enhanced cough reflex sensitivity to capsaicin (26,27) and other tussive agents (28) compared to healthy men. More recently, this gender difference was demonstrated in patients suffering from chronic cough (29), thereby offering a possible explanation for the observed predominance of women among patients seeking medical attention for this complaint (30). The reason for the gender difference in cough reflex sensitivity remains unknown. However, because of this well-documented phenomenon, comparisons of cough reflex sensitivity among different study populations need to be gender specific.

Ethnicity

One study has specifically evaluated cough reflex sensitivity among healthy volunteers of different ethnic groups (31). No differences were noted between Caucasian, Indian, and Chinese subjects when comparisons were gender specific. Among each group, female subjects demonstrated enhanced cough reflex sensitivity compared to males.

Smoking Status

Multiple studies have demonstrated that cigarette smokers have a diminished cough reflex sensitivity compared to that of nonsmoking volunteers (32–34). The elevated cough thresholds in otherwise healthy smokers may reflect chronic cigarette smoke-induced desensitization of cough receptors (34). Alternatively, cigarette smokers may represent a population with inherently diminished cough reflex sensitivity (35). Given this distinction, research studies involving cough challenge need to distinguish smoking status among their subject populations.

Upper Respiratory Tract Infection

A viral upper respiratory tract infection (URI) will induce transient cough receptor hyperresponsiveness to capsaicin (16). Therefore, investigators wishing to study a subject's baseline cough reflex sensitivity should not perform capsaicin cough challenge for at least 4 weeks after the occurrence of symptoms consistent with URI.

Asthma

Cough and bronchoconstriction are separate phenomena controlled by distinct neural pathways (36). Consequently, multiple studies have demonstrated no difference in cough reflex sensitivity between healthy volunteers and stable asthmatics without cough (37–40). However, in the subgroup of asthmatics in whom cough is the sole or predominant complaint (cough-variant asthma), cough reflex sensitivity to capsaicin is significantly enhanced (41). This observation suggests that individuals with cough-variant asthma represent a distinct subgroup of patients with cough receptors that are hypersensitive relative to those of healthy volunteers and subjects with the typical form of asthma.

Chronic Obstructive Pulmonary Disease (COPD)

Previous studies have reported contrasting results in terms of capsaicin sensitivity in subjects with COPD. Using the single-breath method of aerosol administration, one group of investigators demonstrated enhanced sensitivity to capsaicin in subjects with COPD relative to healthy controls (42), whereas another trial, while failing to show hyperresponsiveness to capsaicin, demonstrated enhanced sensitivity to citric acid (43). Presumably, both the heterogeneity of the study populations as well as differences in cough challenge methodology contribute to the discordant data.

Capsaicin Cough Challenge Testing in Children

As in adults, studies in children have shown capsaicin cough challenge testing to be well tolerated, highly reproducible, affected by inspiratory flow rate, and devoid of significant short-term tachyphylaxis (44). Furthermore, pediatric data mirror those of adult studies in demonstrating enhanced cough receptor sensitivity in subjects with pathologic cough (45) and with cough associated with asthma (46). Studies comparing objectively measured cough frequency and cough reflex sensitivity in children with recurrent cough showed only a weak relationship between the two parameters (47). Similarly, the relation between cough reflex sensitivity and subjective cough scores was poor (47).

Specific Issues Relevant to the Use of Capsaicin Cough Challenge Testing in Clinical Research

Placebo Effects

Clinical trials evaluating antitussive therapies and employing subjectively or objectively-measured cough frequency and/or cough severity as end points have shown that a majority of the reduction in cough associated with URI is attributable to treatment with placebo, and only a minority attributable to the active ingredient (48). Possible explanations for this phenomenon include a demulcent effect of the placebo if it is in the form of a syrup; an antitussive effect of endogenous opioids; and the natural recovery from the acute, self-limiting URI (48). A placebo effect has been described in studies using citric acid as the tussive stimulus (49) but, to the author's knowledge, capsaicin-induced cough has not been specifically investigated in this regard.

Voluntary Suppression of Induced Cough

Since cough is to a certain degree under voluntary control, investigators must ensure that subjects participating in cough challenge studies do not voluntarily suppress their cough. As discussed above, clear instruction in this regard should be provided at the outset of the trial. Studies investigating the relevance of voluntary suppression of capsaicin-induced cough have demonstrated that, even though subjects can suppress cough and may be aware of their degree of voluntary control, this did not influence the results and reproducibility of studies in which subjects did not deliberately suppress cough (19). One hypothesis proposes that human cough is a mixture of voluntary cough controlled by higher centers such as the cerebral cortex, and reflex cough controlled by the brainstem (50).

Lack of Antitussive Effect in Healthy Volunteers Does Not Preclude a Therapeutic Effect in Patients

As with most pharmaceuticals, antitussives often undergo initial evaluation in healthy volunteers. This is an appropriate strategy since any new, potential antitussive agent should be evaluated both in terms of its effect on cough receptors in health, as well as in their hypersensitive (hypertussive) disease state. That being said, however, investigators should be cognizant of the fact that the absence of demonstrable inhibition of induced cough by an investigational drug in normal control subjects does not imply a lack of antitussive effect in patients. For example, the leukotriene receptor antagonist zafirlukast, although quite effective in suppressing subjective cough and inhibiting capsaicin-induced cough in patients with cough-variant asthma, did not affect cough reflex sensitivity in healthy volunteers or in stable asthmatics without cough (41).

Inhibition of Induced Cough Does Not Guarantee Suppression of Pathologic Cough

The initial evaluation of a potential antitussive often begins with an assessment of its effect on cough reflex sensitivity in healthy volunteers. Successful inhibition of experimentally induced cough, however, does not imply that a drug will effectively treat pathologic cough. For example, codeine, which has been demonstrated to inhibit capsaicin-induced cough (51,52) was nonetheless shown to be ineffective in cough associated with URI (53).

References

1. Widdicombe JG. Neurophysiology of the cough reflex. Eur Respir J 1995; 8:1193–1202.
2. Karlsson J-A, Fuller RW. Pharmacological regulation of the cough reflex-from experimental models to antitussive effects in man. Pulm Pharmacol Ther 1999; 12:215–228.
3. Caterina MJ, Schumacher MA, Tominaga M, Rosen TA, Levine JD, Julius D. The capsaicin receptor: a heat activated ion channel in the pain pathway. Nature 1997; 389:816–824.
4. Bickerman HA, Barach AL, Itkin SE, Drimmler F. The experimental production of cough in human subjects induced by citric acid aerosols. Preliminary studies on the evaluation of antitussive agents. Am J Med Sci 1954; 228: 156–163.
5. Collier JG, Fuller RW. Capsaicin inhalation in man and the effects of sodium cromoglycate. Br J Pharmacol 1984; 81:113–117.
6. Midgren B, Hansson L, Karlsson J-A, Simonsson BG, Persson CGA. Capsaicin-induced cough in humans. Am Rev Respir Dis 1992; 146:347–351.
7. Morice AH, Higgins KS, Yeo WW. Adaptation of cough reflex with different types of stimulation. Eur Respir J 1992; 5:841–847.
8. O'Connell F, Thomas VE, Pride NB. Adaptation of cough reflex with different types of stimulation [letter]. Eur Respir J 1992; 5:1296–1297.
9. Fuller RW, Dixon CMS, Barnes PJ. Bronchoconstrictor response to inhaled capsaicin in humans. J Appl Physiol 1985; 58:1080–1084.
10. Fujimura M, Kamio Y, Hashimoto T, Matsuda T. Cough receptor sensitivity and bronchial responsiveness in patients with only chronic nonproductive cough: in view of effect of bronchodilator therapy. J Asthma 1994; 31:463–472.
11. Dicpinigaitis PV, Dobkin JB. Antitussive effect of the GABA-agonist baclofen. Chest 1997; 111:996–999.
12. Opec SE, DeBellis RJ, Irwin RS. Chemical analysis of freshly prepared and stored capsaicin solutions: implications for tussigenic challenges. Pulm Pharmacol Ther 2002; 15:529–534.
13. Morice AH, Kastelik JA, Thompson R. Cough challenge in the assessment of cough reflex. Br J Clin Pharmacol 2001; 52:365–375.
14. Nejla S, Fujimura M, Kamio Y. Comparison between tidal breathing and dosimeter methods in assessing cough receptor sensitivity to capsaicin. Respirology 2000; 5:337–342.

15. Barros MJ, Zammattio SL, Rees PJ. Effect of changes in inspiratory flow rate on cough responses to inhaled capsaicin. Clin Sci 1991; 81:539–542.
16. O'Connell F, Thomas VE, Studham JM, Pride NB, Fuller RW. Capsaicin cough sensitivity increases during upper respiratory infection. Respir Med 1996; 90:279–286.
17. Dicpinigaitis PV. Short- and long-term reproducibility of capsaicin cough challenge testing. Pulm Pharmacol Ther 2003; 16:61–65.
18. Hansson L, Wollmer P, Dahlback M, Karlsson J-A. Regional sensitivity of human airways to capsaicin-induced cough. Am Rev Respir Dis 1992; 145:1191–1195.
19. Hutchings HA, Morris S, Eccles R, Jawad MSM. Voluntary suppression of cough induced by inhalation of capsaicin in healthy volunteers. Respir Med 1993; 87:379–382.
20. Morice AH. Inhalation cough challenge in the investigation of the cough reflex and antitussives. Pulm Pharmacol 1996; 9:281–284.
21. Whale C, Singh D, Woodcock AA. Reproducibility of capsaicin induced cough challenges [abstr]. Am J Respir Crit Care Med 2001; 163:A629.
22. American Thoracic Society. Guidelines for methacholine and exercise challenge testing—1999. Am J Respir Crit Care Med 2000; 161:309–329.
23. Fujimura M, Kamio Y, Sakamoto S, Bando T, Myou S, Matsuda T. Tachyphylaxis to capsaicin-induced cough and its reversal by indomethacin in patients with sinobronchial syndrome. Clin Auton Res 1992; 2:397–401.
24. Fujimura M, Sakamoto S, Kamio Y, Matsuda T. Effects of methacholine-induced bronchoconstriction and procaterol-induced bronchodilation on cough receptor sensitivity to inhaled capsaicin and tartaric acid. Thorax 1992; 47:441–445.
25. Nieto L, DeDiego A, Perpina M, Compte L, Garrigues V, Martinez E, Ponce J. Cough reflex testing with inhaled capsaicin in the study of chronic cough. Respir Med 2003; 97:393–400.
26. Fujimura M, Kasahara K, Kamio Y, Naruse M, Hashimoto T, Matsuda T. Female gender as a determinant of cough threshold to inhaled capsaicin. Eur Respir J 1996; 9:1624–1626.
27. Dicpinigaitis PV, Rauf K. The influence of gender on cough reflex sensitivity. Chest 1998; 113:1319–1321.
28. Fujimura M, Sakamoto S, Kamio Y, Matsuda T. Sex difference in the inhaled tartaric acid cough threshold in non-atopic healthy subjects. Thorax 1990; 45:633–634.
29. Kastelik JA, Thompson RH, Aziz I, Ojoo JC, Redington AE, Morice AH. Sex-related differences in cough reflex sensitivity in patients with chronic cough. Am J Respir Crit Care Med 2002; 166:961–964.
30. Irwin RS, Boulet L-P, Cloutier MM, Fuller R, Gold PM, Hoffstein V, Ing AJ, McCool FD, O'Byrne P, Poe RH, Prakash UBS, Pratter MR, Rubin BK. Managing cough as a defense mechanism and as a symptom: a consensus panel report of the American College of Chest Physicians. Chest 1998; 114: 133S–181S.
31. Dicpinigaitis PV, Allusson VRC, Baldanti A, Nalamati JR. Ethnic and gender differences in cough reflex sensitivity. Respiration 2001; 68:480–482.

32. Millqvist E, Bende M. Capsaicin cough sensitivity is decreased in smokers. Respir Med 2001; 95:19–21.
33. Schmidt D, Jorres RA, Magnussen H. Citric acid-induced cough thresholds in normal subjects, patients with bronchial asthma, and smokers. Eur J Med Res 1997; 2:384–388.
34. Dicpinigaitis PV. Cough reflex sensitivity in cigarette smokers. Chest 2003; 123:685–688.
35. Lalloo UG. The cough reflex and the "healthy smoker." Chest 2003; 123: 660–662.
36. Karlsson J-A, Sant'Ambrogio G, Widdicombe JG. Afferent neural pathways in cough and reflex bronchoconstriction. J Appl Physiol 1988; 65:1007–1023.
37. Choudry NB, Fuller RW. Sensitivity of the cough reflex in patients with chronic cough. Eur Respir J 1992; 5:296–300.
38. Millqvist E, Bende M, Lowhagen O. Sensory hyperreactivity: a possible mechanism underlying cough and asthma-like symptoms. Allergy 1998; 53:1208–1212.
39. Fujimura M, Kamio Y, Hashimoto T, Matsuda T. Airway cough sensitivity to inhaled capsaicin and bronchial responsiveness to methacholine in asthmatics and bronchitic subjects. Respirology 1998; 3:267–272.
40. Dicpinigaitis PV. Capsaicin responsiveness in asthma and COPD [letter]. Thorax 2001; 56:161.
41. Dicpinigaitis PV, Dobkin JB, Reichel J. Antitussive effect of the leukotriene receptor antagonist zafirlukast in subjects with cough-variant asthma. J Asthma 2002; 39:291–297.
42. Doherty MJ, Mister R, Pearson MG, Calverley PM. Capsaicin responsiveness and cough in asthma and chronic obstructive pulmonary disease. Thorax 2000; 55:643–649.
43. Wong CH, Morice AH. Cough threshold in patients with chronic obstructive pulmonary disease. Thorax 1999; 54:62–64.
44. Chang AB, Phelan PD, Roberts RGD, Robertson F. Capsaicin cough receptor sensitivity in children. Eur Respir J 1996; 9:2220–2223.
45. Chang AB, Phelan PD, Sawyer SM, Robertson CF. Airway hyperresponsiveness and cough-receptor sensitivity in children with recurrent cough. Am J Respir Crit Care Med 1997; 155:1935–1939.
46. Chang AB, Phelan PD, Robertson CF. Cough receptor sensitivity in children with acute and non-acute asthma. Thorax 1997; 52:770–774.
47. Chang AB, Phelan PD, Robertson CF, Roberts RGD, Sawyer SM. Relation between measurements of cough severity. Arch Dis Child 2003; 88:57–60.
48. Eccles R. The powerful placebo in cough studies?. Pulm Pharmacol Ther 2002; 15:303–308.
49. Rostami-Hodjegan A, Abdul-Manap R, Wright CE, Tucker GT, Morice AH. The placebo response to citric acid-induced cough: pharmacodynamics and gender differences. Pulm Pharmacol Ther 2001; 14:315–319.
50. Lee PCL, Cotterill-Jones C, Eccles R. Voluntary control of cough. Pulm Pharmacol Ther 2002; 15:317–320.
51. Fuller RW, Karlsson JA, Choudry NB, Pride NB. Effect of inhaled and systemic opiates on responses to inhaled capsaicin in humans. J Appl Physiol 1988; 65:1125–1130.

52. Dicpinigaitis PV, Dobkin JB, Rauf K. Comparison of the antitussive effects of codeine and the GABA-agonist baclofen. Clin Drug Invest 1997; 14:326–329.
53. Freestone C, Eccles R. Assessment of the antitussive efficacy of codeine in cough associated with the common cold. J Pharm Pharmacol 1997; 49: 1045–1049.

10

Acid Inhalation Cough Challenge

JACK A. KASTELIK

Division of Academic Medicine, Postgraduate Medical Institute,
  University of Hull, Castle Hill Hospital,
East Yorkshire, U.K.

Introduction

Cough is one of the most common respiratory symptoms (1). Epidemiologic studies estimate the prevalence of cough at between 3% and 40% (2–5). These figures derive from questionnaire surveys that assess mainly the presence or absence of cough and its characteristics, for example, productive or nonproductive. In contrast, specifically designed cough questionnaires allow measurement of the effects of cough on an individual's quality of life (6–9). Another way to quantify cough is using cough provocation tests. These are of particular relevance when studying the pathophysiology of the cough reflex and when assessing the effects of antitussive agents and their mechanisms.

The idea of inhalation cough challenge originated from the clinical observation that during the administration of aerosols such as nebulized bronchodilators, patients can experience a sense of irritation of the upper airways resulting in cough. Cough is recognized to be a reflex action with its sensory afferent mediated by the vagus nerve terminating in the airways (10,11). The afferent nerve fibers transmit impulses to the cough center, which is thought to be situated in the medulla and lower pons (12). The efferent limb of the cough reflex is via the phrenic and other spinal nerves to the respiratory muscles. As aerosols can be delivered to the site of afferent nerve endings, cough can be induced using a variety of chemical stimuli. Inhalation of a tussigenic aerosol therefore forms the basis of cough challenge testing.

Inhalation cough challenge testing can be divided into methods that use acid and nonacid tussives. Capsaicin and distilled water cough challenges are the most commonly used agents in nonacid methods. Citric and tartaric acids are the most widely used acid tussigens. This chapter will discuss inhalation cough challenge with acid tussigens.

Historical Aspects

Early assessments of the effectiveness of antitussive medications were based simply on either counting the number of coughs or using diary cards (13). The lack of objectivity and the changing status of the patients were the main confounding aspects of these methods. To provide more unbiased tools to test and compare the antitussive effects of medications, experimental methods were developed to artificially stimulate the cough reflex. These first involved techniques such as spraying a jet of ammonia vapor to elicit cough (14) or direct administration of ether and peppermint into the larynx via an endotracheal tube (15). By the mid-1950s more comprehensive criteria had been proposed to describe the essential characteristics of cough induction methods (16). First, the method should be nontoxic and relatively simple, allowing the test to be performed on a large number of subjects. Second, it should be uniform and consistent with regard to the response of the test subject to the same threshold of stimulating agent, as well as being reproducible in the same individual during the course of the study.

In 1954 Bickerman et al. (16) provided the first detailed description of acid inhalation cough challenge. Over a 2-year period, the authors systematically tested a total of 33 substances—including varying concentrations of citric, tartaric, benzoic, hydrochloric, and sulfuric acids, ethyl alcohol, and ether—in 105 subjects. The substances were delivered using an air compressor-driven Vaponefrin nebulizer with a Y-tube attachment to permit nebulization during inspiration only. The cough responses to citric, tartaric, and benzoic acids were found to be the most consistent, with a 10% concentration of citric acid inducing cough in the highest percentage of subjects. The authors showed a fairly consistent cough response to 5% and 10% citric acid in healthy volunteers and patients with stable asthma. Ten subjects underwent repeated tests with solutions of citric acid ranging between 2.5% and 10%, and the number of coughs was shown to increase in a concentration-dependent manner. Finally, the effects of several potential antitussive agents were tested, among which codeine and Nalline produced significant reductions in cough compared with the control. This experimental work established that cough can be "artificially" induced by inhalation of acid tussigens. The authors described the single-concentration and concentration–response characteristics of acid inhalation cough challenge. In addition, they showed that this method can be used to assess antitussive agents.

In subsequent work, Bickerman et al. (17) formally characterized an inhalation cough challenge method that used varying concentrations (1.25–25%) of citric acid delivered over a predetermined period. The authors defined "cough response" as the number of coughs recorded. They also introduced the term "cough threshold," defined as the concentration of citric acid that evoked a total of not less than four coughs. Since then other methods have been used. For example, some have measured the time from a single inhalation to cough production (18). Others have used a simple method in which the concentration of citric acid is steadily increased until cough is induced (19).

Bickerman et al. (16,17) were aware that inhalation cough challenge may have limitations including the effects of psychological factors on the cough response. However, the relevance of those factors together with other aspects such as the effect of the time of day or the presence of cough reflex adaptation remained unknown for some time. It was not until 1985—almost 30 years since the original description of citric acid cough challenge by Bickerman et al. (16)—that some of these issues were formally addressed. Pounsford and Saunders (20) demonstrated that, similar to airway resistance, cough response to inhaled citric acid shows diurnal variation. In healthy volunteers cough threshold, which the authors defined as the lowest concentration causing cough, was systematically and significantly higher in the afternoon. More recently, the effects of tachyphylaxis and voluntary cough suppression have also been described (21,22). These aspects of the cough reflex response and their relevance to inhalation cough challenge will be discussed later.

The methodology of inhalation cough challenge has gradually been refined and the number of acid tussigenic agents in use narrowed down to only a few. Tartaric acid has become particularly favored by some (23–26) and others have shown preference for acetic acid (27–30). However, citric acid has become the most commonly used agent. In all these inhalation cough challenges, standardization of the means of delivery has become an important issue and this will now be discussed.

Delivery of Acid Tussives

During inhalation cough challenge, tussive agents are delivered in the form of aerosols. Acid tussives are most commonly administered using jet nebulizers driven by low-output air compressors. The aerosol particles produced in this way vary in size and this in turn affects their deposition. Particles 10 μm in diameter are mainly deposited in the mouth and throat, 5–10 μm particles between the throat and the lungs, and particles of <5 μm mainly in the lungs (31). While there is evidence that particle size affects capsaicin-induced cough (32), no such data exist for acid cough challenge. However, citric acid cough is diminished compared with capsaicin cough in patients who have undergone laryngectomy, suggesting perhaps that citric acid-sensitive neurons are more dominant in the larynx (21). Furthermore, there is good evidence that changes in inspiratory flow rate can affect the citric acid cough response, most likely by altering drug deposition (33). Thus, a lower inspiratory flow produces a greater cough response, perhaps through greater laryngeal deposition. Similarly, rapid changes in airway caliber may affect the citric acid-induced cough response (34).

As the methodology of inhalation cough challenge has evolved, major changes have occurred in relation to aerosol delivery. Dosimeter-controlled jet nebulizers have become the preferred delivery systems and are now accepted as the most standardized way to deliver citric acid (35). Inhalation from the dosimeter generates a burst of compressed air that initiates a fixed duration of nebulization. This facilitates accurate calibration of the output, although some variation in the velocity of inhalation may still occur (36,37). The introduction of dosimeter-controlled jet nebulizers to deliver the tussigenic aerosol has greatly reduced the effects of airway caliber and inspiratory flow on the cough response. Although a dosimeter is considered the optimum method to deliver tussigenic agents during inhalation cough challenges, other methodologies have also been used and therefore merit discussion.

Methodology of Acid Inhalation Cough Challenge

Inhalation cough challenge involves the delivery of a tussive stimulus and subsequent recording of the number of induced coughs. The method involving inhalation of a single concentration of acid tussigen is best suited to screen large populations of subjects, for example, to detect those with reproducible cough (38). It has also been used to study the antitussive activity of pharmacologic agents (39–42). Compared with the concentration–response method, the main advantages of the single-concentration cough challenge are its simplicity, speed, and the lower degree of tachyphylaxis (43). The concentration–response method involves the delivery of incremental concentrations of aerosol. Data from this type of cough challenge allow the construction of concentration–response curves and results are most frequently expressed as C2 and C5 values, defined as the lowest concentrations producing two and five coughs per inhalation, respectively. This method has been used to study the effects of gender (44) and of diseases such as chronic obstructive pulmonary disease (COPD) (45) on the cough reflex. However, the most important use of the concentration–response method has been in the investigation of the antitussive properties of pharmacologic agents (35).

Acid inhalation cough challenge can be further divided into fixed-time inhalation and single-breath techniques. The fixed time inhalation involves the subject breathing tidally while inhaling the acid tussigen over an extended period of time. This inhalation time can vary from 15 to 60 sec (24,25,46,47). The 1 min citric acid fixed inhalation method has been used infrequently (46,47). The 15 sec inhalation method has been used more widely, for example, by Fujimura et al. (23–25), in a number of studies. However, the reproducibility and accuracy of the fixed-time inhalation method may be questioned as the amount of aerosol delivered is influenced by factors such as the individual's breathing effort, the tidal volume, and the type of nebulizer used. These factors can lead to a high intersubject variability in delivered dose (48), and single-breath methods are generally considered more accurate. Single-breath methods involve the inhalation of nebulized acid tussigen using a single breath over a short period of time. This is performed using tidal inhalation, as deep inhalation may affect coughing through the recruitment of irritant receptors. The simplest approach, which involves fixed inspiratory maneuvers such as vital capacity volume inhalation, may be less reliable and has as a result been employed infrequently (20). More reproducible methods have used dosimeter-controlled nebulizers (35). The single-breath dosimeter-controlled technique has now become accepted as the most standardized method for inhalation cough challenge.

All methods of acid inhalation cough challenge can be confounded by the diurnal variability of the cough response and by the fact that cough can be consciously suppressed (20,49). The first problem is minimized simply by performing cough challenge testing at the same time of day. To reduce the effects of voluntary suppression of cough and to increase challenge blindness, the use of placebo inhalation has been encouraged. The accuracy of testing can also be improved through repeat testing, as the learning effect is much smaller during repeated cough challenges (16,43).

Consideration should also be given to placebo effects and to gender. The placebo response involves a nonlinear increase in cough suppression which is most pronounced at 4 hr (50). The gender difference in cough response to inhaled acid tussigens is well recognized. There are suggestions that females may cough more frequently and have more rapid adaptation of cough than males. Reports in healthy volunteers have demonstrated a gender-related difference in cough response to both acid and nonacid tussigenic agents (25,38,51). Fujimura et al. (25), for example, reported that healthy female subjects had a lower cough threshold to tartaric acid. Others have shown an increased number of coughs in female healthy volunteers after the inhalation of a fixed dose of citric acid (38). In addition, there is evidence of a gender difference in cough response to citric acid in patients with chronic cough (44). Therefore, both healthy women and female patients with chronic cough display greater cough sensitivity to acid tussigens compared with men. Another important aspect of inhalation cough challenge relates to the fact that when both citric acid and capsaicin cough challenges are performed within a short period of time, the cough response is affected. Thus, the cough response can be diminished by a quarter when citric acid is inhaled after capsaicin and by a third when capsaicin inhalation follows the administration of citric acid (43). Citric acid inhalation challenge is preferred when cough testing needs to be repeated at short intervals, as recovery from cough challenge to capsaicin is slower, particularly with higher concentrations, resulting in greater tachyphylaxis.

In our centre, concentration–response challenge to inhaled citric acid is performed using a compressed air-driven nebulizer controlled by a breath-activated dosimeter (Mefar MB3 CE; Mefar s.p.a. Bresia, Italy), which is preset to limit the nebulization time to 1 sec (44). Solutions are prepared by serial dilution of 1 M citric acid (Production Pharmacy, Royal Hallamshire Hospital, Sheffield, U.K.) in sterile 0.9% saline to obtain concentrations of 1, 3, 10, 30, 100, 300, and 1000 mM. Citric acid is delivered in incremental concentrations, with inhalation of 0.9% saline randomly interspersed to increase challenge blindness. Subjects exhale to functional residual capacity and then inhale through a mouthpiece for 1 sec until the nebulization ceases. The number of coughs in the first 10 sec after inhalation is recorded using a digital audio tape recorder. There is a 30 sec pause between each inhalation and each concentration of tussive agent is inhaled four times. Citric acid is administered in increasing concentrations with two randomly delivered placebo (0.9% saline) doses introduced as a control. Log concentration–response curves are constructed for each test and C2 and C5 values are calculated by linear interpolation.

For a single-concentration inhalation challenge, we use the same system of a compressed air-driven nebulizer controlled by a breath-activated dosimeter preset to limit the nebulization time to 1 sec. Citric acid is diluted in 0.9% saline to obtain a concentration of 10 mM. Subjects exhale to functional residual capacity and then inhale through a mouthpiece for 1 second until the nebulization ceases. We perform five inhalations with 60 second intervals between each inhalation during which the number of coughs are counted (38,40,52). Both concentration–response and single-concentration cough challenges are performed at the same time of the day to avoid the effect of diurnal variability on the cough response.

Mechanisms of Citric Acid-Induced Cough

A number of chemical stimuli, including sulfur dioxide, ammonia, and cigarette smoke, can trigger the sensory endings of afferent nerves (53). Many provocative or tussive agents used in the inhalation cough challenge have been shown to reliably induce cough in the human model. Citric acid, for example, has been reported to induce cough in approximately 90% of healthy subjects (16). This response is rapid but self-limiting. However, the cough response to citric acid does show adaptability over a short period of time and diurnal variability (20,54). Despite advances in our understanding of the cough reflex, the mechanisms by which citric and other acids induce cough are by no means clear.

The afferent nerves regulating the cough reflex originate from receptors that ramify between individual epithelial cells and travel through the fibers of the vagus nerve. These sensory nerve fibers terminate in the larynx, trachea, and extrapulmonary bronchi. At least two types of vagal sensory fibers participate in the initiation of cough (55,56). These are the rapidly adapting receptors (RARs), which are of a low-threshold mechanosensory type, and C-fiber receptors, which are capsaicin-sensitive. There is good evidence that stimulation of irritant receptors in the laryngeal wall and RARs in the tracheobronchial mucosa can directly induce cough (56). In contrast, C-fiber receptors most likely induce cough indirectly through the release of tachykinins, which act on RARs.

An earlier hypothesis proposed that cough induction with citric acid might be related to the change in osmolarity and acidity of the airway fluid surface (34). However, current evidence suggests that citric acid most likely induces cough through a change of pH. Thus, when citric acid is applied to vagal afferent RARs, an immediate response of action potential discharge is observed (57). The cough response is consistent with different acid tussigenic agents, including citric, acetic, and phosphoric acids (58). A pH level of approximately 6.7 is the threshold of proton-induced activation of RARs (57). However, in the context of RARs stimulation the rapid change in pH is of greater importance. C-fibers can also be activated by a change in pH. In addition, they exhibit characteristics of persistent action potential discharge when pH remains below the threshold level. Thus, it is possible that citric and other acids stimulate both RARs and C-fibers through as yet undefined acid-sensing ion channels.

Whereas the action of capsaicin is relatively well understood, the mechanisms by which citric acid induces cough remain to be fully described. Capsaicin, through the afferent neurons of the nonmyelinated C-fibers, opens a nonselective cation channel, the type 1 vanilloid receptor (VR1), by binding to an intracellular site of the receptor resulting in a flow of calcium and sodium down their concentration gradients (56,59,60). This leads to depolarization and neurotransmitter release. Protons can interact with the extracellular domain of VR1 to increase the opening probability of the channel (61). Thus, it is possible that citric acid may also activate VR1, although most likely through the extracellular domain and therefore a different site from that of capsaicin. This is further evidenced by the fact that capsazepine, a competitive inhibitor of capsaicin, partially blocks citric acid-induced cough in guinea pigs (62). In contrast, an aerosol of citric acid does not induce cough in capsaicin-desensitized unanesthetized guinea pigs (63). However, under the same conditions cough can be induced by nicotine or by mechanical stimulation (63). In humans there is evidence of a correlation between citric acid and capsaicin sensitivity in patients with chronic cough (44) but a lack of any such correlation in healthy subjects (58,64). This may perhaps be explained by factors such as airway inflammation, which is frequently present in patients with chronic cough (65–67). It is possible that inflammatory mediators act as endogenous ligands for the putative cough receptor.

The different pattern of cough response stimulation between citric acid and capsaicin is also apparent in the adaptation process observed with these two substances. Citric acid inhalation cough challenge in human subjects reveals the presence of both acute and chronic adaptation (54). Tachyphylaxis with citric acid is seen within 1 min and continues for 40 min. This may perhaps be explained by the presence of central modulation, similar to that described in pain pathways. In contrast, capsaicin inhalation challenge lacks acute adaptation but does exhibit long-term adaptation. In addition, the recovery is much slower with capsaicin compared to that observed with citric acid. Citric acid and capsaicin show cross-tachyphylaxis (54). This would suggest that these tussive agents do not exclusively stimulate one type of nerve fibers but most likely a common pool of receptors that may be modulated at a higher level. Further support for higher-level modulation of the cough response to citric acid derives from the observation of the learning effect (54).

In guinea pigs inhalation of citric acid causes bronchoconstriction, most likely due to tachykinin release from the sensory nerves (68). In contrast, in human subjects no such change in airway caliber has been observed after inhalation of citric acid (54). In patients with asthma in whom airway resistance is increased, cough reflex sensitivity to citric acid is no different compared with healthy subjects (34). However, when airway caliber is changed rapidly, for example, by the administration of bronchodilators, a marked reduction in the cough response to inhaled citric acid occurs (34). Therefore, in the human model, the cough response to citric acid is unlikely to be affected by the static level of airway resistance but is altered by a change in airway caliber, possibly as a result of alteration of neuroreceptor sensitivity (34).

Animal Studies

Animal models have made a major contribution to our understanding of the physiology of the cough reflex and also play an important role in preclinical studies of potential antitussive agents. Using an in vitro preparation of guinea pig trachea and main bronchi with the attached vagus nerve, the properties of single vagal afferent nerve fibers can be examined (69). The isolated guinea-pig vagus nerve behaves in a very similar way to the isolated human vagus nerve (70). Experimental assessment of the cough reflex can also be performed in conscious animals using inhalation of capsaicin or citric acid (55,62,71). Cough studies have been performed in various species with much of the original research undertaken on cats and dogs (72). In conscious rats there have been doubts about whether the cough response produced resembles that of the human. To date, it is the conscious guinea-pig cough model that has acquired widest acceptance (70). The major advantage of this model is its similarity to the human cough model. Laude et al. (71) demonstrated that both guinea pigs and humans respond to similar concentrations of citric acid and that both cough models show a concentration–response relationship. The main disadvantages of the animal model are associated with the difficulties in calculating the actual dose inhaled because of the unknown factors of deposition and respiratory volume. In addition, citric acid can induce dyspnea in guinea pigs, although to a lesser degree than capsaicin (71).

In a typical model, the conscious animal is placed in a transparent chamber allowing for free movement and an aerosol of the acid tussive agent is then delivered into this chamber. The duration of delivery of aerosol differs between centers. Laude et al. (71), for example, delivered the aerosol challenge for 2 min and counted the number of coughs over a 10 min period. Others have delivered citric acid for 10 min, during which period the number of coughs was determined (55). Cough events can be recognized through observation of the animal, by measuring changes in airflow, and by recording cough sounds. By using a pneumotachograph connected to a manometer and recorder, coughs can be distinguished from sneezes or deep breaths. Pretreatment with a bronchodilator has been recommended to minimize respiratory distress without affecting the cough response (62).

The guinea-pig cough model has been extensively used in both physiologic and pharmacologic studies. Forsberg et al. (63) showed that aerosols of citric acid produced bronchoconstriction and a concentration-dependent increase in the number of coughs in unanesthetized guinea pigs. Many studies have examined the role of tachykinins. Girard et al. (73) demonstrated that neurokinin (NK)-2 receptor stimulation plays an important role in the regulation of the cough reflex in the guinea pig. Others have shown that NK-3 receptor inhibition reduces the citric acid cough response (74,75). Moreaux et al. (75) reported that the local application of substance P to the airways of guinea pigs potentiated the frequency of citric acid-induced cough.

More recently, Ricciardolo et al. (68) investigated interactions between tachy-kinins, bradykinin, and nitric oxide (NO) during citric acid-induced bronch-oconstriction in anesthetized guinea pigs. The authors found that tachykinin release from sensory nerves, in part mediated by endogenously released bradykinin, underlies the bronchoconstrictor response. Simultaneous release of NO counteracts tachykinin-mediated bronchoconstriction.

Laude et al. (76) assessed the effects of fenspiride, a nonsteroidal anti-inflammatory agent, on cough and bronchoconstriction in conscious guinea pigs. Aerosolized fenspiride was shown to reverse the citric acid-induced bronchoconstrictor and cough responses. Other authors have investigated the action of aromatic vapors such as menthol, camphor, and cineole on the cough reflex in the conscious guinea pig (77). Menthol inhalation pro-duced the greatest suppression of cough, suggesting that it may have anti-tussive properties. Subsequent human studies have confirmed that inhalation of menthol causes a reduction in cough evoked as a response to citric acid. These studies illustrate how animal experiments can lead to the testing of antitussives in the human model.

Human Studies

Acetic Acid

Acetic acid cough challenge has acquired only limited use to date. Shimizu et al. (29) studied the relationship between cough reflex sensitivity and airway hyperresponsiveness in asthma. The authors found no relationship between the airway responsiveness to histamine and acetic acid cough threshold, sug-gesting that acid-induced cough sensitivity and bronchoconstriction are independently regulated. Acetic acid cough threshold was also unaltered after inhalation of albuterol (29). Acetic acid cough challenge has also been used in pharmacologic studies. Mochizuki et al. (27) reported that furose-mide and amiloride attenuated cough induced by acetic acid inhalation in asthmatic children. Shimizu et al. (30) observed that administration of roxi-thromycin, a semisynthetic macrolide antibiotic, increased the acetic acid cough threshold in asthmatic children. Other examples of pharmacological studies using acid inhalation cough challenge testing are shown in Table 1.

Tartaric Acid

Although by no means the most popular agent in cough challenge testing, tartaric acid has been employed successfully in cough induction for many years. Its use has largely been confined to experimental testing of cough reflex physiology (24–26). Fujimura et al. (24) showed that cough sensitiv-ity to tartaric acid did not correlate with airway responsiveness in healthy or asthmatic subjects. In a study of gender differences, the authors found that healthy nonatopic women had a significantly lower cough threshold

Table 1 Summary of Pharmacologic Studies Involving Acid Inhalation Cough Challenge

Study	Tussigen	Agent tested
Mochizuki et al. (27)	Acetic acid	Furosemide, amiloride
Shimizu et al. (29)	Acetic acid	Albuterol
Shimizu et al. (30)	Acetic acid	Roxithromycin
Fujimura et al. (23)	Tartaric acid	Methacholine
Fujimura et al (78)	Tartaric acid	Mexiletine
Bickerman et al. (16)	Citric acid	Dextromethorphan, nalline
Bickerman et al. (17)	Citric acid	Codeine, narcotine
Calesnick et al. (18)	Citric acid	Codeine
Rees et al. (19)	Citric acid	Codeine, glaucine
Belcher et al. (79)	Citric acid	Pholcodine, albuterol
Morice et al. (80)	Citric acid	Captopril
Poundsford et al. (34)	Citric acid	Albuterol, ipratropium
Dilworth et al. (81)	Citric acid	Opiates
Packman et al. (42)	Citric acid	Diphenhydramine
Morice et al. (40)	Citric acid	Menthol
Grattan et al. (41)	Citric acid	Dextromethorphan
Manap et al. (52)	Citric acid	Dextromethorphan
Di Franco et al. (82)	Citric acid	Beclomethasone

to tartaric acid than men (25). Addington et al. (26) reported that bilateral anesthesia of the superior laryngeal nerve abolished tartaric acid-induced cough and suggested that tartaric acid may be useful to assess the integrity of the laryngeal cough reflex after anesthesia or in patients with neurologic injury at risk of aspiration. There have also been some pharmacologic experiments using the tartaric acid cough challenge. Fujimura et al. (23) showed that methacholine did not affect cough threshold to tartaric acid. More recently, these authors reported that oral mexiletine reduced the cough response to tartaric acid (78).

Citric Acid

Among the acid tussive stimuli, citric acid has acquired the widest application. Citric acid cough challenge has been employed to study the physiology of the cough reflex and to assess the effects of disease on cough reflex sensitivity. Pounsford et al. (83) found that moderate smokers coughed more than nonsmokers, and occasional smokers did not cough at all. Others observed that the cough threshold to citric acid did not differ in smokers with COPD and nonsmoking asthmatics (47). More recently, Wong et al. (45) reported that patients with COPD had a lower citric acid cough threshold compared with healthy controls. In patients with asthma, Di Franco et al. (82) showed that citric acid-induced cough improved after 1 month of therapy with inhaled beclomethasone dipropionate. Although it is clear that COPD, asthma, and cigarette smoking may affect the cough response, the mechanisms underlying these changes are unknown.

Citric acid cough challenge has also been employed to examine the effects of pharmacologic agents. In the earliest description, Bickerman et al. (16,17) studied a number of potential antitussives including codeine, narcotine, Nalline, D-isomethadone, propoxyphene, and dextromethorphan hydrobromide. Codeine, dextromethorphan hydrobromide, and Nalline were all reported to reduce cough significantly compared with placebo (16). Others have confirmed that codeine phosphate can reduce citric acid-induced cough (18,19). However, Rees and Clark (19) found that the antitussive effect of codeine was by no means universal with only a proportion of the subjects showing an increase in cough threshold. Pholcodine has also been reported to suppress citric acid-induced cough in contrast to oral albuterol, which failed to elicit an antitussive effect in healthy volunteers (79). More recently, Packman et al. (42) reported that diphenhydramine reduced citric acid-induced cough sensitivity. Morice et al. (40) studied the effects of inhaled menthol on the citric acid-evoked cough. The authors observed that menthol produced a significant reduction in cough frequency in healthy volunteers. Similarly, Packman and London (84) showed that application of a chest rub, containing a mixture of aromatic oils including menthol, to humans reduced the cough response to citric acid. The antitussive activity of menthol may be related to stimulation of cold receptor nerve ending (85), although there have also been suggestions that menthol exerts its activity by affecting calcium conductance across the sensory neuronal membrane (86).

Although opiates suppress cough, most likely through a central activity, these agents are not devoid of unwanted effects such as sedation. Therefore, there has been a search for antitussive agents that lack such side effects. Dextromethorphan—a centrally acting codeine analog—is an example of one such compound. Dextromethorphan has been shown to reduce citric acid cough response when given orally (41), although significant antitussive effects of oral dextromethorphan were reported only at high doses (52). In contrast, inhaled dextromethorphan does not suppress cough (41). The pharmacokinetics and pharmacodynamics of dextromethorphan have been studied using the citric acid inhalation cough challenge. Using a single-concentration inhalation method, Wright et al. (39) found that dextromethorphan caused a more prolonged inhibition of citric acid-induced cough than its metabolite dextrorphan.

Conclusions

Acid cough challenge testing has unquestionably contributed greatly to our understanding of the cough reflex in health and disease. Important contributions have come from both animal and human models of acid-induced cough. In addition, acid cough challenge testing has played an important role in pharmacologic studies. Unfortunately, some degree of scepticism is required when analyzing the literature on acid cough challenge. Many reports relate to a small number of subjects and the cough challenge methods applied have not always been rigorously validated. The future of acid cough challenge testing will depend on standardization of this type of chemical induction of cough. Decisions are required on whether to abandon acetic and tartaric acid and accept citric acid inhalation as the standard. In addition, agreement is needed on whether in the human model the breath-activated dosimeter-controlled delivery of citric acid should be accepted as the only validated method with consequent cessation of other methods. Standardized guidelines on cough challenge testing, including acid cough challenge, would assist in making these decisions and would greatly benefit the quality of research on induced cough.

References

1. Irwin RS, Boulet LP, Cloutier MM, Fuller R, Gold PM, Hoffstein V, Ing AJ, Mccool FD, O'Byrne P, Poe RH, Prakash UB, Pratter MR, Rubin BK. Managing cough as a defense mechanism and as a symptom. A consensus panel report of the American College of Chest Physicians. Chest 1998; 114: 133S–181S.
2. Loundon RG, Brown LC. Cough frequency in patients with respiratory disease. Am Rev Respir Dis 1967; 96:1137–1143.
3. Di Pede C, Viegi G, Quackenboss JJ, Boyer-Pfersdorf P, Lebowitz MD. Respiratory symptoms and risk factors in an Arizona population sample of Anglo and Mexican-American whites. Chest 1991; 99:916–922.
4. Cullinan P. Persistent cough and sputum: prevalence and clinical characteristics in south east England. Respir Med 1992; 86:143–149.
5. Janson C, Chinn S, Jarvis D, Burney P. Determinants of cough in young adults participating in the European Community Respiratory Health Survey. Eur Respir J 1991; 18:647–654.
6. French CL, Irwin RS, Curley FJ, Krikorian CJ. Impact of chronic cough on quality of life. Arch Intern Med 1998; 158:1657–1661.
7. Thompson R, Kastelik JA, Ojoo JC, et al. Impact of chronic cough on health. Thorax 2001; 56:71iii.
8. French CT, Irwin RS, Fletcher KE, Adams TM. Evaluation of cough-specific quality of life questionnaire. Chest 2002; 121:1123–1131.

9. Birring SS, Prudon B, Carr AJ, Singh SJ, Morgan MD, Pavord ID. Development of a symptom specific health status measure for patients with chronic cough: Leicester Cough Questionnaire (LCQ). Thorax 2003; 58:339–343.

10. Sant'Ambrogio G. Afferent pathways for the cough reflex. Bull Eur Physiopathol Respir 1987; 23(suppl 10):19s–23s.

11. Korpas J, Widdicombe JG. Aspects of the cough reflex. Respir Med 1991; 85(suppl A):3–5.

12. Shannon R, Baekey DM, Morris KF, Lindsey BG. Brainstem respiratory networks and cough. Pulm Pharmacol 1996; 9:343–347.

13. Cass LJ, Frederick WS. Comparative clinical effectiveness of cough medications. Am Pract 1951; 2:844–851.

14. Hoglund NJ, Michaelson M. A method for determining the cough threshold with some preliminary experiments on the effects of codeine. Acta Physiol Scand 1950; 21:168–178.

15. Hillis BR. The assessment of cough-suppressing drugs. Lancet 1952; 1: 1230–1235.

16. Bickerman HA, Barach AL, Itkin S, Drimmer F. Experimental production of cough in human subjects induced by citric acid aerosols. Preliminary studies on the evaluation of antitussive agents. Am J Med Sci 1954; 228:156–163.

17. Bickerman HA, German E, Cohen BM. The cough response of healthy human subjects stimulated by citric acid aerosol. Am J Med Sci 1957; 234:191–205.

18. Calesnick B, Christensen JA. Latency of cough response as a measure of antitussive agents. Clin Pharmacol Ther 1967; 8:374–380.

19. Rees PJ, Clark TJ. Assessment of antitussive effects by citric acid threshold. Br J Dis Chest 1983; 77:94–97.

20. Pounsford JC, Saunders KB. Diurnal variation and adaptation of the cough response to citric acid in normal subjects. Thorax 1985; 40:657–661.

21. Morice AH. Inhalation cough challenge in the investigation of the cough reflex and antitussives. Pulm Pharmacol Ther 1996; 9:281–284.

22. Hutchings HA, Morris S, Eccles R, Jawad MS. Voluntary suppression of cough induced by inhalation of capsaicin in healthy volunteers. Respir Med 1993; 87:379–382.

23. Fujimura M, Sakamoto S, Kamio Y, Matsuda T. Effects of methacholine induced bronchoconstriction and procaterol induced bronchodilation on cough receptor sensitivity to inhaled capsaicin and tartaric acid. Thorax 1992; 47:441–445.

24. Fujimura M, Sakamoto S, Kamio Y, Matsuda T. Cough receptor sensitivity and bronchial responsiveness in normal and asthmatic subjects. Eur Respir J 1992; 5:291–295.

25. Fujimura M, Sakamoto S, Kamio Y, Matsuda T. Sex difference in the inhaled tartaric acid cough threshold in non-atopic healthy subjects. Thorax 1990; 45:633–634.

26. Addington WR, Stephens RE, Goulding RE. Anesthesia for the superior laryngeal nerves and tartaric acid-induced cough. Arch Phys Med Rehabil 1999; 80:1584–1586.

27. Mochizuki H, Shimizu T, Morikawa A, Kuroume T. Inhaled diuretics attenuate acid-induced cough in children with asthma. Chest 1995; 107:413–417.
28. Mochizuki H, Shimizu T, Maeda S, Tokuyama K, Morikawa A, Kuroume T. Relationship between ultrasonically nebulized distilled water-induced bronchoconstriction and acetic acid-induced cough in asthmatic children. J Allergy Clin Immunol 1995; 96:193–199.
29. Shimizu T, Mochizuki H, Tokuyama K, Morikawa A. Relationship between the acid-induced cough response and airway responsiveness and obstruction in children with asthma. Thorax 1996; 51:284–287.
30. Shimizu T, Kato M, Mochizuki H, Takei K, Maeda S, Tokuyama K, Morikawa A. Roxithromycin attenuates acid-induced cough and water-induced bronchoconstriction in children with asthma. J Asthma 1997; 34:211–217.
31. Bates DV, Fish BR, Hatch TF, Mercer TT, Morrow PE. Deposition and retention models for internal dosimetry of the human respiratory tract. Task group on lung dynamics. Health Phys 1966; 12:173–207.
32. Hansson L, Wollmer P, Dahlback M, Karlsson JA. Regional sensitivity of human airways to capsaicin-induced cough. Am Rev Respir Dis 1992; 145: 1191–1195.
33. Barros MJ, Zammattio SJ, Rees PJ. Importance of inspiratory flow rate in the cough response to citric acid inhalation in normal subjects. Clin Sci 1990; 78:521–525.
34. Pounsford JC, Birch MJ, Saunders KB. Effect of bronchodilators on the cough response to inhaled citric acid in normal and asthmatic subjects. Thorax 1985; 40:662–667.
35. Morice AH, Kastelik JA, Thompson R. Cough challenge in the assessment of cough reflex. Br J Clin Pharmacol 2001; 52:365–375.
36. Dennis JH, Avery AJ, Walters EH, Hendrick DJ. Calibration of aerosol output from the Mefar dosimeter: implications for epidemiological studies. Eur Respir J 1992; 5:1279–1282.
37. Chinn S, Arossa WA, Jarvis DL, Luczynska CM, Burney PG. Variation in nebulizer aerosol output and weight output from the Mefar dosimeter: implications for multicentre studies. Eur Respir J 1997; 10:452–456.
38. Thompson R, Wright C, Morice AH. Female gender and enhanced citric acid induced cough response. Thorax 1999; 54:A75.
39. Wright CE, Thompson R, Meller S, Morice AH. Prolonged inhibition of the cough reflex by dextromethorphan: comparison with its metabolite dextrorphan. Thorax 1999; 54:A75.
40. Morice AH, Marshall AE, Higgins KS, Grattan TJ. Effect of inhaled menthol on citric acid induced cough in normal subjects. Thorax 1994; 49:1024–1026.
41. Grattan TJ, Marshall AE, Higgins KS, Morice AH. The effect of inhaled and oral dextromethorphan on citric acid induced cough in man. Br J Clin Pharmacol 1995; 39:261–263.
42. Packman EW, Ciccone PE, Wilson J, Masurat T. Antitussive effects of diphenhydramine on the citric acid aerosol-induced cough response in humans. Int J Clin Pharmacol Ther Toxicol 1991; 29:218–222.
43. Morice AH, Higgins KS, Yeo WW. Adaptation of cough reflex with different types of stimulation. Eur Respir J 1992; 5:841–847.

44. Kastelik JA, Thompson RH, Aziz I, Ojoo JC, Redington AE, Morice AH. Sex-related differences in cough reflex sensitivity in patients with chronic cough. Am J Respir Crit Care Med 2002; 166:961–964.

45. Wong CH, Morice AH. Cough threshold in patients with chronic obstructive pulmonary disease. Thorax 1999; 54:62–64.

46. Godden DJ, Borland C, Lowry R, Higenbottam TW. Chemical specificity of coughing in man. Clin Sci 1986; 70:301–306.

47. Auffarth B, de Monchy JG, van der Mark TW, Postma DS, Koeter GH. Citric acid cough threshold and airway responsiveness in asthmatic patients and smokers with chronic airflow obstruction. Thorax 1991; 46:638–642.

48. Crapo RO, Casaburi R, Coates AL, Enright PL, Hankinson JL, Irvin CG, MacIntyre NR, McKay RT, Wanger JS, Anderson SD, Cockcroft DW, Fish JE, Sterk PJ. Guidelines for methacholine and exercise challenge testing—1999. Am J Respir Crit Care Med 2000; 161:309–329.

49. Hutchings HA, Eccles R, Smith AP, Jawad MS. Voluntary cough suppression as an indication of symptom severity in upper respiratory tract infections. Eur Respir J 1993; 6:1449–1454.

50. Rostami-Hodjegan A, Abdul-Manap R, Wright CE, Tucker GT, Morice AH. The placebo response to citric acid-induced cough: pharmacodynamics and gender differences. Pulm Pharmacol Ther 2001; 14:315–319.

51. Fujimura M, Kasahara K, Kamio Y, Naruse M, Hashimoto T, Matsuda T. Female gender as a determinant of cough threshold to inhaled capsaicin. Eur Respir J 1996; 9:1624–1626.

52. Manap RA, Wright CE, Gregory A, Rostami-Hodjegan A, Meller ST, Kelm GR, Lennard MS, Tucker GT, Morice AH. The antitussive effect of dextromethorphan in relation to CYP2D6 activity. Br J Clin Pharmacol 1999; 48:382–387.

53. Gravenstein JS, Devloo RA, Beecher HK. Effect of antitussive agents on experimental and pathological cough in man. J Appl Physiol 1954; 7:119–139.

54. Morice AH, Higgins KS, Yeo WW. Adaptation to cough reflex with different types of stimulation. Eur Respir J Suppl 1992; 5:841–847.

55. Fox AJ. Modulation of cough and airway sensory fibres. Pulm Pharmacol 1996; 9:335–342.

56. Widdicombe JG. Afferent receptors in the airways and cough. Respir Physiol 1998; 114:5–15.

57. Undem BJ, Carr MJ, Kollarik M. Physiology and plasticity of putative cough fibres in the guinea pig. Pulm Pharmacol Ther 2002; 15:193–198.

58. Wong CH, Matai R, Morice AH. Cough induced by low pH. Respir Med 1999; 93:58–61.

59. Karlsson JA. The role of capsaicin-sensitive C-fibre afferent nerves in the cough reflex. Pulm Pharmacol 1996; 9:315–321.

60. Bevan S, Geppetti P. Protons: small stimulants of capsaicin-sensitive sensory nerves. Trends Neurosci 1994; 17:509–512.

61. Jordt SE, Tominaga M, Julius D. Acid potentiation of the capsaicin receptor determined by a key extracellular site. Proc Natl Acad Sci USA 2000; 97:8134–8139.

62. Lalloo UG, Fox AJ, Belvisi MG, Chung KF, Barnes PJ. Capsazepine inhibits cough induced by capsaicin and citric acid but not by hypertonic saline in guinea pigs. J Appl Physiol 1995; 79:1082–1087.
63. Forsberg K, Karlsson JA, Theodorsson E, Lundberg JM, Persson CG. Cough and bronchoconstriction mediated by capsaicin-sensitive sensory neurons in the guinea-pig. Pulm Pharmacol 1988; 1:33–39.
64. Midgren B, Hansson L, Karlsson JA, Simonsson BG, Persson CGA. Capsaicin-induced cough in humans. Am Rev Respir Dis 1992; 146:347–351.
65. Jatakanon A, Lalloo UG, Lim S, Chung KF, Barnes PJ. Increased neutrophils and cytokines, TNF-alpha and IL-8, in induced sputum of non-asthmatic patients with chronic dry cough. Thorax 1999; 54:234–237.
66. Boulet LP, Milot J, Boutet M, St Georges F, Laviolette M. Airway inflammation in nonasthmatic subjects with chronic cough. Am J Respir Crit Care Med 1994; 149:482–489.
67. McGarvey LPA, Forsythe P, Heaney LG, MacMahon J, Ennis M. Bronchoalveolar lavage findings in patients with chronic nonproductive cough. Eur Respir J 1999; 13:59–65.
68. Ricciardolo FL, Rado V, Fabbri LM, Sterk PJ, Di Maria GU, Geppetti P. Bronchoconstriction induced by citric acid inhalation in guinea pigs: role of tachykinins, bradykinin, and nitric oxide. Am J Respir Crit Care Med 1999; 159:557–562.
69. Fox AJ, Barnes PJ, Urban L, Dray A. An in vitro study of the properties of single vagal afferents innervating guinea-pig airways. J Physiol 1993; 469: 21–35.
70. Belvisi MG, Bolser DC. Summary: animal models for cough. Pulm Pharmacol Ther 2002; 15:249–250.
71. Laude EA, Higgins KS, Morice AH. A comparative study of the effects of citric acid, capsaicin and resiniferatoxin on the cough challenge in guinea-pig and man. Pulm Pharmacol 1993; 6:171–175.
72. Widdicombe JG. Neurophysiology of the cough reflex. Eur Respir J 1995; 8:1193–1202.
73. Girard V, Naline E, Vilain P, EmondsAlt X, Advenier C. Effect of the two tachykinin antagonists, SR 48968 and SR 140333, on cough induced by citric acid in the unanaesthetized guinea-pig. Eur Respir J 1995; 8:1110–1114.
74. Hay DW, Giardina GA, Griswold DE, Underwood DC, Kotzer CJ, Bush B, Potts W, Sandhu P, Lundberg D, Foley JJ, Schmidt DB, Martin LD, Kilian D, Legos JJ, Barone FC, Luttmann MA, Grugni M, Raveglia LF, Sarau HM. Nonpeptide tachykinin receptor antagonists. III. SB 235375, a low central nervous system-penetrant, potent and selective neurokinin-3 receptor antagonist, inhibits citric acid-induced cough and airways hyper-reactivity in guinea pigs. J Pharm Exp Ther 2002; 300:314–323.
75. Moreaux B, Nemmar A, Vincke G, Halloy D, Beerens D, Advenier C, Gustin P. Role of substance P and tachykinin receptor antagonists in citric acid-induced cough in pigs. Eur J Pharmacol 2000; 408:305–312.
76. Laude EA, Bee D, Crambes O, Howard P. Antitussive and antibronchoconstriction actions of fenspiride in guinea-pigs. Eur Respir J 1995; 8:1699–1704.

77. Laude EA, Morice AH, Grattan TJ. The antitussive effects of menthol, camphor and cineole in conscious guinea-pigs. Pulm Pharmacol 1994; 7:179–184.
78. Fujimura M, Kamio Y, Myou S, Hashimoto T. Effect of oral mexiletine on the cough response to capsaicin and tartaric acid. Thorax 2000; 55:126–128.
79. Belcher N, Rees PJ. Effects of pholcodine and salbutamol on citric acid induced cough in normal subjects. Thorax 1986; 41:74–75.
80. Morice AH, Lowry R, Brown MJ, Higenbottam T. Angiotensin converting enzyme and the cough reflex. Lancet 1987; ii:1116–1118.
81. Dilworth JP, Pounsford JC, White RJ. Cough threshold after upper abdominal surgery. Thorax 1990; 45:207–209.
82. Di Franco A, Dente FL, Giannini D, Vagaggini B, Conti I, Macchioni P, Scuotri L, Taccola M, Bacci E, Paggiaro PL. Effects of inhaled corticosteroids on cough threshold in patients with bronchial asthma. Pulm Pharmacol Ther 2001; 14:35–40.
83. Pounsford JC, Saunders KB. Cough response to citric acid aerosol in occasional smokers. Br Med J Clin Res 1986; 293:1528.
84. Packman EW, London SJ. The utility of artificially induced cough as a clinical model for evaluating the antitussive effects of aromatics delivered by inunction. Eur Respir J Suppl 1980; 110:101–109.
85. Hensel H, Zotterman Y. The effect of menthol on the thermal receptors. Acta Physiol Scand 1951; 24:27–34.
86. Swandulla D, Carbone E, Schafer K, Lux HD. Effect of menthol on 2 types of Ca currents in cultured sensory neurones of vertebrates. Eur J Physiol 1987; 409:52–59.

11

Water Aerosols and Cough

GIOVANNI A. FONTANA, FEDERICO LAVORINI, and
MASSIMO PISTOLESI

Dipartimento di Area Critica Medico Chirurgica,
    Università di Firenze,
Firenze, Italy

Introduction

The observation that exposure to natural fog has an impact on airway function was first reported by De Vries et al. in 1964 (1). Subsequently in 1968, two papers published in the United Kingdom (2) and the United States (3) described the use of ultrasonically nebulized distilled water as an experimental means to induce bronchoconstriction in patients with hyperreactive airways. Interestingly, Cheney and Butler (3) also observed in their experiments that "severe coughing occurred in both normal subjects and patients when distilled water was inhaled from the ultrasonic nebulizer," and that "inhalation of normal saline from the ultrasonic nebulizer did not produce coughing in either group." Thereafter, the use of ultrasonically distilled water, also termed "fog," as a provocative agent in bronchial challenges spread rapidly. Allegra and Bianco (4) were the first to propose the clinical use of fog challenge to detect bronchial hyperresponsiveness in asthma and the method was subsequently standardized by Shoeffel et al. (5). However, it was principally bronchoconstriction rather than cough that was of interest to most investigators. Thus, although there is an extensive literature on the evaluation of the bronchoconstrictor response provoked by inhalation of water solutions, relatively little attention has been devoted to the cough response evoked by such solutions.

The purpose of this chapter is to review the principal experimental and clinical aspects of coughing evoked by inhalation or topical administration of water solutions with different osmolarities and ion contents. An attempt will also be made to describe the main features of inhalation cough challenges performed using water solutions in humans.

Physiology of Cough

Coughing can be regarded as a modified respiratory act generated by the same neuronal network subserving normal ventilation (6). Independently of the nature of the sensory stimulus, the act of coughing is initiated after the respiratory neurons implicated in the genesis of the cough motor pattern have received specific stimuli of sufficient intensity. Whilst normal breathing is suspended, an inhalation is followed by a forced expiration against an initially closed glottis which then opens facilitating the explosive exhalation (7). An analysis of the complex cough motor mechanisms is beyond the scope of this chapter, and detailed descriptions of the mechanical events of cough can be found in the literature (7).

Coughing can most readily be provoked by mechanical or chemical stimuli applied to the epithelium of the larynx, trachea, or carina of the main bronchi. Intraepithelial vagal sensory receptors in these sites are located within the paracellular spaces between the epithelial cells (8). Such receptors have been shown to be extremely sensitive to both mechanical and chemical stimuli, and signals travelling in the vagal fibers innervating these receptors can readily be detected after appropriate receptor stimulation (8).

An interesting aspect of airway physiology, supported by many experimental data, is the impact that the composition of the airway surface liquid (ASL) has on various functions, such as the motility of the cilia, mucus transport, receptor activity, and ultimately, reflex responses (9,10). The cough provoked by inhalation or topical administration of water solutions may thus represent a mechanism to protect the respiratory system when harmful alterations in the ionic composition of the ASL and/or the airway epithelium are likely to occur.

Airway Surface Liquid

The ASL is a thin layer of fluid covering the airways that provides an ideal environment in rheologic terms for the capture of foreign substances, viruses, and bacteria and plays a crucial role in airway host defence by maintaining efficient mucociliary clearance to remove entrapped substances (10).

The ASL consists of a layer 15–30 μm thick with a [Cl⁻] of approximately 80 mM (11). Active secretory and absorptive mechanisms that move fluids and electrolytes across the airway epithelium play a critical role in controlling the composition and volume of the ASL (12). Humidity in the inspired air causes a fall in [Na⁺] and [Cl⁻] together with a fall in osmolarity (13) and inhalation of distilled water or other low-chloride aerosols may be expected to reduce [Cl⁻] further (14).

The Airway Epithelium

The airway epithelium has two different cell membranes: the apical membrane, which faces the airway lumen, and the basolateral membrane, which faces the interstitial side of the epithelium (Fig. 1). These two membranes are separated by tight junctions that encircle the cell and serve as a barrier to the movement of solutes and water across the epithelial sheet. The two membranes have different morphologic and functional characteristics (15,16). The apical membrane is characterized by microvilli and cilia and contains specific transport channels for Na⁺ and Cl⁻. The basolateral membrane is characterized by gap junctions and interdigitated lateral intercellular space, is K⁺ selective, and contains two specific ion transport proteins,

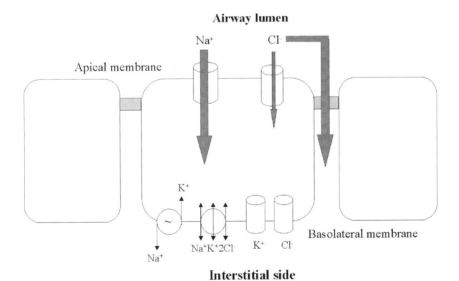

Figure 1 Schematic representation of the airway epithelium structure and the net direction and routes for transepithelial Cl⁻, Na⁺, and K⁺ transport. Shaded blocks represent tight junctions between cells. Ion channels are depicted as cylinders, the Na⁺–K⁺-ATPase pump as a circle with "~" inside, and the Na⁺–K⁺-2Cl⁻ cotransporter as a circle with arrows. See text for further details.

the Na^+–K^+-ATPase pump and the Na^+–K^+-$2Cl^-$ cotransporter (Fig. 1). The localization of these specific ion channels to one or other of the two membranes allows ion transport through the airway epithelium (the cellular pathway). Since the tight junctions have selective permeability to ions, these may also cross the epithelium through the tight junction area between the cells (the paracellular pathway). The net balance between ion transport from one side of the epithelium to the other side controls the movement of fluid by the development of an osmotic gradient (15,16).

In basal conditions, the dominant ion transport process in airway epithelial cells is Na^+ absorption from the lumen into the cell (Fig. 1), whereas Cl^- movement follows Na^+ passively, mainly via the paracellular route or via specific apical channels, to maintain electroneutrality (15,16). Absorption of Na^+ creates an osmotic gradient locally across the epithelium, which results in water absorption. As mentioned earlier, directional transport of ions across the airway epithelium requires the presence of specific transport channels in the apical and basolateral membranes. The Na^+–K^+-ATPase pump maintains intracellular $[Na^+]$ at a low level, thus generating a favorable electrochemical gradient for Na^+ entry into the cell via apically located Na^+ channels. The combination in series of the apical membrane Na^+ channel and the basolateral Na^+–K^+-ATPase pump provides the route for Na^+ absorption via the cellular pathways (Fig. 1). The Na^+–K^+-ATPase pump also raises intracellular $[K^+]$, thus allowing K^+ recycling via a specific basolateral K^+ channel (Fig. 1). The ionic gradients generated by the Na^+–K^+-ATPase pump allows Cl^- to be accumulated above electrochemical equilibrium across the basolateral membrane. The entry of Cl^- into the cell across the basolateral membrane is likely performed by the Na^+–K^+-$2Cl^-$ cotransporter, although other molecular mechanisms, such as Na^+–H^+ or Cl^-–HCO_3^- exchangers, have been proposed (12).

In physiological conditions, Cl^- ion secretion is negligible in human airway epithelium, since Cl^- ions are in electrochemical equilibrium across the apical cell membrane (12). However, active Cl^- secretion can be experimentally induced. For instance, pharmacological blockade of the apical membrane Na^+ channels causes a Cl^- rise above its electrochemical equilibrium across the apical membrane, and transcellular Cl^- secretion into the airway lumen, via the specific apically located Cl^- channel, can occur (12). Because Cl^- is a negatively charged ion, luminal secretion of this ion increases lumen negativity, drawing Na^+ across the tight junction area between the cells. The increase in osmolarity of the airway lumen resulting from the ion secretion provides the driving force for water transport into the lumen. In addition, a specific basolateral Cl^- channel, distinct from those expressed at the apical membrane, has been detected in human airway epithelial cells (12).

Studies aimed at evaluating the response of the airway epithelium to hypertonic solutions have shown that epithelial cell sheets are sensitive to increasing concentrations of solutes on the luminal, but not the interstitial, surface (15). The initial response of the airway epithelium exposed to a hypertonic solution is movement of water from the cells to the airway lumen via the cellular pathway, thus buffering the hypertonicity of the luminal compartment. This compensatory response leads to a rapid reduction in epithelial cell volume (cell shrinkage) and creates a hyperosmolar environment in both the epithelial cells and the submucosa (15). Exposure of the epithelial cells to hypertonic solutions causes a decrease in Na^+ absorption due to the increase in intracellular $[Na^+]$ consequent to cell shrinkage. Furthermore, no net Cl^- movement is observed, since hyperosmolarity of the epithelial surface reduces the permeability of the paracellular pathway and the apically located Cl^- channels (17). This finding seems to suggest that the physiologic epithelial response to hypertonic solutions does not involve Cl^- current.

When airway epithelial cells are exposed to a hypotonic solution, water moves from the airway lumen into the cell, thus leading to a rapid increase in epithelial cell volume (cell swelling). It has been shown that a reduction of extracellular osmolarity may stimulate transepithelial Cl^- secretion through the apically located Cl^- channels, thus suggesting that, at variance with hypertonic solution, exposure to hypotonic solutions stimulates Cl^- current (18).

Stimulation of "Cough Receptors" by Nonisosmolar or Low-Chloride Solutions

It is believed that any nonisosmolar solution, either inhaled or directly applied onto the airway luminal surface or injected into the blood supply to the nerve endings, has the potential to evoke reflex responses because of its effects on the physiology of the airway surface liquid and, hence, on the morphology of the airway epithelium and/or the membrane of the airway sensory nerves. Water-sensitive airway nerves are, for the most part, mechanosensitive endings. Thus, it seems plausible that the response to water and nonisosmotic solutions is simply a response to mechanical deformation of the epithelium (cell shrinkage or swelling) or the neural membrane. Patch–clamp studies have demonstrated opening of mechanosensitive ion channels in various cell types, including nerve membranes, in response to small deviations from isosmolarity (19). Furthermore, hyperosmotic solutions may cause the release of autacoids, such as histamine and prostaglandins, that are known to stimulate airway sensory nerves (20). Non-neurally mediated mechanisms involving release of mediators from osmolarity-sensitive cells of the immune system or release of neuropetides from the terminals of airway sensory nerves may also be implicated (21).

The mechanism of airway receptor stimulation by low [Cl$^-$] in the ASL or interstitial fluid remains poorly defined. It has been suggested that receptor membranes have specific Cl$^-$ binding sites that may need to be occupied to stabilize the nerve (22). Removal of Cl$^-$ might increase the conductance to other ions, notably Na$^+$, with subsequent depolarization and generation of an action potential (22). Indeed, at the laryngeal epithelial level, blocking of the Na$^+$ channels has been shown to reduce responsiveness of a subgroup of water-sensitive endings (23). More simply, it may be that, similarly to other excitable tissues (24), the [Cl$^-$] inside the nerve falls proportionately with decreases in [Cl$^-$] of the surrounding solution. This would result in nerve depolarization with a mechanism similar to that observed in skeletal muscle fibers (25).

The sensory endings involved in the mediation of cough are exclusively vagal in origin. Although cough may thus originate from any vagally innervated territory, the mediation of coughing induced by inhaled tussigenic agents exclusively involves laryngeal and tracheobronchial receptors. The neurophysiology of these receptors has been extensively reviewed (8,26).

Laryngeal Receptors

Receptor Sensitivity

The afferent supply to the larynx is provided mainly by the superior laryngeal nerve (SLN) and, to a minor extent, by the recurrent laryngeal nerve. Several respiratory and airway protective reflexes originate from the larynx and single-fiber recordings from the peripheral cut end of the SLN have been used to characterize receptors likely involved in the mediation of these responses (27). Stimuli such as airflow, transmural pressure, and respiratory movements activate respiratory-modulated endings, whereas others remain silent or display a tonic or random activity during breathing and are termed non-respiratory-modulated receptors (28). The latter are responsive to a variety of irritant and chemical stimuli and are presumed to mediate protective reflexes such as coughing (22,29). These receptors include "irritant" receptors that share similarities with those of the lower airway: they are rapidly adapting and have myelinated fibers. The internal branch of the SLN has a relatively low number of unmyelinated C-fibers (30). The laryngeal "irritant" receptors are normally silent, but respond promptly to a wide range of chemical and mechanical irritants, including distilled water (26,31). With respect to their sensitivity to water solutions, two distinct receptor types have been described and characterized (29). A short latency, short duration discharge, which is dependent on the lack of chloride anions, is probably associated with the activation of the irritant-type receptors; a long latency, long duration response depends on the hyposmolarity of the solution and appears to be mediated by respiration-modulated units

(29).Water-sensitive receptors can also be activated by solutions with a high potassium concentration (22), as well as by strongly acid or alkaline solutions, even when their chloride content is the same as that of plasma (22). The C-fiber receptors are activated by several irritants, particularly capsaicin, and by cooling of the laryngeal lumen (32).

Reflex Responses

Water-induced laryngeal reflex responses have been shown to vary considerably with maturation of the central nervous system. Harding et al. (33) demonstrated that instillation of water into the larynx of the newborn lamb causes startle, arousal, swallowing, apnea, bradycardia, hypertension, and peripheral vasoconstriction. These responses, which are believed to protect the laryngeal airway from liquid aspiration, have been termed the laryngeal chemoreflex (LCR). Similar reflex responses have subsequently been described in other neonatal species (22). Small water boluses instilled in the larynx of human infants were shown to cause prolonged apnea, swallowing and bradycardia (e.g., 34). As the infant matures, swallowing and apnea become less prominent, whereas cough and, possibly, laryngeal closure become more pronounced (35). These maturational changes appear to be related to central neural processing of afferent stimuli rather than reduced sensitivity or altered receptor distribution in the larynx (35).

In awake human adults, the responses evoked by inhalation of aerosolized distilled water or water instillation into the laryngeal lumen have been studied less extensively. Nishino et al. (36) showed that stimulation of the laryngeal mucosa with a small amount of distilled water mainly caused short-lasting responses such as expiration reflex, coughing, and swallowing; other types of reflexes were infrequently observed. In contrast, during light anesthesia, the same stimulus generally caused more sustained but less marked responses. By further increasing the depth of anesthesia, coughing, and the expiration reflex were usually replaced by apnea and laryngeal closure. These findings seem to indicate that both the type and magnitude of the response are influenced by the state of the central nervous system. In another study performed in servoflourane-anesthetized female subjects, Nishino et al. (37) observed that laryngeal water instillation through a laryngeal mask airway evoked coughing, expiration reflex, apnea, and rapid shallow breathing. In these experiments, the incidence of coughing and expiration reflex was unaffected by changing the depth of anesthesia (37). Similar results were obtained by Tagaito et al. (38) in a group of propofol-anesthetized females. These authors also observed that coughing and expiration reflex, but not apnea and laryngospasm, induced by spraying the vocal cord with distilled water, were markedly depressed when propofol-induced anesthesia was supplemented by administration of the opioid agonist fentanyl (38). In heart–lung transplantation patients, coughing provoked by laryngeal water instillation through a bronchoscope could still be evoked in all patients tested, whereas coughing induced by fog inhalation was strikingly reduced (39). Thus, it may be that the larynx is not adequately targeted by fog inhalation (39) and that only direct water instillation onto the laryngeal mucosa represents a stimulus of sufficient intensity to stimulate coughing. This possibility is indirectly supported by the finding that patients breathing through a tracheostomy have cough threshold values to fog inhalation similar to those of control subjects (40).

Tracheobronchial Receptors

Receptor Sensitivity

Of the five main groups (26) of sensory terminals in the airway, the rapidly adapting "irritant" receptors (RARs) with myelinated (Aδ) fibers and the unmyelinated pulmonary and bronchial sensory endings of vagal C-fibers are the most likely candidates for cough receptors (8,20,26). The slowly adapting "stretch" receptors, although known to have a permissive role in cough, do not appear to have chemical sensitivity (26). The sensitivity of tracheobronchial receptors to water solutions seems to vary with the receptor location within the respiratory tract and the location of sensory neurons at the ganglionic level. In experiments aimed at examining the responses of single vagal afferents innervating the isolated guinea pig trachea, application of water or hypertonic saline onto identified receptive fields of the trachea stimulated all of the Aδ- and C-fibers, whilst application of isotonic glucose, a chloride-free solution, stimulated about 70% of the C-fibers and 40% of the Aδ-fibers (41). In dogs, however, only one-third of tracheal RARs appear to be stimulated by water (42). Riccio et al. (43) and Pedersen et al. (44) confirmed that both Aδ- and C-fibers innervating the isolated guinea pig trachea and main stem bronchus are excited by solutions of hypertonic saline. These authors also showed that afferent fiber sensitivity in the guinea pig airway is not homogeneous, so that fibers originating from neurons located in jugular ganglia are much more sensitive to hypertonic saline compared with afferent neurons with cell bodies located in the nodose ganglia (44). Injections of water, hyperosmolar solutions or isosmotic glucose in the dog's lobar bronchus revealed that both the RARs and the sensory terminals of airway C-fibers are sensitive to deviation from isosmolarity, and that none of the RARs tested displayed any consistent response to stimulation by isosmotic glucose solutions (45,46). Previous studies (47) described separate populations of RARs sensitive to either water alone or water and low-chloride solutions. In dogs, the proportion of each receptor type seems to vary down the airway such that several water-sensitive RARs in the larynx are also stimulated by low-chloride solutions (22,29,48), whereas only a minority of tracheal RARs (42) and none of pulmonary RARs (45) are sensitive to both stimuli. Thus, it would appear that true osmotic sensitivity is graded down the airway from the larynx to the intrapulmonary bronchi and that sensitivity to deviations from isosmolarity is particularly prominent at the level of the lower airway. As for the C-fiber receptors, they also appear to be non-homogeneous with respect to their sensitivity to water solutions. In the isolated guinea pig trachea, the majority of water-sensitive C-fiber endings were also stimulated by a low-chloride solution, and only a minority of them (about 30%) by water alone (41). This finding points to the possibility that the stimulatory effect of water on the majority of C-fiber endings can be ascribed to the lack of a permeant anion.

Reflex Responses

At variance with humans (see following text), the airway reflex responses evoked by inhalation or tracheobronchial administration of nonisosmolar and/or chloride-deficient solutions in experimental animals have been less extensively investigated, despite the fact that models for such studies have been made available (46,49–51). In anesthetized dogs, Sullivan et al. (49) studied waking, ventilatory, and reflex tracheal smooth muscle responses to tracheobronchial irritation produced by squirting 0.1–1.0 mL of water into the lower trachea. Airway stimulation generally caused arousal from slow-wave sleep but not from rapid-eye-movement sleep. During wakefulness, water administration caused coughing and tracheal smooth muscle constriction. However, during slow-wave or rapid-eye-movement sleep, these responses occurred only if the stimulus first produced arousal. Thus, cough and airway smooth muscle constriction in response to tracheal irritant stimuli do not occur in the absence of arousal, and arousal responses to such stimuli are depressed in rapid-eye-movement sleep. More peripheral (lobar bronchus) injections of water or hypertonic saline in the anesthetized dog have been shown to cause cardiac depression and apnea, usually followed by rapid shallow breathing, which were consistently associated with tracheal smooth muscle contraction. Furthermore, the amplitude of these reflex responses was shown to vary with the deviation from isosmolarity of the injected solution (46). Additional reflex responses that can be observed in different animal species following injection of nonisosomolar solutions into the airways are represented by changes in local blood flow and ventilation. Tracheal (52) and bronchial (21) instillation of hypertonic solution causes vasodilatation, whereas injection of hyposmotic solutions provokes the opposite effect (52). The participation of the tracheobronchial vasculature in the defence airway responses evoked by nonisosmolar stimuli is of interest since bronchial hyperemia may contribute to airway narrowing in asthma (53). In rabbits, hypertonic saline injected directly into the lung caused small but consistent increases in both the amplitude and frequency of integrated phrenic activity (54). The magnitude of the ventilatory adjustments was positively related to the concentration of injected NaCl and abolished by vagotomy. Increases in minute ventilation and respiratory drive have also been observed in humans during inhalation of tussigenic fog concentrations (55). Thus, it may be speculated that deviation from isosmolarity, rather than hyperosmolarity, represents the actual stimulus to hyperventilation.

Although it has long been known that fog inhalation represents a potent stimulus for cough in normal subjects and for both cough and bronchoconstriction in patients with airway diseases (e.g., 3), the first study aimed at establishing a relationship between cough and bronchoconstriction caused by inhalation of fog in asthmatic patients was carried out by Sheppard et al. in 1984 (56). The authors performed parallel measurements of changes in airway resistance and cough sensitivity during inhalation of serially increasing volumes of fog or normal saline aerosols produced by an ultrasonic nebulizer. Fog inhalation induced cough and bronchoconstriction in virtually all patients tested, whereas saline aerosol did not induce cough and caused only weak changes in airway tone. Subsequently, Eschenbacher et al. (57) demonstrated that the bronchoconstrictor and tussigenic effects of fog can be attributed to two different properties of water, namely hyposmolarity and lack of permeant anions. The authors made clear that inhalation of hyposmolar fluids is a potent stimulus to bronchoconstriction in asthma patients, and that the absence of a permeant anion in an isosmolar aerosol almost selectively stimulates coughing (57). It was also observed that inhalation of hyperosmolar fluids with normal or increased chloride ion concentrations caused cough and bronchoconstriction in asthmatic patients (57), suggesting that hyperosmolarity represents an effective tussigenic stimulus. Subsequent experiments (58,59) confirmed previous observations (3) that normal subjects also cough in response to inhalation of low-chloride solutions, and demonstrated that the magnitude of the evoked cough response, when assessed in terms of cough frequency, is related to the [Cl^-] of the inhaled fluid. In a recent human study (55), inhalation of tussigenic fog concentrations also caused significant increases in minute ventilation and respiratory drive that were accounted for by selective increases in the volume component of the breathing pattern. Since, at variance with asthmatics, normal subjects do not bronchoconstrict in response to fog inhalation (60), the ventilatory changes evoked by fog inhalation do not represent a response to an increase in mechanical load and seem to reflect a link between mechanisms mediating cough and those subserving the control of breathing. In this context, it seems worth recalling that, in normal subjects, susceptibility to the tussigenic effect of hypotonic aerosols is related to the intensity of the ventilatory response to CO_2 rebreathing (61).

Modulation of Coughing Induced by Water Solutions

Several agents of different chemical nature have been assessed for their ability to modulate airway receptor activation or reflex responses evoked by water solutions, in both humans and animal experiments. These agents include bronchodilators (β_2-adrenergic and anticholinergic drugs), antihistamines, cromones, local anesthetics, and diuretics. Lowry et al. (62) demonstrated that prior aerosol administration of both fenoterol and ipratropium bromide significantly reduced the cough response, assessed in terms of cough frequency, provoked by inhalation of low-chloride solutions in normal subjects. It was also found that the magnitude of cough inhibition correlated with the accompanying small but significant degree of bronchodilation (62), and that oral administration of salbutamol and pirenzepine hydrochloride (a drug chemically related to ipratropium) had smaller effects. Similar outcomes were obtained when subjects were premedicated with the anticholinergic drug oxitripium or with a combination of oxitropium plus fenoterol (63). Of note, previous studies indicated that both aerosolized atropine (56) and the β_2-adrenergic drug metaproterenol (57) were ineffective in preventing fog-induced cough in asthmatics, whereas both drugs markedly reduced the bronchoconstrictor response evoked by fog inhalation (57). Conversely, in these experiments, aerosolized lidocaine consistently prevented coughing but not the bronchoconstrictor response provoked by fog inhalation (57). In subsequent studies, aerosol administration of oxitropium bromide failed to significantly reduce fog-induced coughing in patients with respiratory infections (64). Taken together, these results suggest that β_2-adrenergic agents may not represent a homogeneous class of drugs with respect to their actions on the cough reflex, and that the administration route for both β_2-stimulants and anticholinergic agents is of importance in determining their antitussive properties. In addition, the fact that cough and bronchoconstriction can be independently inhibited (57) strongly suggests that these responses involve separate neural pathways (65).

The protective effects of cromolyn and sodium nedocromil, two widely used mast cell stabilizing agents, have been evaluated in two separate studies (55,57). Whilst cromolyn proved to be ineffective in modulating cough sensitivity to fog in asthmatic patients, prior administration of nedocromil in normal subjects was found to induce slight but significant increases in cough threshold and to virtually abolish the ventilatory adjustments evoked by fog inhalation (55).

In normal subjects, Stone et al. (66) demonstrated that coughing response induced by inhalation of a chloride-deficient solution is reduced during infusion of 5-hydroxytryptamine, or its precursor 5-hydroxytryptophan, suggesting a serotoninergic influence on the cough reflex at either the peripheral or central level. In recent years, premedication with oral loratidine was shown to reduce cough frequency during 1-min exposures to fog in patients with chronic cough but not in normal subjects (67).

Pharmacological studies involving the use of diuretics such as furosemide, an agent that inhibits Na^+/Cl^- cotransporter at the level of the ascending loop of Henle, and acetazolamide, a selective inhibitor of carbonic anhydrase, have provided insights into the mechanisms of coughing induced by water solutions. Following the observations that, in asthmatic patients, inhaled furosemide inhibits the bronchoconstriction induced by allergen, exercise, fog, and metabisulfite (68), Ventresca et al. (68) investigated the effects of inhaled furosemide on the cough response evoked by 1-min challenges with isosmolar solutions containing decreasing chloride concentrations ranging from 150 to 0 mM or capsaicin. The tussigenic effect of all water solutions tested were partially but significantly inhibited by prior inhalation of furosemide, whereas capsaicin-induced cough was unaffected (68). The authors concluded that furosemide may act indirectly by preventing local ionic changes in the vicinity of the "cough receptor." The possibility that furosemide could also act as a local anesthetic was ruled out by the lack of effect on capsaicin-induced cough (68). In similar experimental conditions, Foresi et al. (69) demonstrated a stronger protective effect of inhaled acetazolamide, compared with that of furosemide, in a group of normal subjects. It is possible that the protective activity of furosemide and acetazolamide may take place at both the epithelial and receptor membrane level. In facts, both epithelial cells and airway receptor membranes are able to modulate ion gradients by means of ion transport mechanisms that include the Na^+/Cl^- cotransporter and the bicarbonate exchanger, respectively inhibited by furosemide and acetazolamide, controlling both cell volume and resting membrane potential (12). In addition, in isolated guinea pig airways, furosemide has been shown to selectively reduce the response of $A\delta$-fibers to low-chloride solutions, but not water and hyperosmolar solutions (41). This finding would suggest that, at least in this animal model, furosemide partially but specifically blocks the mechanisms implicated in receptor activation by low-chloride solutions.

Cough Challenges with Water Aerosols in the Clinical Setting

Cough inhalation challenge with aerosolized water solutions represents a safe and reliable procedure to evaluate the sensitivity of the cough reflex, to investigate cough motor mechanisms and, as outlined above, to assess the effectiveness of antitussive treatments. In general, cough challenges with aqueous solutions share methodological similarities to those aimed at evaluating bronchial hyperresponsiveness. In the latter case, however, standardized guidelines (70) can be applied, whereas no universal standards for cough challenges are available as yet. Thus, the procedures tend to be laboratory specific and comparisons between study outcomes are difficult. In particular, fluids with different osmolarities and ion contents have been used for cough provocation and different methods have been devised for aerosol delivery and assessment of the evoked cough response (Table 1).

The common feature to all cough inhalation challenges with aqueous solutions is delivery of the tussigenic agent to the sensitive areas of the airways by means of a nebulizer producing sufficient amounts of aerosol to stimulate airway receptors. The use of an ultrasonic nebulizer is mandatory due to its unique ability to produce dense aerosols with droplet sizes within the respirable range. Most ultrasonic nebulizers have a variable power output (74) that determines the density of the aerosol produced. The mass median aerodynamic diameter of aerosol particles generated by different makes of ultrasonic nebulizers has been reported to vary from 4.0 to 7.1 μm (74).

Several different types of water solutions have been used in cough challenges (Table 1), but fog is by far the stimulus most commonly employed. It should be noted, however, that a percentage (15–20%) of subjects do not cough even if exposed to the highest attainable fog output (71), while the same subjects do cough if challenged with other tussigenic stimuli such as capsaicin and citric acid aerosols (authors' unpublished observations). Hyperosmolar saline and water solutions with variable ion content have also been used in studies aimed at assessing the tussigenic effects of either graded increases in osmolarity (59) or decreases in permeant anion content (57).

At variance with stimuli such as capsaicin or citric acid, the conventional method for inhalation of water aerosols is resting tidal breathing. The simplest procedure is the single-concentration inhalation challenge, in which multiple inhalations of a single concentration of the stimulant, usually, but not necessarily (57), corresponding to the maximum attainable

Table 1 Most Frequently Used Types of Water Solutions and Response Assessment Methods

Type of stimulus	Measure of cough sensitivity	References
One-min fog exposure (maximum output)	Cough frequency	(39,62–64,66,67)
Fog with step increases in output	Cough threshold	(40,55,57,71–73)
Variable osmolarity	Cough threshold	(61)
Isosmolar solutions with variable ion content	Cough frequency	(58,62,63,66,69)
	Cough threshold	(57)

output of the nebulizer, are performed. Cough challenges with water aerosols, besides being very effective in provoking cough in the majority of subjects, have additional advantages with respect to other techniques. For instance, at least in the authors' experience, they are particularly well accepted by both normal subjects and patients. In addition, since water aerosols are inhaled during resting tidal breathing, they may be suitable for evaluating the ventilatory adjustments brought about by inhalation of these tussigenic agents (55). In common with other tussigenic agents, cough induced by fog inhalation is subject to a considerable degree of adaptation, so that the number of cough efforts tends to diminish toward the end of the inhalation period (75). Of note, some lines of evidence indicate that cough susceptibility to fog is in part genetically determined (14).

Assessment of Cough

Cough Sensitivity

The most convenient method for assessing cough sensitivity to inhalation of water solutions, as well as any other tussigenic agent, is the measurement of cough threshold. This can be defined as the lowest concentration of an agent reproducibly causing at least one cough effort (71) or a predetermined number of expiratory thrusts (57). The short- and long-term repeatability of cough threshold values in human fog challenges has recently been demonstrated (72).

Cough Response

In most challenges, including those with water solutions, the cough response is assessed in terms of cough frequency (Table 1). Although measurement of this variable has the undeniable advantage of being inexpensive and relatively easy to assess, it is unclear whether it reflects cough sensitivity, the intensity of the evoked motor response, or both. Furthermore, the reproducibility of cough threshold measurements has been shown to be subject to experimental conditions. Trials specifically designed to evaluate the reproducibility of cough frequency during fog challenges demonstrated a low degree of repeatability in response to stimuli of threshold intensity (72). Conversely, for stimuli of suprathreshold intensity, cough frequency measurements displayed a higher degree of repeatability (72).

The intensity of cough can adequately be quantified by recording cough expiratory flow [see (40) for references]. The airflow generated by a subject during voluntary and reflex cough efforts can easily be recorded by means of a large-size pneumotachograph. Several variables that may be important for assessing the intensity of a cough effort can be measured or calculated from a cough flow tracing. These include the cough peak flow, the time that elapses from the onset of flow to peak flow, i.e., the so-called time to peak, and volume acceleration, which is the ratio of cough peak flow to the time to peak. Cough peak flow, however, may be influenced not only by the intensity of the muscle effort produced during coughing, but also by the mechanical properties of the respiratory system, particularly airway resistance. Recordings of flow-related variables measured during voluntary (71,76) and reflex (9,71,77) cough efforts have been used to assess cough frequency in normal subjects during fog challenges (9,77) and to explore cough mechanics and motor pattern during voluntary (71,76,78) and reflex (40) coughing in patients with vocal cord palsy (78) and in laryngectomized patients (40,76).

Cough intensity can also be assessed by means of the integrated electromyographic (IEMG) activity of the abdominal muscles, namely the *obliquus externus* muscle, which has been shown to represent the principal expiratory force generator during voluntary and reflex coughing (73). From IEMG recordings, it is possible to measure the peak amplitude of the IEMG activity (IEMGP), and the time duration of the expiratory ramp, i.e., the cough expiratory time (TEC). The ratio between these two variables (IEMGP/TEC) represents the rate of rise or "slope" of the IEMG activity. The IEMGP is an expression of the total number of recruited motor units and of their maximal frequency of discharge, while IEMGP/TEC reflects the rate of motor unit recruitment as well as the rate of increase in firing frequency (79). Both IEMGP and IEMGP/TEC have been shown to be proportional to the actual tension, or force, developed by the contacting muscles (80). It has recently been shown that, during coughing elicited by inhalation of progressively increasing fog concentrations, both the peak and slope of the IEMG activity correlate with the simultaneously recorded expiratory flow rate in normal subjects (73).

Conclusions

Inhalation and topical administration of water solutions represent useful experimental tools for investigating the sensory and motor components of coughing in both humans and animal preparations. Additional studies will help to clarify how nonisosmolar or chloride deficient stimuli are sensed by the airway receptors and initiate cough. In the clinical setting, quantitative assessments of cough sensitivity and intensity of cough motor responses are of greatest importance to establish disease-related changes and drug-induced modulations of the cough reflex. Finally, there is an obvious need for better standardization of challenge procedures to improve comparability of the results obtained in both patients and normal subjects using the different methodologies presently available.

References

1. De Vries K, Booij-Noord H, Goei JT, et al. Hyperreactivity of the bronchial tree to drugs, chemical and physical agents. In: Orie NGM, Sluiter HJ, eds. Bronchitis II. Assen: Royal Vangorocum, 1964:167–180.
2. Abernathy JD. Effects of inhalation of an artificial fog. Thorax 1968; 23: 421–426.
3. Cheney FW, Butler J. The effects of ultrasonically-produced aerosols on airway resistance in man. Anesthesiology 1968; 29:1099–1106.
4. Allegra L, Bianco S. Nonspecific bronchoreactivity obtained with an ultrasonic aerosol of distilled water. Eur J Respir Dis 1986; 61:41–49.
5. Schoeffel RE, Anderson SD, Altounyan RE. Bronchial hyperreactivity in response to inhalation of ultrasonically nebulised solutions of distilled water and saline. Br Med J 1981; 283:1285–1287.
6. Fontana GA, Bongianni F, Lavorini F, Pantaleo T. Neurobiology and mechanics of cough. In: Dal Negro RW, Geppetti P, Morice AH, eds. Experimental and Clinical Pharmacology of Gastroesophageal Reflux-Induced Asthma. Pisa: Pacini Editore, 2002:34–46.
7. Fontana GA. Motor mechanisms and the mechanics of cough. In: Chung F, Widdicombe J, Boushey H, eds. Cough: Causes, Mechanisms and Therapy. Oxford: Blackwell Publishing Ltd, 2003:193–206.
8. Widdicombe JG. Sensory neurophysiology of the cough reflex. J Allergy Clin Immunol 1996; 98:S84–S90.
9. Higenbottam T. Cough induced by changes of ionic composition of airway surface liquid. Bull Eur Physiopathol Respir 1984; 20:553–562.
10. Widdicombe JH, Widdicombe JG. Regulation of human airway surface liquid. Respir Physiol 1995; 99:3–12.
11. Joris L, Dab I, Quinton PM. Elemental composition of human airway surface fluid in healthy and diseased airways. Am Rev Respir Dis 1993; 148: 1633–1637.
12. Welsh MJ. Electrolyte transport by airway epithelia. Physiol Rev 1987; 67: 1143–1184.
13. Mann SF, Adams GK, Proctor DF. Effects of temperature, relative humidity, and mode of breathing on canine airway secretions. J Appl Physiol 1979; 46: 205–210.
14. Morice AH, Turley AJ, Linton TK. Human ACE gene polymorphism and distilled water induced cough. Thorax 1997; 52:111–113.
15. Boucher RC. Human airway transport. Part one. Am J Respir Crit Care Med 1994; 150:271–283.
16. Widdicombe JH. Ion transport by airway epithelia. In: Crystal RG, West JB, eds. The Lung: Scientific Foundations. 2nd ed. Philadelphia: Lippincott–Raven Publisher, 1997:573–584.
17. Willumsen JN, Davis CW, Boucher RC. Selective response of human airway epithelia to luminal but not serosal solution hypertonicity. Possible role for proximal airway epithelia as an osmolality transducer. J Clin Invest 1994; 94:779–787.

18. McCann JD, Li M, Welsh MJ. Identification and regulation of whole-cell chloride currents in airway epithelium. J Gen Physiol 1989; 94:1015–1036.
19. Morris CE. Mechanosensitive ion channels. J Membr Biol 1990; 111:93–107.
20. Coleridge HM, Coleridge JCG. Reflexes evoked from tracheobronchial tree and lungs. In: Handbook of Physiology. The Respiratory System. Control of Breathing. Section 3. Part 1. Chapter 12. Vol. II. Bethesda, MD: American Physiological Society, 1986:395–429.
21. Zimmerman MP, Pisarri TE. Bronchial vasodilation evoked by increased lower airway osmolarity in dogs. J Appl Physiol 2000; 88:425–432.
22. Boggs DF, Bartlett D. Chemical specificity of a laryngeal apneic reflex in puppies. J Appl Physiol 1982; 53:455–462.
23. Ghosh TK, Van Scott MR, Mathew OP. Epithelial modulation of afferent nerve endings: differential effects of amiloride on afferent subtypes. J Appl Physiol 1995; 78:2235–2240.
24. Fenn WO, Cobb DM, Hegnauer AH, Marsh BS. Electrolytes in nerve. Am J Physiol 1934; 110:74–96.
25. Hodgkin AL, Horowitz P. Influence of potassium and chloride ions on the membrane potential of single muscle fibers. J Physiol 1959; 148:127–160.
26. Widdicombe J. Airway receptors. Respir Physiol 2001; 125:3–15.
27. Sant'Ambrogio G, Sant'Ambrogio FB. Role of larynx in cough. Pulm Pharmacol 1996; 9:379–382.
28. Sant'Ambrogio G, Mathew OP, Fisher JT, Sant'Ambrogio FB. Laryngeal receptors responding to transmural pressure, airflow and local muscle activity. Respir Physiol 1983; 54:317–330.
29. Anderson JW, Sant'Ambrogio FB, Mathew OP, Sant'Ambrogio G. Water-responsive laryngeal receptors in the dog are not specialized endings. Respir Physiol 1990; 79:33–43.
30. Chung K, Sant'Ambrogio FB, Sant'Ambrogio G. The fiber composition of the superior laryngeal nerve. FASEB J 1993; 7:A402.
31. Sant'Ambrogio G, Sant'Ambrogio FB. Role of laryngeal afferents in cough. Pulm Pharmacol 1996; 9:309–314.
32. Jammes Y, Nail B, Mei N, Grimaud CH. Laryngeal afferents activated by phenyldiguanide and their response to cold air or helium-oxygen. Respir Physiol 1987; 67:379–389.
33. Harding R, Johnson P, McCelland ME. Liquid-sensitive laryngeal receptors in the developing sheep, cat and monkey. J Physiol 1978; 277:409–422.
34. Davies AM, Koenig JS, Thach BT. Characteristics of upper airway chemoreflex prolonged apnea in human infants. Am Rev Respir Dis 1988; 139:668–673.
35. Thach BT. Maturation and transformation of reflexes that protect the laryngeal airway from liquid aspiration from fetal to adult life. Am J Med 2001; 111:69s–77s.
36. Nishino T, Tagaito Y, Isono S. Cough and other reflexes on irritation of airway mucosa in man. Pulm Pharmacol 1996; 9:285–292.
37. Nishino T, Kochi T, Ishii M. Differences in respiratory reflex responses from the larynx, trachea, and bronchi in anesthetized female subjects Anesthesiology 1996; 84:70–74.

38. Tagaito Y, Isono S, Nishino T. Upper airway reflexes during a combination of propofol and fentanyl anesthesia. Anesthesiology 1998; 88:1459–1466.
39. Higenbottam T, Jackson TM, Woolman P, Lowry R, Wallwork J. The cough response to ultrasonically nebulized distilled water in heart-lung transplantation patients. Am Rev Respir Dis 1989; 140:58–61.
40. Fontana GA, Pantaleo T, Lavorini F, Mutolo D, Polli G, Pistolesi M. Coughing in laryngectomized patients. Am J Respir Crit Care Med 1999; 160: 1578–1584.
41. Fox AJ, Barnes PJ, Dray A. Stimulation of guinea-pig tracheal fibres by non-isosmotic and low-chloride stimuli and the effect of frusemide. J Physiol 1995; 42:179–187.
42. Lee B, Sant'Ambrogio G, Sant'Ambrogio FB. Afferent innervation and receptors of the canine extrathoracic trachea. Respir Physiol 1992; 90:55–65.
43. Riccio MM, Myers AC, Undem BJ. Immunomodulation of afferent neurons in guinea-pig isolated airway. J Physiol 1996; 491:499–509.
44. Pedersen KE, Meeker SN, Riccio MM, Undem BJ. Selective stimulation of jugular ganglion afferents in guinea pig airways by hypertonic saline. J Appl Physiol 1998; 84:499–506.
45. Pisarri TE, Jonzon A, Coleridge HM, Coleridge JCG. Intravenous injection of hypertonic NaCl solution stimulates pulmonary C-fibers in dogs. Am J Physiol 1991; 260:H1522–H1530.
46. Pisarri TE, Jonzon A, Coleridge HM, Coleridge JCG. Vagal afferents and reflex responses to changes in surface osmolarity in lower airways of dogs. J Appl Physiol 1992; 73:2305–2313.
47. Boushey HA, Richardson PS, Widdicombe JG, Wise JGM. The response of laryngeal afferent fibres to mechanical and chemical stimuli. J Physiol 1974; 240:153–175.
48. Tsubone H, Sant'Ambrogio G, Anderson JW, Orani G. Laryngeal afferent activity and reflexes in the guinea pig. Respir Physiol 1991; 86:215–231.
49. Sullivan CE, Kozar LF, Murphy E, Phillipson EA. Arousal, ventilatory, and airway responses to bronchopulmonary stimulation in sleeping dogs. J Appl Physiol 1979; 47:17–25.
50. Lalloo UG, Fox AJ, Belvisi MG, Chung KF, Barnes PJ. Capsazepine inhibits cough induced by capsaicin and citric acid but not by hypertonic saline in guinea pigs. J Appl Physiol 1995; 79:1082–1087.
51. Chapman RW, House A, Skeans S, Lamca J, Egan RW, Celly C, Hey JA. A simple non-invasive method to measure the cough reflex in dogs. J Pharmacol Toxicol Methods 2001; 46:21–26.
52. Prazma J, Coleman CC, Shockley WW, Boucher RC. Tracheal vascular response to hypertonic and hypotonic solutions. J Appl Physiol 1994; 76: 2275–2280.
53. McFadden ER Jr. Microvasculature and airway responses. Am Rev Respir Dis 1992; 145:s42–s43.
54. Yu J, Zhang JF, Fletcher EC. Stimulation of breathing by activation of pulmonary peripheral afferents in rabbits. J Appl Physiol 1998; 85:1485–1492.

55. Lavorini F, Fontana GA, Pantaleo T, Camiciottoli G, Castellani W, Maluccio NM, Pistolesi M. Fog-induced respiratory responses are attenuated by nedocromil sodium in humans. Am J Respir Crit Care Med 2001; 163:1117–1120.

56. Sheppard D, Rizk NW, Boushey HA, Bethel RA. Mechanism of cough and bronchoconstriction induced by distilled water aerosol. Am Rev Respir Dis 1983; 127:691–694.

57. Eschenbacher WL, Boushey HA, Sheppard D. Alteration in osmolarity of inhaled aerosols cause bronchoconstriction and cough, but absence of a permeant anion causes cough alone. Am Rev Respir Dis 1984; 129:211–215.

58. Godden DJ, Borland C, Lowry R, Higenbottam TW. Chemical specificity of coughing in man. Clin Sci (Lond) 1986; 70:301–306.

59. Lowry RH, Wood AM, Higenbottam TW. Effects of pH and osmolarity on aerosol-induced cough in normal volunteers. Clin Sci (Lond) 1988; 74:373–376.

60. Chadha TS, Birch S, Allegra L, Sackner MA. Effects of ultrasonically nebulized distilled water on respiratory resistance and breathing pattern in normals and asthmatics. Bull Eur Physiopathol Respir 1984; 20:257–262.

61. Banner AS. Relationship between cough due to hypotonic aerosol and the ventilatory response to CO_2 in normal subjects. Am Rev Respir Dis 1988; 137: 647–650.

62. Lowry R, Higenbottam T, Johnson T, Godden D. Inhibition of artificially induced cough in man by bronchodilators. Br J Clin Pharmacol 1987; 24: 503–510.

63. Lowry R, Wood A, Johnson T, Higenbottam T. Antitussive properties of inhaled bronchodilators on induced cough. Chest 1988; 93:1186–1189.

64. Lowry R, Wood A, Higenbottam T. The effect of anticholinergic bronchodilator therapy on cough during upper respiratory tract infections. Br J Clin Pharmacol 1994; 37:187–191.

65. Karlsson JA, Sant'Ambrogio G, Widdicombe J. Afferent neural pathways in cough and reflex bronchoconstriction. J Appl Physiol 1988; 65:1007–1023.

66. Stone RA, Worsdell YM, Fuller RW, Barnes PJ. Effects of 5-hydroxytryptamine and 5-hydroxytryptophan infusion on the human cough reflex. J Appl Physiol 1993; 74:396–401.

67. Tanaka S, Hirata K, Kurihara N, Yoshikawa J, Takeda T. Effect of loratadine, an H1 antihistamine, on induced cough in non-asthmatic patients with chronic cough. Thorax 1996; 51:810–814.

68. Ventresca PG, Nichol GM, Barnes PJ, Chung KF. Inhaled furosemide inhibits cough induced by low chloride content solutions but not by capsaicin. Am Rev Respir Dis 1990; 142:143–146.

69. Foresi A, Cavigioli G, Pelucchi A, Mastropasqua B, Marazzini L. Effect of acetazolamide on cough induced by low-chloride-ion solutions in normal subjects: comparison with furosemide. J Allergy Clin Immunol 1996; 97: 1093–1099.

70. Joos GF, O'Connor B, Anderson SD, Chung F, Cockcroft DW, Dahlen B, DiMaria G, Foresi A, Hargreave FE, Holgate ST, Inman M, Lotvall J,

Magnussen H, Polosa R, Postma DS, Riedler J. ERS Task Force Indirect airway challenges. Eur Respir J 2003; 21:1050–1068.

71. Fontana GA, Pantaleo T, Lavorini F, Boddi V, Panuccio P. A noninvasive electromyographic study on threshold and cough intensity in humans. Eur Respir J 1997; 10:983–989.

72. Fontana GA, Pantaleo T, Lavorini F, Maluccio NM, Mutolo D, Pistolesi M. Repeatability of cough-related variables during fog challenges at threshold and suprathreshold stimulus intensity in humans. Eur Respir J 1999; 13: 1447–1450.

73. Fontana GA, Pantaleo T, Lavorini F, Benvenuti F, Gangemi S. Defective motor control of coughing in Parkinson's disease. Am J Respir Crit Care Med 1998; 158:458–464.

74. Sterk PJ, Plomp A, van de Vate JF, Quanjer PH. Physical properties of aerosols produced by several jet- and ultrasonic nebulizers. Bull Eur Physiopathol Respir 1984; 20:65–72.

75. Morice AH, Higgins KS, Yeo WW. Adaptation of cough reflex with different types of stimulation. Eur Respir J 1992; 5:841–847.

76. Murty GE, Smith MCF, Lancaster P. Cough intensity in the laryngectomee. Clin Otolaryngol 1991; 16:25–28.

77. Higenbottam T. The ionic composition of airway surface liquid and coughing. Bull Eur Physiopathol Respir 1987; 23(suppl 10):25s–27s.

78. Murty GE, Lancaster P, Kelly PJ. Cough intensity in patients with a vocal cord palsy. Clin Otolaryngol 1991; 16:248–251.

79. Desmedt JE, Godaux E. Ballistic contractions in man: characteristic recruitment pattern of single motor units of the tibialis anterior muscle. J Physiol 1977; 264:673–693.

80. Bigland B, Lippold OCJ. The relation between force, velocity and integrated electrical activity in human muscles. J Physiol 1954; 123:214–224.

12

Acute Cough: Epidemiology, Mechanisms, and Treatment

RONALD ECCLES

Common Cold Centre, Cardiff School of Biosciences, Cardiff University, Cardiff, U.K.

Definition of Acute Cough

Estimating the duration of cough is the first step in diagnosis. Obviously all types of cough have an onset and hopefully an end, therefore by definition all types of cough must go through an initial acute stage at the time of onset. Irwin and Madison (1) categorize cough on the basis of duration; acute cough lasting less than 3 weeks, subacute 3–8 weeks, and chronic lasting more than 8 weeks. Most cases of acute cough will not be seen by specialists as the self-limiting nature of the condition means that the cough is likely to have resolved before the patient can obtain an appointment to see the specialist. Morice (2) defines cough into only two diagnostic groups; acute cough that is usually due to viral respiratory tract infection and chronic cough that may be arbitrarily defined as lasting longer than 8 weeks. It is the latter definition by Morice (2) that will be used in the present discussion and acute cough will be defined as caused by acute upper respiratory tract viral infection. Irwin et al. (3) list other common causes of acute cough such as acute bacterial sinusitis, pertussis, exacerbation of chronic obstructive pulmonary disorder (COPD), allergic rhinitis, and exposure to environmental irritants; and lists less common causes of acute cough as asthma, congestive heart failure, pneumonia, aspiration syndromes, and pulmonary embolism. The present discussion will be limited to acute cough associated with viral infection of the upper respiratory tract.

Epidemiology

Incidence

Irwin and Madison (1) state "there have been no studies of the spectrum and frequency of causes of acute cough." However, since it is generally accepted that acute upper respiratory tract viral infection (URTI) is the most common cause of acute cough, an estimate of the incidence of URTI could provide an indication of the incidence of acute cough. One problem in using this approach is that cough is not always a symptom of URTI. In a study on patients with naturally acquired URTI and complaint of sore throat pain it was reported that cough as a symptom was present in around 50% of this population (4). The most common symptoms of URTI found in this study were runny nose and sneezing with an incidence of 60–70%. The incidence of cough associated with URTI may vary according to the virus as in studies in which healthy volunteers were infected with different strains of rhinovirus, coronavirus and respiratory syncytial virus (RSV) the incidence of cough in the subjects varied from 9% to 64% (5). In this viral challenge study, cough was usually a late symptom and developed 4–5 days after challenge, compared to runny nose, which was a common symptom 1 day after challenge.

URTI may be defined as separate diseases on the basis of the infectious agent or as a familiar syndrome of common cold symptoms. The common viruses associated with URTI are rhinovirus, coronavirus, respiratory syncytial virus (RSV), influenza virus, parainfluenza virus, adenovirus, enterovirus, and a variety of less common viruses (6). As a group the rhinoviruses are the most common cause of colds in children and adults. Common colds occur at rates of two to five per person per year, with school children suffering between 7 and 10 colds per year (6). If one accepts the lowest rate of infection of only two colds per person per year then this translates into a very conservative estimate of 120 million colds per year in the United Kingdom (double the population to get the incidence of colds in any community). If one further assumes that the lowest incidence of cough as a symptom is 10% of those with colds then this means that there will be at least 12 million cases of acute cough per year in the United Kingdom.

Quantifying the global significance of acute cough is difficult because the condition is benign and self-limiting and many patients do not seek medical attention. One measure of the incidence of acute cough is the sale of nonprescription liquid cough medicines that grossed £96.5 millions in 2001 in the United Kingdom (7). This sales figure is an underestimate of total sales as it is for sales from pharmacy and grocery outlets only, and does not include sales from many outlets such as supermarkets and convenience stores. The two figures, of an estimated 12 million cases of acute cough and an expenditure of £96 million on cough medicines indicate an expenditure of around £8 per case of acute cough. With cough medicines averaging £3–4 per unit, the above estimate of 12 million cases per year may be an underestimate of the cases of acute cough, and that the true incidence of acute cough of sufficient symptom severity to trigger purchase of a cough medicine may be at least 24 million cases per year in the United Kingdom.

Seasonality

Acute upper respiratory viral infections exhibit seasonality and this causes seasonality in the incidence of acute cough and sales of cough medicines (8). It is common knowledge that the incidence of URTI such as common cold and influenza exhibit seasonal fluctuations. In the more northerly and southerly parts of the hemisphere there is a peak of respiratory illness during the winter months. Winter seasonality has been reported for a wide range of URTI caused by over 200 different viruses belonging to six families: orthomyxoviruses (influenza), paramyxoviruses (RSV, parainfluenza), coronaviruses, picornaviruses (common cold), herpes viruses, and adenoviruses (9). Lower respiratory tract diseases such as pneumonia which may be viral or bacterial in etiology also show a similar seasonal pattern with the peak of illness in winter (10,11). The nose is the entrance to the lower airways and URTI predisposes to lower airway infection with viruses and bacteria. Life-threatening lower airway infections often start as a URTI, especially in the elderly. Annual vaccination programs against influenza can help to protect those at risk of lower airway infection, but there is at present no protection from the hundreds of viruses responsible for the common cold syndrome.

Every year in the United Kingdom the decrease in air temperature in winter is associated with a great increase in mortality and morbidity. For every degree centigrade decrease in average temperature there is an increase in the number of winter deaths by around 8000 (12). For every degree centigrade decrease in mean temperature below 5°C there is a 10.5% increase in all respiratory consultations (13). Respiratory infections are a major cause of seasonal mortality and illness, and they place a great seasonal burden on the health service. Around 33% of the seasonal increase in mortality is associated with respiratory disease associated with infection (14), and there is increasing evidence that some of the seasonal increase in mortality associated with cardiovascular disease may be related to respiratory infection (15).

The seasonal increase in cough associated with URTI is associated with a seasonal increase in acute cough due to other causes such as exacerbation of asthma, and cough due to exacerbation of bronchitis and other respiratory disease. URTI often progresses to more serious respiratory infection as the viral infection weakens respiratory defences and predisposes to secondary bacterial infection of the lower respiratory tract.

The seasonality of URTI has been commonly explained as due to increased crowding in winter and poor ventilation of working and living spaces (16). At the start of the 21st century the crowding theory persists in textbooks of human virology as an explanation for the seasonality of respiratory infection and there are some signs that any link with climate is now lost. In a summary on the seasonality of viral respiratory infections Collier and Oxford (9) state that "[t]he precise conditions that result in seasonal spread are not known with certainty but may be attributed more to changes in social behaviour with the seasons e.g. overcrowding in cold weather, than with variations in humidity and temperature" (9). The seasonal increase in URTI and cough may be caused by seasonal cooling of the upper airway as inhalation of cold air causes cooling of the nasal epithelium sufficient to inhibit respiratory defences against infection such as mucociliary clearance and the phagocytic activity of leukocytes (17).

In winter we protect our core body temperature by wearing thicker winter clothes but our nose and upper airways are still directly exposed to cold air. Heating, clothing, and food are obvious ways to promote winter health, but it is surprising that the idea of some form of respirator to conserve respiratory heat loss, has not been developed. A simple facemask has been shown to reduce the incidence of asthma induced by cold air (18). Even a simple woollen scarf has been shown to halve the bronchoconstrictor response to inhaling cold air (19). Perhaps the simple precaution of wearing a scarf over the nose and mouth, could provide similar protection against nasal airway cooling and susceptibility to URTI and cough, especially in the elderly, when they are obliged to be exposed to cold air in winter.

Children

Acute cough in children associated with URTI is a very common problem and the cause of many primary care consultations. Acute cough in the majority of cases needs no more than symptomatic treatment and patience for natural resolution of the disease but unfortunately there is much pressure on the primary care physician to prescribe antibiotics. Since acute cough is viral in origin in the overwhelming majority of patients, the routine prescription of antibiotics cannot be justified. In a review on acute cough in children aged between 0 and 4 years Hay and Wilson (20) report, "At one week, 75% of children may have improved but 50% may be still coughing and/or have a nasal discharge. At two weeks up to 24% of children may be no better. Within two weeks of presentation, 12% of children may experience one or more complication, such as rash, painful ears, diarrhoea, vomiting, or progression to bronchitis/pneumonia." Their review indicates that parents and clinicians need to have more realistic expectations about the course of acute cough and that with patience the condition will resolve with only symptomatic treatment.

Mechanisms

Cough is a protective reflex that has two main functions, first to prevent the entry of food and fluid into the lower airways, and second to help expel mucus from the lower airways. The first function is mainly achieved by mechanical and chemical stimulation of sensory nerves in the larynx and trachea, the second by mechanical stimulation of sensory nerves in the tracheobronchial tree. Cough is not a common occurrence in healthy persons, cough occurs when food or fluid "goes down the wrong way." There are no data to my knowledge on the frequency of cough in healthy persons. The cough frequency in health must be extremely low, perhaps one or two coughs a day, otherwise it would be extremely difficult to perform cough challenge studies on healthy persons. The most common cause of an increase in cough frequency is acute cough associated with URTI.

Origin of Cough Associated with URTI

Despite the fact that acute cough is the most common type of cough, it is surprising that very little is known about the mechanism of this type of cough. It is assumed that the normal protective cough reflex is exaggerated in some way during URTI so that cough occurs spontaneously instead of in response to food or fluid entering the airway. In order to understand how cough may be initiated from the upper airways it is important to understand the sensory innervation of the upper airways in relation to the cough reflex.

Sensory Innervation of the Upper Airways

The term upper airways is not a strict anatomical term, but is used more in a functional way, to include the nasal passages, paranasal sinuses, Eustachian tube and middle ear air space, pharynx (nasopharynx, oropharynx, laryngopharynx), larynx, and the extra thoracic portion of the trachea as illustrated in Fig. 1 (21). The sensory nerve supply to the upper airways is provided by the first, fifth, seventh, ninth, and tenth cranial nerves (I, olfactory; V, trigeminal; VII, facial; IX, glossopharyngeal; X, vagus) as illustrated in Fig. 2 (22,23). The olfactory nerve enters the nasal cavity through the cribriform plate and forms a distinct olfactory area in the roof of the nasal cavity. The facial nerve supplies gustatory fibers to the tongue. The

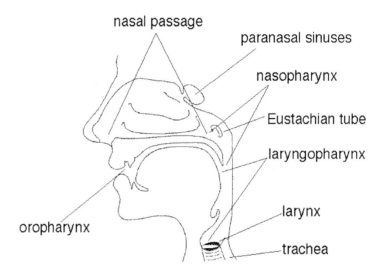

Figure 1   Anatomy of the upper airways.

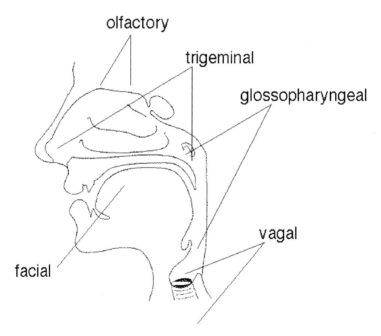

Figure 2   Sensory innervation of the upper airways. The areas of the upper airways served by the different cranial nerves are illustrated.

maxillary and ophthalmic divisions of the trigeminal nerve supply the nasal passages, paranasal sinuses, and anterior parts of the nasopharynx and oropharynx. The glossopharyngeal nerve supplies sensory fibers to the posterior areas of the nasopharynx and oropharynx, supplying the tympanic cavity, Eustachian tube, fauces, tonsils, uvula, inferior surface of the soft palate, and posterior third of the tongue. The vagus nerve supplies the larynx and trachea with sensory fibers, and via a small auricular branch also supplies sensory fibers to the external acoustic meatus and tympanic membrane.

Apart from the specialized sensory receptors of the olfactory and gustatory areas it appears that all of the remaining sensory supply to the lining of the upper airway consists of bare nerve endings without any specialized form of terminal receptor. Despite this lack of specialized structure the bare nerve endings serve as transducers for a wide range of stimuli such as physical and chemical stimulation, changes in temperature and pressure, and stimuli that cause tissue damage.

The cough reflex is believed to be mediated by sensory receptors in the epithelium of the airway from the larynx to the bronchi (24). Widdicombe (25) makes no mention of the upper airways in the neuroregulation of cough and states that "[c]ough is caused by excitation of sensory receptors in the walls of the respiratory tract, from larynx down to bronchi." The reflexes associated with mechanical stimulation of the upper airways are illustrated in Fig. 3. The nose, paranasal sinuses, and most of the upper airways are innervated by branches of the trigeminal nerves. Mechanical or chemical stimulation of the trigeminal nerves causes the protective sneeze reflex (22). The glossopharyngeal nerves are primarily involved in the gag and swallowing reflexes and there is no evidence that this cranial nerve is involved in cough.

Widdicombe (26) states that "cough has never been directly initiated from the pharynx or other upper airway structure above the larynx" and that "the origin of cough is unique to structures innervated by the vagus nerve." If cough is a purely vagal phenomenon related to the larynx and lower airways how does upper airway infection trigger cough? URTI is usually defined as a rhinosinusitis and the larynx and bronchi are not usually involved in the infection, otherwise the infection would cause laryngitis and bronchitis.

Role of Infection and Inflammation

If one accepts that cough can only be initiated by stimulation of vagal nerve endings then acute cough associated with URTI must in some way involve the lower airways from the larynx downwards. Infection of the upper airway causes inflammation and the generation of inflammatory mediators such as bradykinin, prostaglandins, and tachykinins. The excitability of the sensory

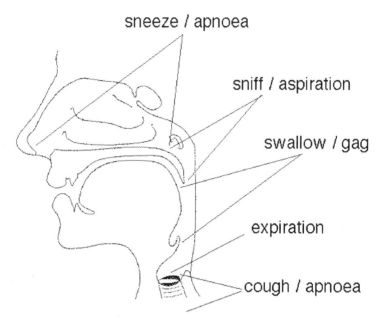

sneeze / apnoea

sniff / aspiration

swallow / gag

expiration

cough / apnoea

Figure 3   Reflexes initiated from the different areas of the upper airways. Note that cough can only be initiated from the larynx and below.

receptors in the airway that normally mediate cough can be increased by the presence of these inflammatory mediators. Carr and Ellis (27) state that "[t]he activation of airway afferent neurons initiates a variety of reflexes including cough and bronchoconstriction. Like somatic afferent neurons involved in inflammation-induced hyperalgesia, the excitability of airway afferent neurons is not fixed but, rather can be increased by the action of a variety of mediators produced during inflammation." This theory of inflammation causing airway hyperreactivity similar to the hyperalgesia of somatic pain is generally accepted by those involved in cough research (25,28,29). The problem with developing a similar mechanism for acute cough associated with URTI is that the site of inflammation in the nose and paranasal sinuses may be physically separate from the sensory receptors that mediate cough in the larynx, trachea, and bronchi.

As discussed in the preceding text, not all cases of URTI are associated with cough and the dominant symptoms are of rhinosinusitis. In those cases of URTI associated with cough there may be some inflammation of the lower airways that predisposes to hyperreactivity of the airway sensory receptors mediating cough. Three different mechanisms involving inflammatory mediators in the generation of acute cough associated with URTI are illustrated in Fig. 4.

Mechanism (1) has already been discussed as the local effects of mediators. The inflammatory response of the upper airway to viral infection may extend to include the larynx and trachea. This may or may not involve viral infection of the larynx and trachea. Because of the close proximity of the larynx and trachea to the nose and upper airway it is reasonable to expect that these organs will be affected by the inflammatory response tracking along the airway. Cough is usually a late symptom of URTI and it may take some days of infection before the inflammation and infection spreads from the nose towards the lower airway.

Mechanism (2) involves humoral effects of inflammatory mediators on the lower airways. The mediators generated in the upper airway in response to viral infection enter the blood stream and are transported to the lower airways where they may initiate an inflammatory response.

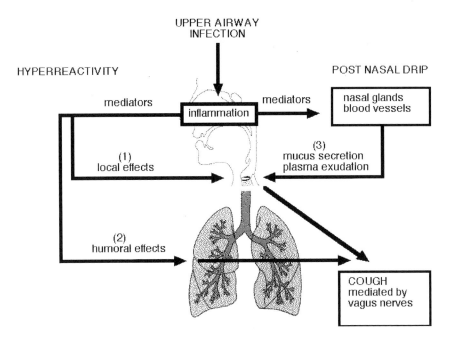

Figure 4 Mechanisms of cough. Infection of the upper airways causes inflammation and the generation of inflammatory mediators. The mediators may cause cough by three mechanisms. (**1**) Inflammation of the upper airway spreads to the larynx and trachea and mediators cause hyperreactivity of sensory receptors that mediate cough. (**2**) Inflammatory mediators circulate in the blood from the site of inflammation in the upper airway to the lower airways and cause hyperreactivity of sensory receptors that mediate cough. (**3**) Inflammatory mediators cause secretion of a viscous mucus that mechanically stimulates the larynx to induce cough, often referred to as postnasal drip syndrome (PNDS).

Humoral effects of inflammatory mediators of viral infection on the central nervous system are well documented, such as the development of fever associated with cytokines released from white cells at the site of infection (30,31). URTI has been associated with an increase in the production of the inflammatory marker nitric oxide (NO) in the lower airways (32). The increase in lower airway NO associated with URTI has been explained by circulation of inflammatory mediators from the nose to lungs and this has been proposed as a mechanism of airway hyperreactivity (33). Circulation of inflammatory mediators such as cytokines from the upper to the lower airway may cause a condition of airway hyperreactivity and cough.

Mechanism (3) involves post nasal drip. The inflammatory mediator associated with URTI cause the secretion of mucus and the generation of a plasma exudates (31). Postnasal drip syndrome (PNDS) has been proposed as a major cause of acute cough associated with URTI. Irwin and coauthors (3) state that PNDS is the most common cause of cough in cases of URTI in the United States. However, Morice (2) gives a different picture of PNDS in the United Kingdom and suggests that the condition is not as common as in the United States, and goes so far as to propose that a better term for the disorder is "cough associated with rhinosinusitis" or even "cough-variant rhinitis." The mechanism of cough production in PNDS is unclear but the term implies direct mechanical stimulation of the larynx with mucus, perhaps in the form of viscous strings of mucus that are difficult to clear from the nasopharynx. Morice (2) is sceptical about this mechanism of cough with PNDS and suggests that "it is possible that disease in the upper airways merely reflects the inflammation occurring in the lower airways."

Dry vs. Productive Cough

Cough associated with URTI is often classified as either "dry" or "productive" with productive cough often referred to as a "chesty" cough. Nonprescription cough medicines are often targeted to treat either dry cough or chesty cough. The mechanisms by which URTI produces dry or chesty cough are not known but it is possible to relate this cough classification to the mechanisms described previously and illustrated in Fig. 4. Dry cough may be related to mechanism (1) with hyperreactivity of the larynx and trachea being the cause of cough, or possibly to mechanism (3) with PNDS causing mechanical stimulation of the larynx with throat clearing and cough. A productive or chesty cough may be related to mechanism (2) with inflammation of the lower airways triggering mucus production and cough. URTI can present as a syndrome of cough and phlegm and these symptoms may cause some clinicians to diagnose a condition of bacterial bronchitis and prescribe antibiotics. However, Irwin and Madison (1) state that "in the absence of chronic obstructive pulmonary disease, the failure to diagnose bronchitis when it is present will probably not adversely affect the patient, because most acute respiratory infections are viral."

Treatment

Acute cough associated with viral URTI is a self-limiting condition that will resolve spontaneously in almost all cases. However, cough can be a disturbing symptom and many patients will seek some form of treatment to alleviate the symptom. Viral infection triggers an immune response and inflammation. The inflammatory process causes the sensitization of airway sensory receptors that mediate cough, and coughing occurs spontaneously, or in response to stimuli that would not normally trigger coughing, e.g., exposure to cold air. The various treatment options are illustrated in Fig. 5. The treatments can be targeted at different sites along the chain of interactions from viral infection through to cough.

Antiviral Treatments

Antiviral treatments are available for influenza A and B but at present there are no antiviral treatments for the large number of viruses associated with URTI. Antiviral treatments such as neuraminidase inhibitors and amantadines for the treatment of influenza are unlikely to be of any benefit for the treatment of cough since cough is a late symptom and usually develops 4–5 days after viral challenge, whereas antiviral medicines need to be taken within 48 hr of the development of symptoms in order to combat the early stages of viral replication (34,35).

Anti-inflammatory Treatments

Infection causes a complex immune response that triggers the generation of inflammatory mediators such as bradykinin, prostaglandins, tachykinins, and cytokines (31). The mediators act on nerve endings, glands, and blood vessels to cause the familiar symptoms of URTI including cough. Medicines that inhibit the inflammatory response by inhibiting the generation of mediators or antagonizing their effects will reduce the severity of symptoms such as cough. Because of the complex soup of mediators generated with inflammation, and because of overlap in their effects, knocking out a single mediator is unlikely to abolish cough. The mediators may sensitize or stimulate airway sensory receptors that mediate cough. Bradykinin is generated in response to URTI and this mediator may be involved in the stimulation of cough receptors in the airway (27,29). At present there is no medication that inhibits the generation of bradykinin or antagonizes its effects but this may be a useful area for future research in cough medicines.

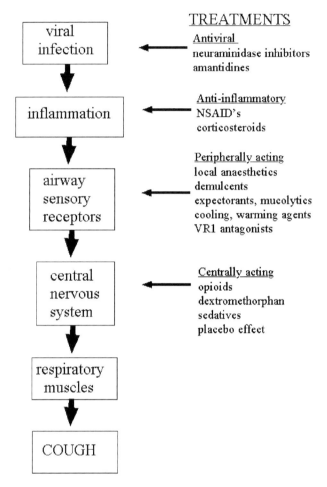

Figure 5 Treatments for acute cough. The figure illustrates the series of processes from viral infection to cough, and at which levels the various treatments act.

Nonsteroidal Anti-inflammatory Drugs

The effect of bradykinin on sensory nerve endings such as pain nerve endings is enhanced by prostaglandins and this may be the basis for the hyperreactivity of pain nerve endings, allodynia or hyperalgesia (36). There are many similarities between allodynia and cough hyperreactivity, and medications that influence allodynia (25) may be effective cough medicines (36). Medications that inhibit prostaglandin synthesis such as nonsteroidal anti-inflammatory drugs (NSAIDs) are effective analgesics but at present there is limited evidence that this class of medicine has any effect on acute cough caused by URTI. In a study on URTI caused by rhinovirus challenge subjective scores of cough severity were significantly reduced by treatment with the NSAID naproxen compared to placebo treatment (37). Despite the beneficial effects of NSAID treatment in this study by Sperber et al. in 1992 (37), a search of the literature has failed to find any other support for the effects of NSAIDs on acute cough associated with URTI. However, NSAIDs have been shown to be of use in the treatment of cough associated with angiotensin converting enzyme inhibition (ACEI) (38,39).

Corticosteroids

Cough associated with asthma responds well to treatment with corticosteroids that inhibit the inflammatory response (40) but these medicines are not usually used to treat acute cough associated with URTI, perhaps because the inhibition of inflammation in the case of infection may not be beneficial.

Peripherally Acting Treatments

Local Anesthetics

The airway sensory receptors that mediate cough play a central role in the generation of cough. Mechanical stimulation of the airway from the larynx down will cause coughing and this type of cough is routinely abolished by the application of local anaesthetics during endoscopy of the airway. Inhalation of local anesthetic abolishes cough in humans (41). Local anesthetics should similarly inhibit or abolish cough associated with URTI, but the safety problems associated with their use prevents the development of any local anesthetic treatment. The problem being that inhalation of a local anesthetic aerosol into the airway causes numbness of the throat and impairment of the swallowing reflex with the risk of aspiration (42). Local anesthetics may also cause a hypersensitivity reaction and may inhibit mucociliary clearance (42).

Demulcents

Since the majority of cough medicines are sugar-based syrups, there has been some speculation that a demulcent effect of the sugar may make a major contribution to the antitussive activity of the medicine (43). Such a demulcent effect would be in addition to any pharmacological and placebo effects of the medicine. The demulcent action of the syrup may exert its antitussive effect by at least three mechanisms according to Fuller and Jackson (43).

1. The sugar content of the cough mixture encourages saliva production and swallowing; the act of swallowing may interfere with the cough reflex.

2. The sugar solution may coat sensory nerve endings in the epi-
    pharynx and cause their stimulation; this stimulation may sup-
    press cough by a "gating" process.
3. The sugar solution may act as a protective barrier to sensory
    receptors that can either produce cough or heighten the cough
    reflex.

The demulcent effect of antitussive medicines is exploited to the
maximum in cough syrups that contain sapid substances, such as sugar
and honey, and bitter tasting substances such as lemon and citric acid.
These sapid substances promote salivation and may also promote secretion
of airway mucus. Gustatory rhinorrhea has been shown to occur after eating spicy foods and this observation demonstrates a link between gustation
and airway secretion of mucus (44). Many cough medicines contain capis-
cum which is a potent gustatory stimulus and which may also promote
airway secretions. The fact that almost all cough medicines are formulated
as sapid syrups indicates that the demulcent action of the syrup may contribute to the antitussive activity of the treatment. The demulcent effect
may be termed a "physiological" effect of a cough syrup as it is related
to physiological effects such as salivation and stimulation of airway mucus
secretions. The physiological effect of a cough syrup may exhibit similar
characteristics to a pharmacological effect, with a time course of action,
peak effect, cumulative effect, and carry over effect, but at present there
is no information on the pharmacodynamics of any physiological effect
of treatment on cough. In the case of cough medicines, there is likely
to be a large physiological effect with a cough syrup, but little if any physiological effect with a tablet or capsule formulation.

Other medicines apart from cough medicines may have a physiological effect that can be distinguished from a pharmacological or placebo
effect. The efficacy of throat lozenges for the treatment of sore throat is
mainly related to the stimulation of salivation, and in this respect there is
some similarity between the effects of throat lozenges and cough syrups.
Many treatments for common cold are taken as a hot tasty drink, and this
mode of treatment may have a physiological effect by stimulating salivation
and airway secretions.

Expectorants and Mucolytics

Expectorants such as guaiphenesin are found in a wide range of common
cold medications often in combination with an antitussive such as dextromethorphan. The rationale behind such a combination is not always clear
but many of these combination medications are aimed at treatment of a
"chesty" productive cough. By reducing the viscosity of respiratory tract
mucus, guaiphenesin is believed to increases the efficacy of the cough reflex
and mucociliary clearance, in removing accumulated mucus from the

trachea and bronchi. The pharmacology of guaiphenesin is poorly understood and it is not clear how the drug acts. Guaiphenesin may act as a gastric irritant and promote salivation and airway mucus secretions. There is little clinical evidence to support the use and efficacy of any expectorant medication in the treatment of cough associated with URTI (45).

Mucolytics such as carbocysteine are sometimes included in over the counter (OTC) cough medicines but there is little evidence that mucolytics provide any benefit to patients with cough associated with URTI.

Cooling and Warming Agents

Cooling and warming agents are often added to give extra sensations to the cough treatment and these agents may influence the activity of cold and warm sensory receptors in the airway and digestive tract. Cooling agents such as menthol are sometimes included as flavouring agents in cough medicines although menthol may also have pharmacological activity as a local anesthetic (46). The cooling properties of menthol and other cooling agents could also be considered as a pharmacological component of treatment, as there is evidence that cooling properties are determined by interaction with a menthol type of pharmacological receptor on sensory nerves (46). Although menthol is usually declared as a flavoring agent in cough medicines there is some evidence that it may have specific antitussive activity (47).

Vanilloid VR1 Receptor Antagonists

The inflammation associated with URTI is believed to stimulate or sensitize airway sensory receptors and initiate cough. In a prospective study on healthy volunteers it was shown that the cough sensitivity to inhaled capsaicin was increased when the volunteers were studied whilst suffering from URTI (48). Similar increase in cough sensitivity associated with URTI has also been found when using inhaled citric acid (49) or nebulized distilled water (50) to induce cough. Empey et al. (49) have proposed that the increase in cough sensitivity during URTI may be due to an increased sensitivity of the rapidly adapting sensory receptors in the airway. The activation of airway sensory receptors that initiate cough may be related to the activation of a pharmacological receptor sensitive to capsaicin, the vanilloid VR1 receptor (29). If there was some way of returning the sensitivity of airway sensory receptors back towards a normal level then this would be likely to reduce or abolish the coughing associated with URTI but still leave the protective reflex of cough intact. With the identification of the vanilloid pharmacological receptor as a key receptor interacting with inflammatory mediators the development of peripherally acting antitussive medicines is now a feasible goal (25,29) and there is now much interest in developing antagonists to the vanilloid VR1 receptor. However, at present there are no peripherally acting antitussives available for use in patients.

Centrally Acting Treatments

Cough is regulated from the "cough center" in the brain stem. The cough center is not a discrete nucleus but a diffuse network of neurones in the respiratory area of the brainstem that integrates and modulates the sensory input from the vagal innervation of the airway, and acts as a pattern generator for cough. In recent years there has been a great increase in our knowledge about the neuropharmacology of the control of cough (51), but of necessity this knowledge is based on induced cough in animal models, and the results of these studies may not relate to acute human cough associated with URTI. Another problem associated with the development of centrally acting cough medicines is that they are likely to influence the activity of other control areas in the brain apart from cough. This inevitably means that side effects may influence the safety and usefulness of any centrally acting antitussive medicine.

Opioids

Opioids such as morphine and codeine are believed to inhibit cough by inhibition of the cough center, and this inhibitory effect is more specific than the depression induced by general anesthesia as the antitussive effect occurs at doses that do not have a general inhibitory effect on respiratory control centers and breathing. Although there is much evidence from animal experiments and from human studies on chronic and induced cough that codeine has antitussive activity (52), there is no convincing evidence that codeine is an effective antitussive for the treatment of acute cough associated with URTI (53).

Dextromethorphan

Because of the problems of abuse and addiction with codeine, nonopioid antitussives such as dextromethorphan are preferred for the treatment of acute cough. Cough medicines containing dextromethorphan are widely used and freely available without prescription. "In the United Kingdom alone there are 16 over the counter (OTC) cough products containing dextromethorphan, and in the USA, dextromethorphan accounts for 75% of OTC sales of antitussives" (54). A 30 mg dose of dextromethorphan is the standard OTC dose and a meta-analysis of six clinical studies using this dose has shown that dextromethorphan is on average 15% more effective than placebo treatment in reducing cough counts (54). However, other clinical studies have failed to demonstrate any superiority of dextromethorphan above placebo (55) and the efficacy of this medication is at best marginally superior to placebo (56).

Sedatives

Cough can be abolished by general anesthesia (57) and medications such as first-generation antihistamines may inhibit cough by their sedative effects. Alcohol is a common constituent in cough medicines and it may inhibit cough by its sedative action, especially in nighttime cough remedies. Overdose of any sedative, including alcohol, may cause depression of the cough reflex, that may lead to life-threatening aspiration of stomach contents into the airway.

First-generation antihistamines such as diphenhydramine are often included in OTC cough medicines but there is little clinical evidence to support their efficacy as antitussives in the treatment of cough associated with URTI. Curley et al. (58) reported that a combination of antihistamine and decongestant "reduced postnasal drip and significantly decreased the severity of cough, nasal obstruction, nasal discharge, and throat clearing during the first few days of a common cold." Any antitussive efficacy of antihistamines is likely to be due to central sedation and peripheral anticholinergic activity causing a decrease in airway secretions and inhibition of the cough reflex. There is no evidence that histamine has any significant role in the etiology of cough associated with URTI.

Placebo Effect

Treatment with antitussive medicines is usually associated with a large placebo response as illustrated in Fig. 6, which illustrates the large decrease in cough frequency after treatment with either a single 30 mg dose of dextromethorphan or matched placebo capsule (55). The reduction in cough frequency associated with placebo treatment may be due to at least two factors; spontaneous recovery due to rest, and a true placebo response related to belief in the efficacy of the treatment, perhaps influencing voluntary control of cough (59). The large placebo response associated with cough treatment has many similarities with the placebo response associated with analgesics and this has led to a hypothesis that endogenous opioids may be involved in the placebo response of cough and analgesic medications (56). This would explain why potent analgesics such as morphine and codeine are also antitussives, as exogenously administered opioids may mimic the effects of endogenous opioids that modulate the cough reflex and the sensation of pain.

Most of the treatments for acute cough are self-prescribed OTC cough medicines. Because of safety considerations the dose of active medication in most OTC medicines is at the lowest possible level and antitussive efficacy is often minimal. In a recent review of OTC cough medicines the authors concluded that "[o]ver the counter cough medicines for acute cough cannot be recommended because there is no good evidence for their effectiveness. Even when trials had significant results, the effect sizes were

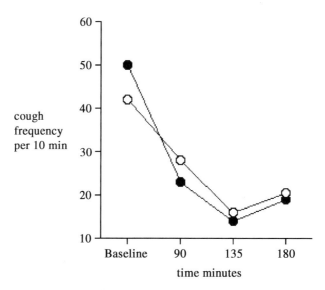

Figure 6 Median cough frequency before and after treatment with placebo (*unshaded symbols*) $n = 22$, and 30 mg dextromethorphan (*shaded symbols*) $n = 21$, treatment groups. Medication was given in a hard gelatin capsule with the placebo capsule containing lactose powder. (Redrawn from Ref. 55.)

small and of doubtful clinical relevance" (60). This statement can be challenged, as it is likely that all OTC medicines provide benefit in the treatment of acute cough by means of placebo and demulcent effects. This will make it very difficult to demonstrate any superiority of antitussive activity above placebo in clinical trials. In placebo-controlled clinical trials where the placebo medicine is a syrup, perhaps containing cooling and menthol agents as flavoring ingredients, the placebo is likely to have much antitussive activity. The small average difference of 15% greater antitussive activity of dextromethorphan compared to placebo in a series of clinical trials reported by Pavesi et al. (54) may be explained by 85% of the antitussive activity being due to a placebo effect (56).

Conclusions

Acute cough associated with URTI is the most common form of cough yet there is little knowledge about the mechanisms involved in this type of cough. The lack of research in this area may be due to the self-limiting nature of this type of acute cough or because of difficulties in studying an acute and variable disease state. PNDS is reported to be the main mechanism involved in the generation of acute cough associated with URTI but there is a scarcity of evidence to support this hypothesis. A wide range of medicines is freely available to treat acute cough but most are little more effective than placebo treatment. Fortunately, placebo treatment is a very effective treatment for acute cough and simple demulcent cough syrups can provide relief.

References

1. Irwin RS, Madison JM. The diagnosis and treatment of cough. N Engl J Med 2000; 343:1715–1721.
2. Morice AH. Epidemiology of cough. Pulm Pharmacol Ther 2002; 15:253–259.
3. Irwin RS, Boulet LP, Cloutier MM, Fuller R, Gold PM, Hoffstein V, Ing AJ, McCool FD, Obyrne P, Poe RH, Prakash UBS, Pratter MR, Rubin BK. Managing cough as a defence mechanism and as a symptom—a consensus panel report of the American College of Chest Physicians. Chest 1998; 114: S133–S181.
4. Eccles R, Loose I, Jawad MS, Nyman L. Effects of acetylsalicylic acid on sore throat pain and other pain symptoms associated with acute upper respiratory tract infection. Pain Med 2003; 4:118–124.
5. Tyrrell DA, Cohen S, Schlarb JE. Signs and symptoms in common colds. Epidemiol Infect 1993; 111:143–156.
6. Johnston S, Holgate S. Epidemiology of viral respiratory infections. In: Myint S, Taylor-Robinson D, eds. Viral and Other Infections of the Human Respiratory Tract. London: Chapman & Hall, 1996:1–38.
7. Annual review and report. London: Proprietary Association of Great Britain (PAGB), 2002.
8. Loudon RG. Weather and cough. Am Rev Respir Dis 1963; 89:352–359.
9. Collier L, Oxford J. Human Virology. Oxford: Oxford University Press, 2000:231–232.
10. Smillie WG, Caldwell EL. A study of pneumonia in a rural area in southern Alabama. J Exp Med 1929; 50:233–244.
11. Lieberman D, Friger MD. Seasonal variation in hospital admissions for community-acquired pneumonia: a 5-year study. J Infect 1999; 39:134–140.
12. Alderson M. Season and mortality. Health Trends 1985; 17:87–96.
13. Hajat S, Haines A. Associations of cold temperatures with GP consultations for respiratory and cardiovascular disease amongst the elderly in London. Int J Epidemiol 2002; 31:825–830.
14. Curwen M. Excess winter mortality in England and Wales with special reference to the effects of temperature and influenza. In: Charlton J, Murphy M, eds. The Health of Adult Britain 1841–1994. Vol. 1. Chap. 13. London: The Stationery Office, 1997:205–216.
15. Stout R, Crawford V. Seasonal variations in fibrinogen concentrations among elderly people. Lancet 1991; 338:9–13.
16. Hill L, Clemen M. Common Colds, Causes and Preventive Measures. London: William Heinemann, 1929:126.
17. Eccles R. An explanation for the seasonality of acute upper respiratory tract viral infections. Acta Otolaryngol (Stockholm) 2002; 122:183–191.

18. Millqvist E, Bake B, Bengtsson U, Lowhagen O. A breathing filter exchanging heat and moisture prevents asthma induced by cold-air. Allergy 1995; 50: 225–228.

19. Millqvist E, Bake B, Bengtsson U, Lowhagen O. Prevention of asthma induced by cold-air by cellulose-fabric face mask. Allergy 1995; 50:221–224.

20. Hay AD, Wilson AD. The natural history of acute cough in children aged 0–4 years in primary care: a systematic review. Br J Gen Pract 2002; 52: 401–409.

21. Proctor DF. The upper airway. In: Proctor DF, Andersen I, eds. The Nose. Upper Airway Physiology and the Atmospheric Environment. Amsterdam: Elsevier, 1982:23–43.

22. Eccles R. Neurological and pharmacological considerations. In: Proctor DF, Andersen I, eds. The Nose, Upper Airways Physiology and the Atmospheric Environment. Amsterdam: Elsevier, 1982:191–214.

23. Widdicombe J. Reflexes from the upper respiratory tract. In: Cherniack N, Widdicombe J, eds. Hand Book of Physiology. The Respiratory System. Section 3. Chapter 11. Vol. II. Bethesda, MD: American Physiological Society, 1986:363–394.

24. Widdicombe J. Airway receptors. Respir Physiol 2001; 125:3–15.

25. Widdicombe J. Neuroregulation of cough: implications for drug therapy. Curr Opin Pharmacol 2002; 2:256–263.

26. Widdicombe JG. Neurophysiology of the cough reflex. Eur Respir J 1995; 8: 1103–1202.

27. Carr MJ, Ellis JL. The study of airway primary afferent neuron excitability. Curr Opin Pharmacol 2002; 2:216–219.

28. Spina D, Page CP. Pharmacology of airway irritability. Curr Opin Pharmacol 2002; 2:264–272.

29. Hwang SW, Oh U. Hot channels in airways: pharmacology of the vanilloid receptor. Curr Opin Pharmacol 2002; 2:235–242.

30. Netea MG, Kullberg BJ, Van der Meer JW. Circulating cytokines as mediators of fever. Clin Infect Dis 2000; 31(suppl 5):S178–S184.

31. Eccles R. Pathophysiology of nasal symptoms. Am J Rhinol 2000; 14:335–338.

32. Kharitonov SA, Yates D, Barnes PJ. Increased nitric oxide in exhaled air of normal human subjects with upper respiratory tract infections. Eur Respir J 1995; 8:295–297.

33. Ferguson EA, Eccles R, James A. Changes in upper and lower airway nitric oxide concentration associated with upper respiratory tract infection—a possible naso-bronchial link? J Physiol (Lond) 1997; 504:P203–P204.

34. Fleming DM. The management of influenza in people of working age. Occup Med (Lond) 2002; 52:259–263.

35. Ross A, Kai J, Ross J, Fleming D. Presentation with influenza-like illness in general practice: implications for use of neuraminidase inhibitors. Commun Dis Public Health 2000; 3:256–260.

36. Ma W, Eisenach JC. Morphological and pharmacological evidence for the role of peripheral prostaglandins in the pathogenesis of neuropathic pain. Eur J Neurosci 2002; 15:1037–1047.

37. Sperber SJ, Hendley JO, Hayden FG, Riker DK, Sorreentino JV, Gwaltney JM. Effects of naproxen on experimental rhinovirus colds. Ann Intern Med 1992; 117:37–41.

38. Fogari R, Zoppi A, Tettamanti F, Malamani GD, Tinelli C, Salvetti A. Effects of nifedipine and indomethacin on cough induced by angiotensin-converting enzyme inhibitors: a double-blind, randomized, cross-over study. J Cardiovasc Pharmacol 1992; 19:670–673.

39. Tenenbaum A, Grossman E, Shemesh J, Fisman EZ, Nosrati I, Motro M. Intermediate but not low doses of aspirin can suppress angiotensin-converting enzyme inhibitor-induced cough. Am J Hypertens 2000; 13:776–782.

40. Chung KF. Assessment and measurement of cough: the value of new tools. Pulm Pharmacol Ther 2002; 15:267–272.

41. Cross BA, Guz A, Jain SK, Archer S, Stevens J, Reynolds F. The effect of anaesthesia of the airway in dog and man: a study of respiratory reflexes, sensations and lung mechanics. Clin Sci Mol Med 1976; 50:439–454.

42. Karlsson JA. Airway anaesthesia and the cough reflex. Bull Eur Physiopathol Respir 1987; 23(suppl 10):29s–36s.

43. Fuller RW, Jackson DM. Physiology and treatment of cough. Thorax 1990; 45:425–430.

44. Choudry NB, Harrison AJ, Fuller RW. Inhibition of gustatory rhinorrhea by intranasal ipratropium bromide. Eur J Clin Pharmacol 1992; 42:561–562.

45. Kuhn JJ, Hendley O, Adams KF, Clark JW, Gwaltney JM. Antitussive effect of guaifenesin in young adults with natural colds. Chest 1982; 82:713–718.

46. Eccles R. Menthol and related cooling compounds. J Pharm Pharmacol 1994; 46:618–630.

47. Morice AH, Marshall AE, Higgins KS, Grattan TJ. Effect of inhaled menthol on citric acid induced cough in normal subjects. Thorax 1994; 49:1024–1026.

48. O'Connell F, Thomas VE, Studham JM, Pride NB, Fuller RW. Capsaicin cough sensitivity increases during upper respiratory infection. Respir Med 1996; 90:279–286.

49. Empey DW, Laitinen LA, Jacobs L, Gold WM, Nadel JA. Mechanisms of bronchial hyperreactivity in normal subjects after upper respiratory tract infection. Am Rev Respir Dis 1976; 113:131–139.

50. Lowry R, Wood A, Higenbottam T. The effect of anticholinergic bronchodilator therapy on cough during upper respiratory tract infections. Br J Clin Pharmacol 1994; 37:187–191.

51. Karlsson JA, Fuller RW. Pharmacological regulation of the cough reflex—from experimental models to antitussive effects in man. Pulm Pharmacol Ther 1999; 12:215–228.

52. Eddy NB, Friebel H, Hahn KJ, Halbach H. Codeine and its alternates for pain and cough relief. Bull World Health Organ 1969; 40:425–454.

53. Eccles R. Codeine, cough and upper respiratory infection. Pulm Pharmacol Ther 1996; 9:293–297.

54. Pavesi L, Subburaj S, Porter-Shaw K. Application and validation of a computerized cough acquisition system for objective monitoring of acute cough—a meta- analysis. Chest 2001; 120:1121–1128.

55. Lee PCL, Jawad MSM, Eccles R. Antitussive efficacy of dextromethorphan in cough associated with acute upper respiratory tract infection. J Pharm Pharmacol 2000; 52:1137–1142.

56. Eccles R. The powerful placebo. Pulm Pharmacol Ther 2002; 15:303–308.

57. Nishino T, Tagaito Y, Isono S. Cough and other reflexes on irritation of airway mucosa in man. Pulm Pharmacol Ther 1996; 9:285–292.

58. Curley FJ, Irwin RS, Pratter MR, Stivers DH, Doern GV, Vernaglia PA, Larkin AB, Baker SP. Cough and the common cold. Am Rev Respir Dis 1988; 138:305–311.

59. Lee P, Cotterill-Jones C, Eccles R. Voluntary control of cough. Pulm Pharmacol Ther 2002; 15:317–320.

60. Schroder K, Fahey T. Systematic review of randomised controlled trials of over the counter cough medicines for acute cough in adults. Br Med J 2002; 324:1–6.

13

Systematic Evaluation of Chronic Cough

CAROLINE F. EVERETT

Postgraduate Medical Institute, University of Hull, Castle Hill Hospital, Hull, U.K.

ALYN H. MORICE

Division of Academic Medicine, University of Hull, Hull, U.K.

Introduction

Chronic cough can be differentiated from acute cough by an arbitrary cutoff of 8 weeks (1). This distinction is helpful in clinical practice as the etiology and epidemiology of chronic cough are quite different from those of acute cough. However, when faced with a chronic cough patient, determining which of the possible underlying causes is to blame can be far from easy. Community-based data on chronic cough reveal a suboptimally managed population whose median duration of cough is 6.5 years, despite a high rate of medical consultations in both primary and secondary care (2). In contrast, data from specialist cough clinics, where a more systematic approach to diagnosis and management is usually employed, support very high treatment success rates (3). This is because cough may arise from anywhere along the distribution of the vagus nerve and therefore the possibility of disease in a variety of different systems must be considered in a logical and structured way. Indeed, one of the important reasons for misdiagnosis of chronic cough in both primary and secondary care is the failure to consider common extrapulmonary causes (4).

237

The difficulty in reaching a diagnosis is further exacerbated by the fact that the presentation of the underlying cause of chronic cough is often atypical. For example, it is not uncommon to encounter patients with cough-predominant asthma or with reflux-associated cough in whom obvious symptoms such as wheeze and heartburn are absent, although more subtle clues to diagnosis are often available in the history. The use of a systematic approach to the evaluation and management of chronic cough, which takes into account common causes such as asthma, gastroesophageal reflux, and rhinitis, will lead to a successful outcome in the vast majority of cases.

Anatomic Diagnostic Protocol

In 1981, Irwin et al. (5) published an "anatomic diagnostic" protocol for the investigation of chronic cough. This was based on the premise that investigations should be targeted to evaluate the known locations of receptors and afferent nerves of the cough reflex. Patients were initially assessed with a clinical history, physical examination, and chest radiograph followed by further investigations, such as blood count, pulmonary function tests, sinus imaging, sputum examination, bronchoscopy, and upper gastrointestinal studies as was clinically indicated. Diagnoses would then be confirmed according to symptomatic response to targeted therapy. This methodology was adopted by many specialist centers and the resulting reports in the literature certainly demonstrated much better success rates (3), in terms of diagnostic yield and treatment outcomes, than those from clinics which lacked a logical diagnostic pathway (4,6).

The precise methodology employed clearly has an important role to play in the eventual outcome of this type of investigational approach. Multiple causes of cough were found in more than 60% of subjects when a large number of diagnostic tests were performed (7), whereas this figure was reduced to 26% when investigations were tailored to the presenting symptoms (8). Indeed, several European centers, using a more conservative attitude to the investigational protocol, have established a single cause of chronic cough in over 89% of patients (9–11). This reduction in multiple diagnoses seems, however, to be associated with a concomitant increase in the number of patients with idiopathic cough, with diagnostic yields dropping as low as 82% when a more conservative approach is employed (9,12,13).

Since the anatomic diagnostic model was proposed, our knowledge of the conditions causing cough and the mechanisms by which the cough reflex is stimulated has evolved. Recently described causes of chronic cough, such as eosinophilic bronchitis (10,14) and esophageal dysmotility (15,16), may have been labeled as idiopathic in the past and it is likely that patients who are currently classified as having idiopathic cough actually have syndromes that are yet to be described. An updated management pathway for an investigational diagnostic protocol is presented in Fig. 1.

Clinical Protocol

More recently, a clinical approach to the diagnosis of chronic cough has been proposed. This has arisen out of the observation that many of the investigations employed do not accurately predict response to therapy. Indeed, the anatomic protocol requires that a diagnosis that is identified by an abnormal test result is confirmed by a positive response to specific therapy. In the case of gastroesophageal reflux-related cough, for example, positive 24 hr pH monitoring does not always predict a good response of the cough to antireflux therapy, nor does a negative test preclude it (16–18). For this reason an empirical trial of antireflux therapy has been advocated (19).

The clinical protocol for evaluation of chronic cough simply takes this pragmatic approach one step further by using trials of therapy rather than investigations to confirm the diagnosis, once a basic initial assessment with clinical history, physical examination, spirometry, and chest radiograph has been performed (Fig. 2). The aim is to accurately and successfully diagnose and treat chronic cough without resorting to large numbers of investigations, which can be expensive and sometimes uncomfortable for the patient. This protocol has been shown by Ojoo et al. (20) to result in successful management of the majority of patients, without resort to more detailed investigations.

Initial Clinical Assessment

A careful initial assessment is essential to the success of any schema for the evaluation of chronic cough. It should provide a reliable screening process for significant intrapulmonary pathology, such as lung cancer and interstitial lung disease, and should pick up the diagnostic clues necessary to guide further management. The main components of the initial assessment are listed below.

Clinical History

The most important component of the initial assessment is, without doubt, the clinical history. Carefully elicited, it may provide important diagnostic clues that will allow for targeted trials of therapy without the need for further investigation. As with any thorough history, details of respiratory symptoms and risk factors should be obtained. Any significant or worrying symptoms can then be investigated and managed as appropriate. What follows here is a summary of key aspects in the clinical history of chronic cough that aid diagnosis.

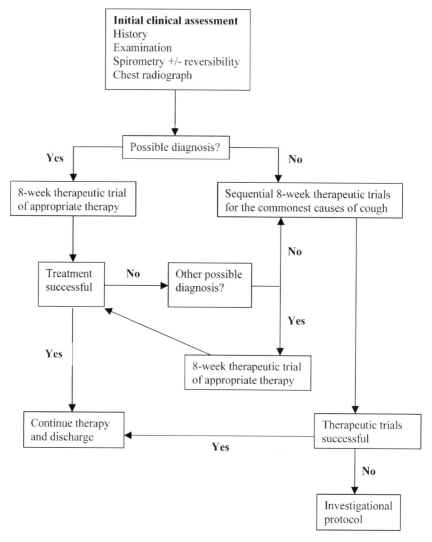

Figure 1   Investigative protocol management pathway.

Sputum production is a relatively common complaint in patients with chronic cough and this symptom should be explored in some depth before deciding on its clinical significance. Copious production of purulent or mucopurulent sputum may suggest bronchiectasis but other causes of cough may also present with phlegm. For example, patients with rhinosinusitis and postnasal drip may expectorate mucus that originates from the nose, not the bronchi. Those with gastroesophageal reflux-related cough

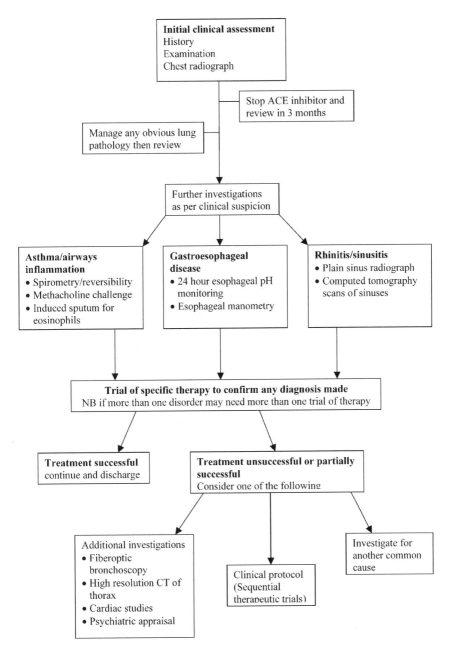

Figure 2 Clinical protocol management pathway.

often complain of one of two patterns of expectoration. Some patients describe moderate volumes of watery mucoid secretions, especially after a severe bout of coughing, which is probably a variation of "water-brash." Others complain of a sensation of thick mucus in the throat, which can only be expectorated in very small volumes and with great difficulty, if at all. This is a symptom of laryngeal inflammation associated with reflux and is often accompanied by persistent throat clearing.

Symptoms such as wheeze, dyspnea, and chest tightness are classical of asthma but may occur during a severe bout of coughing due to any cause. Therefore, they should be considered to be of greater diagnostic significance when they occur independently of the cough. In addition, one must bear in mind that certain forms of asthma, such as cough-predominant asthma and eosinophilic bronchitis, may occur in the absence of wheeze and breathlessness (10,21).

Similarly, when considering a diagnosis of reflux-related cough, symptoms of reflux into the distal esophagus such as heartburn and dyspepsia are helpful if present but do not exclude the diagnosis if absent (22). Chronic cough can also be caused by supra-esophageal reflux of gastric juices, often termed laryngopharyngeal reflux, which is characterized by symptoms of laryngeal irritation (23). These include hoarse voice, transient aphonia, globus (a sensation of a lump in the throat), and persistent throat clearing.

The third common cause of chronic cough is rhinosinusitis. This is suggested by symptoms of inflammation and/or infection in the nasal cavity and paranasal sinuses. These include nasal obstruction, congestion, rhinorrhea, anosmia, postnasal drip, and facial pain. Although cough can be the sole presenting symptom of both asthma and reflux, it is rare for rhinosinusitis to present without at least one of these typical symptoms.

In the many cases where more classical symptoms are absent, the most reliable way to distinguish a problem arising from the upper gastrointestinal tract from one due to airways inflammation is to take a history of the timing and precipitating factors of the cough. For example, reflux-related cough is more likely to occur in association with relaxation of the lower esophageal sphincter and knowledge of its physiology provides important clues to the diagnosis (24). Thus, cough during or shortly after meals or in association with eating certain foods such as chocolate or curry is often noted. It is useful to know that the sphincter also closes on recumbency at night, reopening to allow for belching on rising in the morning. Although some patients with reflux cough say that it is worse on first lying down, the majority are not woken from sleep by the cough once they have settled. This is one of the most useful ways in the history to distinguish between reflux and asthma. In asthma which is not optimally controlled, symptoms are often worse at night and in the early hours of the morning as we know from the diurnal variability of peak expiratory flow and "morning dipping," which is commonly seen. Cough that actually wakes the patient up, either during the night or in the morning, is therefore more likely to be due to one of the asthma syndromes. Conversely, patients who wake without cough in the morning and then start coughing on movement are more likely to have gastroesophageal reflux. This distinction is a subtle but important one as it can sometimes be the only reliable diagnostic clue available in the history. It is well worth pressing the patient to be very specific about the exact timing of cough symptoms in the mornings.

Another relatively common complaint is cough brought on by singing, laughing, or speaking. This is because the crural diaphragm forms part of the mechanism that maintains closure of the lower esophageal sphincter. Movement of the diaphragm during phonation can therefore disrupt the sphincter and cause reflux, which in turn triggers a cough. This phenomenon is often exacerbated by an increase in the intra-abdominal pressure and typically comes on when the patient is sitting talking, for example, on the telephone.

When discussing triggers for the cough it is common for factors such as exercise, smoky atmospheres, perfumes, and changing atmospheres to be identified. These types of stimuli are remarkably nonspecific when making a diagnosis, as they are simply mild causes of airway irritation. The sensitivity of the cough reflex is heightened in nearly all patients with chronic cough, regardless of the cause (11,25) They are therefore much more sensitive to these nonspecific stimuli than individuals with a normal cough reflex, possibly due to upregulation of the VR1 putative cough receptor (26).

In the drug history it is important to ask about angiotensin converting enzyme (ACE) inhibitor therapy. ACE inhibitors cause a dry cough in up to 15% of people. The cough may come on some time after commencing therapy and may take several months to resolve once it has been discontinued. This is because it acts by increasing the sensitivity of the cough reflex (27) and can take some time to alter. In addition, ACE inhibitors should be discontinued even in patients whose symptoms predate the start of therapy, because their effect on the cough reflex will only exacerbate any underlying mechanism for cough. Indeed, the patient may give a good history of reflux cough, which abates when the ACE inhibitor is withdrawn. Presumably, cough reflex upregulation by the ACE inhibitor causes previously subclinical reflux to become symptomatic.

Finally, it is useful to document some sort of measure of the severity of the cough when eliciting the history. This will help in judging the progress of symptoms and response to trials of therapy in the future. A simple and relatively sensitive way of doing this is to ask the patient to give the cough a score on a scale of nought to 10, where nought equates to "no symptoms" and 10 indicates "unbearable symptoms." Other symptoms, if present, can also give an indication of the severity of the cough. Paroxysms of coughing that induce cough syncope, incontinence, or vomiting are usually more severe than those that do not.

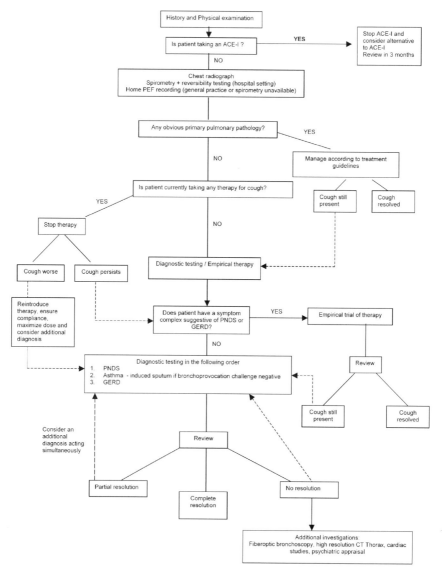

Figure 3 Combined investigative and clinical pathway as recommended by the European Respiratory Society Taskforce on Chronic Cough.

Physical Examination

Physical examination is usually unremarkable in patients with chronic cough, but is nevertheless important in ruling out significant pathology. Signs of airflow obstruction, digital clubbing, coarse crepitations, or wheeze may indicate an underlying cause, but in practice it is rare to find them. In rhinitis it may be possible to visualize a postnasal drip or a "cobblestone" appearance of the oropharyngeal mucosa but this is easier to appreciate with rhinoscopy. Similarly, if appropriate equipment is available to examine the larynx, signs of erythema, edema, or hypertrophy may indicate laryngopharyngeal reflux.

Chest Radiography

It is not unusual to find minor abnormalities on the chest radiograph in chronic cough patients as they do tend to represent an older population with mean age between 45 and 55 years (28). However, these do not usually add significantly to the diagnosis. Nevertheless, it is imperative that a plain chest radiograph is performed early in the evaluation of chronic cough as a screening tool for significant pathology, which requires a different management strategy.

Conclusion

The differential diagnosis of chronic cough is a wide-ranging one, spanning several different specialties of medicine. A systematic approach to evaluation of this common and debilitating symptom is therefore advocated in order that common causes are not missed. Whether one particular approach to diagnosis is superior to another is not clear. Indeed, the European Respiratory Society Taskforce on Chronic Cough has recommended a combination of investigative and clinical approaches (Fig. 3).

References

1. Morice AH. Epidemiology of cough. Pulm Pharmacol Ther 2002; 15:253–259.
2. Everett CF, Ojoo JC, Thompson RH, Morice AH. A questionnaire survey of individuals complaining of chronic cough (abstract). Am J Respir Crit Care Med 2003; 167:A316.
3. Morice AH, Kastelik JA. Chronic cough in adults. Thorax 2003; 58:901–907.
4. McGarvey LPA, Heaney LG, MacMahon J. A retrospective survey of diagnosis and management of patients presenting with chronic cough to a general chest clinic. Int J Clin Pract 1998; 52:158–161.
5. Irwin RS, Corrao WM, Pratter MR. Chronic persistent cough in the adult: the spectrum and frequency of causes and successful outcome of specific therapy. Am Rev Respir Dis 1981; 123:413–417.
6. Puolijoki H, Lahdensuo A. Causes of prolonged cough in patients referred to a chest clinic. Ann Med 1989; 21:425–427.
7. Palombini BC, Villanova CA, Araújo E, et al. A pathogenic triad in chronic cough: asthma, postnasal drip syndrome, and gastroesophageal reflux disease. Chest 1999; 116:279–284.

8. Irwin RS, Curley FJ, French CL. Chronic cough. The spectrum and frequency of causes, key components of the diagnostic evaluation, and outcome of specific therapy. Am Rev Respir Dis 1990; 141:640–647.
9. Marchesani F, Cecarini L, Pela R, Sanguinetti CM. Causes of chronic persistent cough in adult patients: the results of a systematic management protocol. Monaldi Arch Chest Dis 1998; 53:510–514.
10. Brightling CE, Ward R, Goh KL, Wardlaw AJ, Pavord ID. Eosinophilic bronchitis is an important cause of chronic cough. Am J Respir Crit Care Med 1999; 160:406–410.
11. O'Connell F, Thomas VE, Pride NB, Fuller RW. Capsaicin cough sensitivity decreases with successful treatment of chronic cough. Am J Respir Crit Care Med 1994; 150:374–380.
12. Poe RH, Harder RV, Israel RH, Kallay MC. Chronic persistent cough. Experience in diagnosis and outcome using an anatomic diagnostic protocol. Chest 1989; 95:723–728.
13. McGarvey LP, Heaney LG, Lawson JT, et al. Evaluation and outcome of patients with chronic non-productive cough using a comprehensive diagnostic protocol. Thorax 1998; 53:738–743.
14. Fujimura M, Ogawa H, Yasui M, Matsuda T. Eosinophilic tracheobronchitis and airway cough hypersensitivity in chronic non-productive cough. Clin Exp Allergy 2000; 30:41–47.
15. Fouad YM, Katz PO, Hatlebakk JG, Castell DO. Ineffective esophageal motility: the most common motility abnormality in patients with GERD-associated respiratory symptoms. Am J Gastroenterol 1999; 94:1464–1467.
16. Kastelik JA, Redington AE, Aziz I, et al. Abnormal oesophageal motility in patients with chronic cough. Thorax 2003; 58:699–702.
17. Ours TM, Kavuru MS, Schilz RJ, Richter JE. A prospective evaluation of esophageal testing and a double-blind, randomized study of omeprazole in a diagnostic and therapeutic algorithm for chronic cough. Am J Gastroenterol 1999; 94:3131–3138.
18. Kiljander TO, Salomaa ER, Hietanen EK, Terho EO. Chronic cough and gastro-oesophageal reflux: a double-blind placebo-controlled study with omeprazole. Eur Respir J 2000; 16:633–638.
19. Irwin RS, Madison JM. The diagnosis and treatment of cough. N Engl J Med 2000; 343:1715–1721.
20. Ojoo JC, Mulrennan SA, Kastelik JA, Thompson R, Redington AE, Morice AH. Utility of history in the diagnosis of chronic cough (abstract). Thorax 2002; 57(Suppl 3):iii72.
21. Corrao WM, Braman SS, Irwin RS. Chronic cough as the sole presenting manifestation of bronchial asthma. N Engl J Med 1979; 300:633–637.
22. Irwin RS, Zawacki JK, Curley FJ, French CL, Hoffman PJ. Chronic cough as the sole presenting manifestation of gastroesophageal reflux. Am Rev Respir Dis 1989; 140:1294–1300.
23. Belafsky PC, Postma GN, Koufman JA. Validity and reliability of the reflux symptom index (RSI). J Voice 2002; 16:274–277.
24. Mittal RK, Balaban DH. The esophagogastric junction. N Engl J Med 1997; 336:924–932.

25. Kastelik JA, Thompson RH, Aziz I, Ojoo JC, Redington AE, Morice AH. Sex-related differences in cough reflex sensitivity in patients with chronic cough. Am J Respir Crit Care Med 2002; 166:961–964.
26. Trevisani M, Milan A, Gatti R, et al. Iodo-resiniferatoxin is a potent antitussive drug in guinea pigs. Thorax 2004; 59:769–772.
27. Morice AH, Lowry R, Brown MJ, Higenbottam T. Angiotensin converting enzyme and the cough reflex. Lancet 1987; 2:1116–1118.
28. Morice AH. Epidemiology of cough. In: Chung KF, Widdicombe JG, Boushey HA, eds. Cough: Causes, Mechanisms and Therapy. 1st ed. Oxford: Blackwell Publishing, 2003:11–16.
29. Morice AH, et al. European Respiratory Society Task Force: The diagnosis and management of chronic cough. Eur Respir J. 2004; 24:481–492.

14

The Pathogenesis of Cough in Gastroesophageal Reflux Disease

ALVIN J. ING

University of Sydney, Concord Hospital,
Concord, New South Wales, Australia

Gastroesophageal Reflux

The primary event in gastroesophageal reflux (GER) is the movement of acid, pepsin, and other noxious substances from the stomach into the esophagus (1). In healthy individuals, reflux is a normal, mostly asymptomatic event. Gastroesophageal reflux disease (GERD) is defined as occurring when reflux leads to symptoms or physical complications. In most patients this occurs when there is excessive exposure of the distal esophageal mucosa to refluxed gastric contents resulting in heartburn, epigastric or retrosternal discomfort, and chest pain (2). Prolonged exposure can lead to esophagitis, esophageal ulceration and its complications such as bleeding or stricture formation. However, esophageal reflux symptoms can also occur without esophagitis, and there can be significant reflux without classical symptoms (3).

GER has long been associated with pulmonary symptoms and diseases, many of which present with cough. These range from bronchopulmonary dysplasia in the newborn, bronchial asthma, chronic persistent cough, chronic bronchitis, and diffuse pulmonary fibrosis, through to the pulmonary aspiration syndromes, including lung abscess, bronchiectasis, aspiration pneumonitis, recurrent pneumonia, and eventually respiratory failure (4). Pulmonary complications may result from either direct micro- and/or macroaspiration, as well as from both local and centrally mediated reflex mechanisms.

As a cause of chronic cough, GERD has been documented in many series to be one of the most common etiologies across all age groups (5–7).

The Normal Antireflux Barrier

The lower esophageal sphincter (LES), crural diaphragm, and the phreno-esophageal ligament are considered to be the anatomic structures that play a major role in the normal antireflux barrier (1). The intraluminal pressure at the gastroesophageal junction reflects the strength of the antireflux barrier, and reflux occurs only when this pressure is reduced.

The LES is 2.5–3.5 cm in length, and is probably part intra-abdominal and part intrathoracic. It consists of a zone of thickened muscle with evidence of higher neuronal density than that of the adjacent esophagus in animals. The end-expiratory pressure at the gastroesophageal junction at rest is due to the smooth muscle activity of the LES, but the LES pressure can also fluctuate with the migrating motor activity of the stomach. The circular muscle of the LES can generate tonic activity, which is influenced by neurogenic, hormonal, and myogenic factors (8,9).

The crural diaphragm, phrenooesophageal ligament, and LES form an anatomical and physiological antireflux barrier which prevents GER under both resting conditions and when increased intra-abdominal pressure occurs. The transdiaphragmatic pressure (Pdi) or the pressure difference between the stomach and the esophagus is +4–6 mmHg during tidal volume expiration, while it is +10–18 mmHg during tidal volume inspiration. During maximal inspiratory effort, e.g., to total lung capacity, the Pdi can reach values of 60–80 mm Hg (1). However, GER does not result from raised transdiaphragmatic pressure alone. This is because as Pdi increases during inspiration, esophagogastric junction pressure increases due to contraction of the crural diaphragm. For GER to occur, therefore, there must be significant defects in the normal antireflux barrier since increases in Pdi and intra-abdominal pressure are effectively counteracted by intact antireflux mechanisms.

Pathogenesis of Gastroesophageal Reflux Disease

It is currently thought that LES dysfunction is the major cause of defective gastroesophageal competence and thus reflux, with nonsphincteric mechanisms having a secondary role (2). The majority of patients with GERD have normal basal LES tone. Reflux occurs, however, because of transient relaxation of this tone, a phenomenon termed transient LES relaxation (TLESR) by Dent and colleagues (10).

Simultaneous measurements of esophageal pH and motility have shown that, under resting conditions, LES sphincter pressure has to be absent for reflux to occur in normal subjects, and both adults and children with reflux (10–12). In the majority of reflux episodes this is due to TLESR, with only a minority of episodes due to chronic absence of LES pressure or reduced basal LES tone. TLESR is likely to be neurally (vagally) mediated, and triggered by gastric distension, and perhaps pharyngeal activity (13). There are also nonsphincteric factors related to occurrence of pathological GER. Of particular interest in patients with chronic persistent cough is increased Pdi during the inspiratory phase of cough, and raised intra-abdominal pressure during the compressive and expiratory phases of cough. In healthy subjects, increased Pdi provokes GER only if basal LES pressure is less than or equal to 4 mm Hg (14), normal resting pressure being 10–26 mmHg. Reflux was not demonstrated when LES was normal, and only occurred in the presence of raised Pdi when there was TLESR or swallowing (10).

Reduced basal LES tone is unusual in patients with chronic cough, but has been documented. Tomonaga et al. (15) found that 16 (12%) of 133 patients with upper respiratory symptoms, including cough, and GER symptoms had proximal reflux and reduced basal LES pressures. Nocturnal cough predicted proximal acid reflux on dual-probe esophageal pH monitoring and reduced basal LES tone. However, these patients were in the minority and most patients with cough and GER had distal reflux only and normal basal LES tone.

The relationship between cough and esophageal reflux, with regards to mechanisms by which cough may aggravate or precipitate reflux episodes, has not been fully studied. There is no doubt that raised Pdi occurs as a result of chronic cough, but this alone is not sufficient to produce reflux on a background of normal basal LES tone (1,10). Possible mechanisms by which cough may precipitate reflux includes cough stimulating either TLESR or swallow-induced sphincter relaxation. As yet neither has been proven although some animal studies are suggestive. Autonomic dysfunction may also play a role and has been reported in patients with bronchial asthma (16). However, this has not been investigated in patients with unexplained chronic persistent cough.

The Role of Gastroesophageal Reflux in the Pathogenesis of Cough

Chronic persistent cough has been the most widely studied entity when investigating the role of GERD in the pathogenesis of cough. It is defined as cough persisting for at least 3 weeks, in patients with a normal chest x-ray and not on angiotensin converting enzyme inhibitors (17). In multiple series, GER has been documented to be a cause of chronic persistent cough (either solely or in combination with bronchial asthma and postnasal drip) in 38–82% of patients (3,5–7,17–20). GERD, bronchial asthma, and postnasal drip account either singly or in combination for over 90% of patients with chronic persistent cough.

Chronic cough secondary to GER has been associated with a wide range of disease entities. These may be categorized based on the pathogenesis of the cough.

Aspiration of Gastric Contents

Aspiration implies that a significant volume of gastric refluxate ascends past the proximal esophagus, penetrates the larynx, and enters the tracheobronchial tree. Aspiration has been considered a likely mechanism in a number of pulmonary pathologies associated with cough, including recurrent aspiration pneumonia, pulmonary abscess, bronchiectasis (21), pulmonary fibrosis including idiopathic pulmonary fibrosis (IPF), and progressive systemic sclerosis (22–26), and obliterative bronchiolitis in heart lung transplant recipients (27). However, studies accurately assessing the presence and degree of gastric refluxate in the tracheobronchial tree have been lacking. Most studies assessing the role of aspiration of gastric contents have looked at surrogate markers of aspiration. These include proximal esophageal pH monitoring, assessment of esophageal motility and the presence of hiatus hernia. Tobin et al. (23), for example, performed proximal and distal esophageal pH monitoring in patients with IPF and in patients with interstitial lung disease as a result of other etiologies (including sarcoidosis and systemic lupus erythematosis). They found that patients with IPF had a higher prevalence of both distal and proximal esophageal acid exposure times. This implies that aspiration may be important in the pathogenesis of IPF but no direct measurements of acid or pepsin were taken from the tracheobronchial tree.

In patients with chronic persistent cough, initial studies have shown that cough correlates with and has a temporal association with distal esophageal reflux but not proximal reflux (3,18). However, in a more recent study, Tomonaga et al. (15) performed 24 hr esophageal pH monitoring with proximal and distal pH probes, as well as manometric measurements of the upper and lower esophageal sphincters. In 133 patients they found that 79 (59%) had no acid reflux, 38 (29%) had distal acid reflux and 16 (12%) had evidence of proximal acid reflux as well. The authors found that nocturnal cough predicted proximal reflux, suggesting that nocturnal cough implied more severe GERD including reduced basal LES tone and aspiration. Previous studies (3,18) have found that proximal reflux and nocturnal cough in patients with chronic persistent cough and proven GER was unusual and that the normal reflex which increases basal LES tone when in the supine position was generally maintained (Fig. 1) (18). However, the study of Tomonaga et al. suggests that proximal reflux and by implication aspiration may occur in a minority of patients.

Reflex Mechanisms

Vagally mediated distal esophageal–tracheobronchial reflex mechanisms have been documented in patients with chronic persistent cough with otherwise asymptomatic reflux (28) and in patients with bronchial asthma (29).

In patients with chronic persistent cough whose cough is unexplained after a standard diagnostic evaluation, including history and examination, chest x-ray, laryngoscopy, paranasal sinus x-rays, lung function testing, bronchial provocation testing, and home peak flow monitoring, cough is commonly associated with GER (17). In this setting, cough has been shown to be a result of gastric acid stimulating a distal esophageal–tracheobronchial reflex mechanism with little evidence of microaspiration or proximal esophageal reflux (28,30). In 22 patients with chronic persistent cough and proven GER on esophageal pH testing, Ing et al. (28) performed distal esophageal acid testing using 0.1 M HCl in a randomized blinded controlled fashion. Compared with control subjects, patients experienced a significantly greater number of coughs, increased cough amplitude, and decreased cough latency. This cough was inhibited by the esophageal instillation of local anesthetic (4% topical lidocaine), and by nebulized ipratropium bromide (28). The authors concluded that a distal esophageal–tracheobronchial reflex mechanism was likely to exist with the afferent pathway originating from acid sensitive esophageal receptors (and inhibited by lidocaine), and the efferent pathway being inhibited by ipratropium bromide. This reflex arc was considered the likely mechanism by which GER leads to cough in patients with chronic persistent cough, although intraoesophageal acid may not be the sole mediator (30).

The nature of this reflex arc has not been fully elucidated in patients with cough, although in patients with bronchial asthma, there is evidence that GER may initiate airway inflammation from the esophagus via axonal reflexes (31). Axonal reflexes are mediated by nociceptive afferent nerves that release neurotransmitters which act to trigger an inflammatory response. Tachykinins including substance P and neurokinin A are associated with nociceptive afferent nerves and are potent mediators of bronchospasm and mucus secretion. Whether local axonal reflexes such as this have a role in the pathogenesis of cough associated with GER is unknown, although it is likely to play a role in the development of cough secondary to GER in patients with asthma.

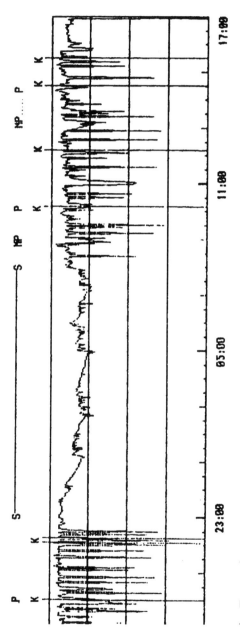

Figure 1 Twenty-four-hour ambulatory distal esophageal pH monitoring in a patient with chronic persistent cough. Lack of acid reflux in the supine position is demonstrated. *Y* axis, esophageal pH; *X* axis, time over 24 hr. *Abbreviations:* S, supine position; K, cough event. (From Ref. 18.)

There is also growing evidence that central reflexes may be important in the pathogenesis of GER-induced cough in patients with chronic persistent cough. An animal model has been developed using Wistar rats, showing that stimulation of the esophagus by acid and pepsin resulted in an increase in c-Fos immunoreactvity in brainstem regions (32). In a randomized controlled fashion, Suwanprathes and colleagues (32) perfused the oesophagus of 10 rats with 0.1M HCl and pepsin (3200–4500 IU/ml). The brainstem was then processed immunohistochemically for detection of c-Fos protein, an immediate-early gene with low basal central nervous system (CNS) expression, which is detected maximally in CNS neurons 30–45 min after stimulation. This study found that c-Fos immunoreactivity was significantly increased in a number of brainstem regions in rats including the nucleus of the solitary tract, medial part (mNTS), Kolliker–Fuse nucleus (KF), central amygdala nucleus (CeC), nucleus ambiguus (Amb), retroambiguus nucleus (ra) and paratrigeminal nucleus (PTN). These areas represent the dorsomedial medulla (mNTS), dorsolateral medulla (PTN), ventrolateral medulla (Amb and RA), and forebrain (CeC). Other studies have found that vagal efferent pathways originate from the RA and Amb, and that the PTN is the initial processing center for afferent signals, with a subpopulation of secondary neurons projecting onto the NTS and then the RA and Amb which possibly represent the cough efferent center. These studies therefore suggest that acid and pepsin in the distal esophagus may stimulate afferent pathways which project to the brainstem "cough center" (including the PTN, NTS, Amb, and RA), which in turn may activate srinicough efferent pathways (Fig. 2). The applicability of this in humans remains unknown. However, this animal model may be invaluable in assessing the efficacy of antitussive agents, particularly those with purported central mechanisms of action.

Cough Threshold and Responsiveness

Cough responsiveness as measured by capsaicin testing has also been found to be increased in patients with GERD. Wu et al. (33) performed distal esophageal acid perfusion testing with 0.1 M HCl and capsaicin challenge testing in seven patients with bronchial asthma. Cough responsiveness as measured by the lowest concentration of capsaicin eliciting three coughs (PD$_3$) significantly increased during periods of distal esophageal HCl perfusion when compared with saline perfusion (Fig. 3). There were no changes in FEV$_1$, FVC, or PEF. Wu et al. concluded that GER may increase cough responsiveness in asthmatic patients via reflex mechanisms, and that this may occur without demonstrable changes in lung function. This, however, has not been shown yet in patients with chronic persistent cough without bronchial asthma.

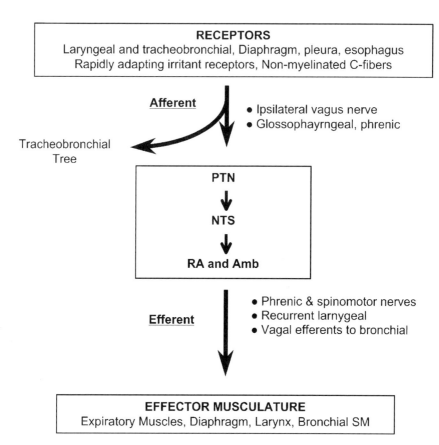

Figure 2 Anatomy of the cough reflex incorporating central pathways. *Abbreviations*: PTN, paratrigeminal nucleus; NTS, nucleus, solitary tract; RA, retro-ambiguus nucleus; Amb: nucleus ambiguous.

Benini et al. (34) studied 21 patients with reflux esophagitis, who were nonsmokers. Patients underwent esophageal pH monitoring, manometry, endoscopy, laryngoscopy, methacholine challenge, and capsaicin challenge. Cough responsiveness was measured by the dose of inhaled capsaicin producing five coughs (PD_5) and was determined at baseline, after five days of omeprazole therapy, and when esophageal and laryngeal damage had healed. In all 21 patients, baseline spirometry and methacholine challenge testing were normal. Thirteen patients had posterior laryngitis and eight had cough. Twenty patients showed enhanced cough responsiveness, which improved both after 5 and 60 days of antireflux therapy. The severity of esophagitis did not influence PD_5, and the improvement in cough threshold (decreased responsiveness) was greater in patients with proven laryngitis.

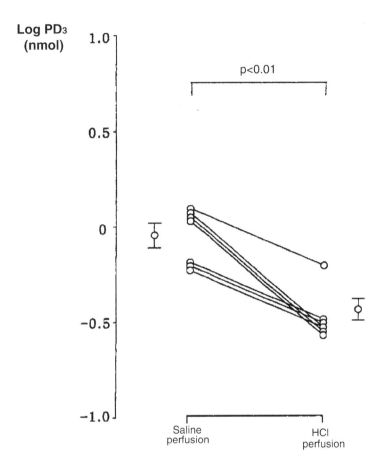

Figure 3 Changes in cough responsiveness (PD$_3$) to inhaled capsaicin during distal esophageal saline or HCl perfusion in patients with asthma. (From Ref. 33).

Benini et al. (34) concluded that patients with GERD and reflux esophagitis had decreased cough threshold and this was related to laryngeal inflammation but not severity of esophagitis. Omeprazole improved respiratory and GERD symptoms as well as cough threshold.

Both Wu et al. (33) and Benini et al. (34) studies reveal that GER may decrease cough threshold and increase cough responsiveness. Wu et al.'s paper suggests that this is via reflex mechanisms, and Benini et al.'s paper suggests it is via aspiration (micro or macro) and laryngeal inflammation. There is thus evidence to suggest that no matter what the predominant mechanism by which GER is involved in the pathogenesis of cough, it is responsible for increasing cough responsiveness. This could be via either reflex mechanisms (the likely majority of patients with chronic cough), aspiration, and direct mucosal injury to the upper respiratory tract, or a combination of both.

Further evidence that laryngeal pathology may be important in a minority of patients with chronic persistent cough and GER is found in research utilizing the technique of fiberoptic endoscopic evaluation of swallowing with sensory testing (FEESST). Utilizing measured air pulses delivered onto the arytenoid cartilage during nasolaryngoscopy, researchers (35–37) have used the induced laryngeal adductor reflex (LAR) to reflect laryngeal sensitivity. In normal subjects an air pressure pulse of 2.5–4.0 mmHg will elicit the LAR, a transient adduction of the true vocal cords. However, in patients with proven GERD, including proven proximal acid reflux on dual-probe pH testing, air pressures of >9.0 mmHg are often required to elicit the same reflex. These findings imply that in patients with proximal GER and laryngeal involvement laryngeal sensitivity is impaired and the risk of aspiration is significantly increased.

Autonomic Dysfunction

TLESR accounts for the majority of acid reflux episodes in patients with chronic persistent cough (2,10,11). These are vagally mediated and are influenced by numerous factors including drugs, pharyngeal activity, esophageal motility, and gastric emptying. TLESR is also influenced by autonomic neural activity and a number of authors have investigated the role of autonomic function in patients with cough.

Lodi et al. (38) investigated 15 nonsmoking asthmatic patients with proven GER and compared results to 23 age-matched control subjects. All patients and control subjects underwent autonomic function testing including heart rate and blood pressure measurements during an 80° passive tilt, Valsalva maneuver, quiet and deep breathing, handgrip, and an echo stress test of cortical arousal. Each autonomic function test was analyzed and defined as normal, hypervagal, hyperadrenergic, or mixed (a combination of hypervagal and hyperadrenergic responses). All asthmatics with GER had at least one autonomic function test display a hypervagal response. Overall, eight of 15 patients had a predominant hypervagal response, and seven had a mixed response. Of the seven who had a mixed response score, two had a hypervagal predominant response. Lodi et al. concluded that asthmatics with GER have evidence of autonomic dysfunction and that heightened vagal tone may be partially responsible for the heightened airway responsiveness to esophageal acidification in asthmatics with reflux.

The implication from this study is that a hypervagal response may have a role in influencing control of TLESR, and may potentially worsen GERD if increased TLESR is a result of autonomic dysfunction. This study has not been repeated in patients with chronic cough without asthma, however, and the role of asthma and cough in the pathogenesis of autonomic dysfunction has not been investigated.

The role of autonomic dysfunction in the pathogenesis of chronic persistent cough and GER has also been raised in a recent report of a new syndrome, hereditary sensory neuropathy type I (HSN I) with cough and GER (39,40). Kok et al. (39) have described a new form of HSN I associated with cough and GER with a locus on chromosome 3p22–p24pHSN I has autosomal dominant inheritance and two large families with HSN I associated with GER induced cough are described (Fig. 4). Eight members (of 27) from the first family and two members (of 11) from the second family were classified as affected. Linkage to chromosome 3p22–p24 has been found in both families with no evidence for linkage to other known loci for HSN I. These families represent a genetically novel variant of HSN 1, with cough and GER as predominant features.

Affected individuals presented initially with paroxysmal cough, with half having cough syncope. The mean age of onset of cough was 30.5

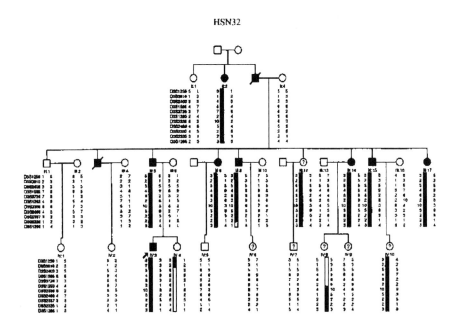

Figure 4 Haplotype analysis of markers from chromosome 3p22–p24 in family HSN32 with autosomal dominant HSN 1 with cough and GER. The haplotype segregating with the disease is indicated (*blackened bar*). The markers are presented in order from telomere (*top*) to centromere (*bottom*). Blackened symbols denote affected individuals, unblackened symbols denote unaffected individuals, and individuals with unknown clinical status are denoted by a question mark. (From Ref. 39).

(10.0) years, whereas the mean onset of sensory neuropathy symptoms was 47.7 (12.8) years. All affected individuals had abnormal 24 hr ambulatory esophageal pH monitoring, with evidence of distal reflux and a temporal association between cough and acid reflux episodes. Three patients had evidence of proximal acid reflux, and this correlated with abnormal FEESST findings, laryngeal inflammation and a hoarse voice. Half of affected individuals also had sensorineural hearing loss, and all had sensory axonal neuropathy on nerve conduction studies. Autonomic function and sweat testing revealed a number of abnormalities including distal hypohidrosis, decreased sweating in the upper limbs, absent sympathetic skin response, and peripheral adrenergic impairment. Overall, five of 10 affected individuals tested had abnormalities of autonomic function, although none had evidence of gastroparesis. Esophageal manometry revealed abnormal esophageal motility in four of five patients tested.

These studies describe a rare syndrome, but the onset of cough many years prior to the onset of neuropathic symptoms is intriguing. It is likely that GER is important in the pathogenesis of the cough given its presence in all patients, and the documented temporal relationship. It appears that reflex mechanisms are more likely to be important than aspiration in the development of cough but, as in chronic persistent cough not associated with HSN I, aspiration is likely to have some role in a minority of patients. What is more difficult to explain, however, is the role of HSN I in the development of GER and cough. There are abnormalities of esophageal motility present, but these are often seen as a result of GERD and may reflect this rather than being a cause of GERD (41). Moreover, esophageal motility was not abnormal in all patients. Gastroparesis was not present, and other abnormalities of autonomic function were minor only. All hemodynamic measurements were normal.

Kok et al.'s paper (39) thus highlights the importance of GER in the pathogenesis of chronic cough, but remains unclear on the role of autonomic dysfunction and its effect on TLESR.

Esophageal Motility

Patients with chronic persistent cough and proven GER have been found to have esophageal motility abnormalities of varying severity. Ing et al. (41) described impaired esophageal clearance of acid in such patients and raised the likelihood that such abnormalities may increase the distal esophageal acid exposure time, and thus increase mucosal abnormalities that may increase cough responsiveness via reflex mechanisms. Subsequent research (42) has revealed that patients with chronic cough had increased abnormal esophageal motility, including increased retrograde contractions and nonpropulsive contractions. Kastelik et al. (43) performed esophageal manometry and 24 hr esophageal pH monitoring in 43 patients with chronic cough, 34 of whom had symptoms of GERD. Results were compared with 21 healthy subjects. Nine patients had normal manometry and pH monitoring, 11 (32%) had abnormal manometry alone, 5 (15%) had abnormal pH monitoring alone, and 18 (53%) had both tests abnormal. Only one control subject had abnormal esophageal manometry. Kastelik et al. concluded that there was a high prevalence of abnormal esophageal manometry in patients with chronic cough, and that esophageal dysmotility may be important in the pathogenesis of cough.

The important finding in this study is that abnormal esophageal motility was documented in some patients with chronic cough without GER. This implies that motility abnormalities may be independent of GERD and may be important in the pathogenesis of GERD rather than just being a result of it. The implications of this are potentially far reaching. In patients with chronic cough and esophageal dysmotility without GER, dysmotility may be a result of cough, given that cough has been associated with increased swallowing and increased swallow-related LES relaxation (42,44,45). The potential role of autonomic dysfunction in the pathogenesis of esophageal dysmotility also needs further investigation. In turn, esophageal dysmotility may lead to abnormalities in TLESR and/or basal LES tone completing a cough–reflux feedback cycle.

The Cough–Reflux Self-Perpetuating Cycle (Fig. 5)

GER may precipitate cough via the mechanisms described in the preceding text. These include local and central reflex mechanisms and aspiration. A number of investigators have proposed a self-perpetuating positive feedback cycle between cough and esophageal reflux, whereby cough from any cause may precipitate further reflux (17,18,46). The mechanisms by which GER is worsened or triggered by cough are still being elucidated. However, the role of cough in TLESR, autonomic dysfunction, and esophageal dysmotility may be important. Evidence for the existence of this cycle is found in studies showing that the antitussive action of antireflux therapy is prolonged and is present long after the antireflux therapy is ceased (42,46). The other implication of this cycle is that chronic cough from whatever cause may trigger GER, and that therapy for GER may be required for refractory cough even if other specific etiologies are identified (17).

Summary

- GERD is one of the three most common causes of chronic persistent cough.
- TLESR is the most common reason for defective gastroesophageal competence and thus development of GER. Reduced basal LES

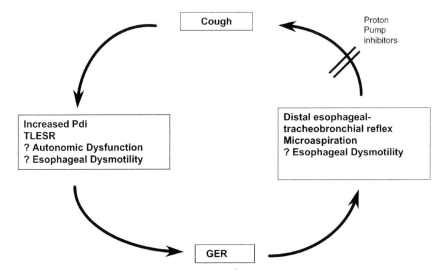

Figure 5   Cough–reflux positive feedback cycle.

tone does occur but is less common and is usually associated with proximal reflux and more severe GERD.

- GERD most commonly precipitates cough via reflex mechanisms that have local and central projections.
- GERD may less commonly trigger chronic cough via aspiration of gastric contents, and this is usually associated with nocturnal cough, proximal acid reflux, laryngeal inflammation, and impaired laryngeal sensitivity.
- GERD may result in increased cough responsiveness and decreased cough threshold as a result of both reflex mechanisms and aspiration.
- Patients with chronic cough may have autonomic dysfunction, but it remains unclear as to whether cough is causal, or if autonomic dysfunction is important in the pathogenesis of GERD.
- A cough–reflux positive feedback cycle is likely to exist whereby cough from any cause may precipitate GERD. The mechanism remains uncertain, but esophageal motility disorders and increased TLESR may be important.

References

1. Mittal RK. Current concepts of the antireflux barrier. Gastroenterol Clin North Am 1990; 19:501–517.

2. Dent J. Recent views on the pathogenesis of gastro-oesophageal reflux disease. Bailliere's Clin Gastroenterol 1987; 1(4):727–745.
3. Irwin RS, Zawacki JK, Curley FJ, French CL, Hoffman PJ. Chronic cough as the sole presenting manifestation of gastroesophageal reflux. Am Rev Respir Dis 1989; 140:1294–1300.
4. Mansfield LE. Gastro-esophageal reflux and respiratory disorders: a review. Ann Allergy 1989; 62:158–163.
5. Irwin RS, Curley FJ, French CL. Chronic cough. The spectrum and frequency of causes, key components of the diagnostic evaluation, and outcome of specific therapy. Am Rev Respir Dis 1990; 141:640–647.
6. Palombi BC, Villanova CAC, Araújo E, Gastal OL, Alt DC, Stolz DP, Palombini CO. A pathogenic triad in chronic cough: asthma, postnasal drip syndrome, and gastroesophageal reflux disease. Chest 1999; 116:279–284.
7. McGarvey LP, Forsythe P, Heaney LG, McMahon J, Ennis M. Bronchoalveolar lavage findings in patients with chronic nonproductive cough. Eur Respir J 1999; 13:59–65.
8. Liebermann-Meffert D, Allgower M, Schmid P. Muscular equivalent of the lower esophageal sphincter. Gastroenterology 1979; 76:31–38.
9. Tottrup A, Forman A, Uldbjerg N, et al. Mechanical properties of isolated human esophageal smooth muscle. Am J Physiol 1990; 21:G329–G337.
10. Dent J, Dodds WJ, Friedman RH, et al. Mechanisms of gastroesophageal reflux in recumbent asymptomatic human subjects. J Clin Invest 1980; 65:256–267.
11. Mittal RK, McCallum RW. Characteristics of transient lower esophageal sphincter relaxation in humans. Am J Physiol 1987; 252:G636–G641.
12. Dent J, Holloway RH, Toouli J, Dodds WJ. Mechanisms of lower oesophageal sphincter incompetence in patients with symptomatic gastro-oesophageal reflux. Gut 1988; 29:1020–1028.
13. Holloway RH, Dent J. Pathophysiology of gastroesophageal reflux: lower esophageal sphincter dysfunction in gastroesophageal reflux disease. Gastroenterol Clin North Am 1990; 19:571–535.
14. Stanciu C, Bennett JR. Esophageal acid clearing. One factor in production of reflux oesophagitis. Gut 1974; 15:852–857.
15. Tomonaga T, Awad ZT, Filipi CJ, Hinder RA, Selima M, Tercero F Jr, Marsh RE, Shiino Y, Welch R. Symptom predictability of reflux-induced respiratory disease. Dig Dis Sci 2002; 47:9–14.
16. Lodi U, Harding SM, Coghlan HC, Guzzo NR, Walker LH. Autonomic regulation in asthmatics with gastroesophageal reflux. Chest 1997; 111:65–70.
17. Managing cough as a defense mechanism and as a symptom—a consensus panel report of the American College of Chest Physicians. Chest 1998; 114:133S–181S.
18. Ing AJ, Ngu MC, Breslin ABX. Chronic persistent cough and gastro-oesophageal reflux. Thorax 1991; 46:479–483.
19. Irwin RS, Corrao WM, Pratter MR. Chronic persistent cough in the adult. The spectrum and frequency of causes and successful outcome of specific therapy. Am Rev Respir Dis 1981; 123:413–417.

20. Poe RH, Harder RV, Israel RH, Kallay MC. Chronic persistent cough: experience in diagnosis and outcome using an anatomic diagnostic protocol. Chest 1989; 95:723–728.
21. Pasteur MC, Helliwell SM, Houghton SJ, Webb SC, Foweraker JE, Coulden RA, Flower CD, Bilton D, Keogan MT. An investigation into causative factors in patients with bronchiectasis. Am J Respir Crit Care Med 2000; 162: 1277–1284.
22. Mays EE, Dubois JJ, Hamilton GB. Pulmonary fibrosis associated with tracheobronchial aspiration. A study of the frequency of hiatal hernia and gastro-oesophageal reflux in interstitial pulmonary fibrosis of obscure etiology. Chest 1976; 69:512–515.
23. Tobin RW, Pope CE II, Pellegrini CA, et al. Increased prevalence of gastroesophageal reflux in patients with idiopathic pulmonary fibrosis. Am J Respir Crit Care Med 1998; 158:1804–1808.
24. Johnson DA, Drane WE, Curran J, et al. Pulmonary disease in progressive systemic sclerosis. A complication of gastroesophageal reflux and occult aspiration? Arch Intern Med 1989; 149:589–593.
25. Troshinsky MB, Kane GC, Varga J, et al. Pulmonary function and gastroesophageal reflux in systemic sclerosis. Ann Intern Med 1994; 121:6–10.
26. Lock G, Pfeifer M, Straub RH, et al. Association of esophageal dysfunction and pulmonary function impairment in systemic sclerosis. Am J Gastroenterol 1998; 93:341–345.
27. Reid KR, McKenzie FN, Menkis AH, et al. Importance of chronic aspiration in recipients of heart–lung transplants. Lancet 1990; 336:206–208.
28. Ing AJ, Ngu MC, Breslin ABX. Pathogenesis of chronic persistent cough associated with gastroesophageal reflux. Am J Respir Crit Care Med 1994; 149:160–167.
29. Harding SM. The role of gastroesophageal reflux in chronic cough and asthma. Chest 1997; 111:1389–1402.
30. Irwin RS, French CL, Curley FJ, Zawacki JK, Bennett FM. Chronic cough due to gastroesophageal reflux. Clinical, diagnostic, and pathogenetic aspects. Chest 1993; 104:1511–1517.
31. Canning BJ. Role of nerves in asthmatic inflammation and potential influence of gastroesophageal reflux disease. Am J Med 2001; 111(suppl 8A):13S–17S.
32. Suwanprathes P, Ngu M, Ing A, Hunt G, Seow F. c-Fos immunoreactivity in the brain after esophageal acid stimulation. Am J Med 2003; 115(suppl 3A):31S–38S.
33. Wu D-N, Yamauchi K, Kobayashi H, Tanifuji Y, Kato C, Suzuki K, Inoue H. Effects of esophageal acid perfusion on cough responsiveness in patients with bronchial asthma. Chest 2002; 122:505–509.
34. Benini L, Ferrari M, Sembenini C, Olivieri M, Micciolo R, Zuccali V, Bulighin GM, Fiorino F, Ederle A, Cascio VL, Vantini I. Cough threshold in reflux oesophagitis: influence of acid and of laryngeal and oesophageal damage. Gut 2000; 46:762–767.
35. Aviv JE, Liu H, Parides M, Kaplan ST, Close LG. Laryngopharyngeal sensory deficits in patients with laryngopharyngeal reflux and dysphagia. Ann Otol Rhinol Laryngol 2000; 109:1000–1006.

36. Phua SY, McGarvey LP, Breslin ABX, Ing AJ. Fibreoptic endoscopic evaluation of laryngeal sensitivity (FEELS)—a new method of assessing patients with chronic lung disease and gastroesophageal reflux (GER) [abstr]. Am J Respir Crit Care Med 2001; 163:A184.

37. Phua SY, McGarvey LPA, Peters MJ, Breslin ABX, Ing AJ. Assessing laryngeal sensitivity of patients with chronic cough and gastroesophageal reflux (GER) using fibreoptic endoscopic evaluation of laryngeal sensitivity (FEELS)[abstr]. Am J Respir Crit Care Med 2002; 165:A406.

38. Lodi U, Harding SM, Coghlan HC, Guzzo MR, Walker LH. Autonomic regulation in asthmatics with gastroesophageal reflux. Chest 1997; 111:65–70.

39. Kok C, Kennerson ML, Spring PJ, Ing AJ, Pollard JD, Nicholson GA. A locus for hereditary sensory neuropathy with cough and gastroesophageal reflux on chromosome 3p22–p24. Am J Hum Genet 2003; 73:632–637.

40. Spring PJ, Kok C, Nicholson GA, Ing AJ, Spies J, Bassett ML, Cameron J, Kerlin P, Bowler S, Tuck R, Polland JD. Autosomal dominant hereditary sensory neuropathy with gastro-oesophageal reflux-induced cough: clinical features in two families linked to chromosome 3p22–p24. J Neurol Sci 2002; 199(suppl 1):S64.

41. Ing AJ, Ngu MC, Breslin ABX. Chronic persistent cough and clearance of esophageal acid. Chest 1992; 102:1668–1671.

42. Ing AJ. Cough and gastroesophageal reflux. Am J Med 1997; 103:91S–96S.

43. Kastelik JA, Redington AE, Aziz I, Buckton GK, Smith CM, Dakkak M, Morice AH. Abnormal oesophageal motility in patients with chronic cough. Thorax 2003; 58:699–702.

44. Ing AJ, Ngu MC, Breslin ABX. Impaired oesophageal motility in patients with chronic persistent cough associated with gastro-oesophageal reflux [abstr]. Am Rev Respir Dis 1993; 147:A456.

45. Ing AJ, Ngu MC, Breslin ABX. Chronic persistent cough may precipitate gastro-oesophageal reflux. Am Rev Respir Dis 1993; 147:A968.

46. Kiljander TO, Salomaa ERM, Hietanen EK, Terho EO. Chronic cough and gastro-oesophageal reflux: a double blind placebo controlled study with omeprazole. Eur Respir J 2000; 16:633–638.

15

Management of Gastroesophageal Reflux Disease-Related Chronic Cough

CHRISTOPHER J. ALLEN

Firestone Institute for Respiratory Health, St. Joseph's
    Healthcare—McMaster University,
Hamilton, Ontario, Canada

Introduction

In patients with chronic cough who are systematically evaluated the cause is one or more of postnasal drip syndrome, cough-variant asthma, or gastroesophageal reflux disease (GERD) in 90% (1,2). There have been major advances in the diagnosis and management of GERD in recent years and there is now consensus in the management of many aspects of this very common condition (3–5). The management of patients with cough due to GERD, however, remains a challenging problem requiring an understanding of management of both cough and gastroesophageal reflux. The more difficult patients are best managed by a multidisciplinary team with a pulmonary physician, a gastroenterologist, and an experienced esophageal surgeon capable of performing laparoscopic surgery. This chapter will present an overview of the current approach to the diagnosis and management of GERD based on recent consensus documents and systematic overviews, discuss the currently available literature regarding the treatment of gastroesophageal reflux in patients with chronic cough, and finally present a practical approach to the assessment and treatment of these patients.

Gastroesophageal Reflux Disease: The Current Approach to Diagnosis and Treatment

Symptoms

Heartburn is the most common symptom of reflux disease. It occurs in at least 75% of patients, and is usually diagnostic of GERD if it occurs on 2 or more days a week (3). However, the word heartburn is frequently misinterpreted by patients (3). Recommended definitions of heartburn include: "a burning feeling rising from the stomach or lower chest up towards the neck" (3) or "a substernal burning occurring shortly after meals or upon bending over and is relieved with antacids or other over the counter agents" (6). The other typical, or classical, symptom of GERD is regurgitation which can be defined as "the spontaneous return of gastric contents into the esophagus or mouth" (6). When both heartburn and regurgitation occur together a diagnosis of GERD can be established with a greater than 90% certainty (6). Therefore, if a careful history is taken, and the symptoms are typical, this may be highly specific for the presence of GERD (4,5).

There is poor correlation between symptoms and the presence of esophagitis—neither the presence nor the frequency of symptoms predict the degree of damage to the distal esophagus (6), and endoscopic erosion or ulceration are absent in more than 50% of individuals who have heartburn two or more times a week (3). Among patients in primary care with typical symptoms, as few as 5% may have esophagitis on endoscopy (3). Thus many patients have typical reflux symptoms, increased acid exposure on 24 hr pH monitoring, but negative endoscopy. This variant of GERD has been termed NERD (nonerosive reflux disease) or "symptomatic GERD" (7). This has led to an increasing emphasis on symptom assessment in patients with suspected reflux and it is now considered appropriate to offer a trial of empirical therapy to patients with symptoms consistent with GERD and to assume a diagnosis of GERD in patients who respond to appropriate therapy (4). A recommended treatment trial is a full dose of proton pump inhibitor (PPI) (40 mg omeprazole, 30 mg lansoprazole, 40 mg pantoprazole, or 20 mg rabeprazole) twice daily for 1 month (3).

Diagnosis

Barium Swallow

The barium swallow can be used to identify disorders that may mimic GERD (8). Such disorders include: esophageal spasm, achalasia, esophageal neoplasms, and rings. The barium esophagogram is the best way to demonstrate a hiatal hernia and the majority of patients with reflux symptoms can be shown to have a hiatal hernia. However, the presence of a hiatal hernia does not predict the presence of esophagitis or GERD. A barium swallow has a very low sensitivity and specificity for GERD diagnosed either by esophagoscopy (9) or 24 hr pH monitoring (8). Free reflux is seen in up to 30% of normal subjects and may be absent in up to 60% of patients with positive 24 hr pH monitoring (10). In a study of 125 patients with reflux who underwent both a 24 hr pH study and a barium swallow the sensitivities of spontaneous reflux and hiatus hernia, respectively, identified on the barium examination for reflux defined by abnormal pH monitoring were low (26% and 43%), and specificities were modest (77% and 65%) (11). This is consistent with earlier studies which gave a pooled sensitivity of 33% for the diagnosis of GERD (8). If barium refluxes into the esophagus while the patient is swallowing water in the supine position this is a positive water-siphon test (8,12). The addition of a positive water-siphon test gave a sensitivity of 92%, but the specificity was zero (11). This very low specificity arises because swallowing relaxes the lower esophageal sphincter (LES), the normal reflux barrier created by the LES is abolished, and therefore reflux can be obtained in virtually all patients (8). There are no trials to evaluate the significance of reflux to the thoracic inlet or higher and no evaluation using a proximal pH electrode in the upper esophagus (6). Thus it has been concluded that "The barium swallow should not be used as the first line of investigation for GERD. The demonstration of reflux of barium is of questionable significance because it may be present in asymptomatic persons and is not always demonstrated in severely symptomatic patients. A barium swallow is of little use in the investigation of uncomplicated GERD" (5).

Twenty-Four-Hour pH Monitoring

This is the best way to demonstrate that symptoms are associated with acid reflux. However, to be successful this requires that the patient keep an accurate diary and use the event marker. There is only one study that has been able to simultaneously record coughs using ambulatory manometry and esophageal pH and this showed that only 10% of manometrically recognized single coughs were recognized by patients and only 23% of "bursts" of coughing (13). It is also apparent that the specificity of 24 hr pH monitoring is a problem. Normal acid exposures are found in up to 29% of patients with typical reflux esophagitis and about 35% of patients with endoscopy-negative reflux disease have a negative pH test (3,4). Thus the 24 hr pH study is invaluable in the analysis of symptoms (especially atypical symptoms such as cough) but cannot be used as a gold standard for the diagnosis of GERD. If patients have failed an adequate trial of maximal medical therapy a 24 hr pH study on medication can be helpful because it will document whether or not the gastric acid secretion has been adequately suppressed and whether symptoms are due to residual acid reflux (14).

The acid perfusion test was first described by Bernstein and Baker (15). In a seated subject a catheter is inserted 35 cm (many authors use 30 cm) from the nose and perfused with saline for 15 min. Without cueing the subject, the infusion is changed to 0.1 M hydrochloric acid and the test is considered positive if the subject's symptoms are reproduced. If the subject's symptoms are provoked by acid and not by normal saline, the test is highly specific for GERD, but much less sensitive. The Bernstein test may establish that a patient's symptoms are related to GERD, but cannot exclude reflux (4). In patients with asthma this test may provoke bronchoconstriction (16) or cough in patients with chronic cough (17). Recently, we have reported the utility of a randomized double blind Bernstein test in the evaluation of patients with chronic cough who are being considered for antireflux surgery (18). Patients with a positive Bernstein for cough had a greater improvement in cough after surgery. We have found this test to be of particular value in patients with cough and borderline 24 hr acid exposure.

Antireflux Therapy

Diet and Lifestyle

There are many studies that have shown that various diet and lifestyle factors are associated with reflux (19). Often, patients will recognize this for themselves. Dealing with these factors makes good clinical sense, but there is a paucity of data in this area from controlled clinical trials. All trials of medical therapy in patients with esophagitis show a substantial 20–30% improvement with placebo therapy (20) which some authors have attributed to diet and lifestyle factors (4). Expert opinion supports the education of patients regarding diet and lifestyle factors (3).

Most reflux is postprandial (21,22) so patients should avoid lying down after meals (23,24). Foods that exacerbate reflux include: fatty foods (25), chocolate (26), peppermint (27), coffee either caffeinated or decaffeinated (28), onions and garlic (29). Alcohol (30) and smoking (31–33) should be discouraged but the importance of weight loss is controversial (34). If symptoms are present at night there is objective evidence that the rate of healing of esophagitis is enhanced by bed elevation (35) and reflux is also reduced by lying on the left side (36).

Drug Therapy—Acid Suppression

The cornerstone of antireflux therapy is control of gastric pH. Antacids provide symptomatic relief but are more effective when combined with alginate (37). There is evidence of benefit from combinations of antacid and alginate (Gaviscon) (38–46), these medications provide an effective self-help therapy (47), and after healing of mild to moderate esophagitis with either an H2 receptor antagonist or a PPI 76% of patients remained in remission on alginate–antacid (48).

There are three pharmacological pathways that lead to acid secretion by the gastric parietal cells: neural (cholinergic) via the vagus, endocrine—the secretion of gastrin by duodenal and antral G cells, and paracrine—the release of histamine from the enterochromaffin cells (49). The cholinergic and gastrin pathways act directly on the parietal cell inducing gastric acid secretion by the membrane bound H^+, K^+-ATPase proton pump through a calcium dependent pathway. Gastrin also induces secretion of histamine from the enterochromaffin cells which acts on the H2 receptor on the parietal cell which induces adenylyl cyclase to activate a cyclic AMP dependent pathway which in turn acts on the proton pump. The H2 receptor antagonists (cimetidine, ranitidine, famotidine, and nizatidine) block the histamine-driven pathway but also blunt the responses to gastrin and acetylcholine. Thus the H2 receptor blockers reduce both gastric acid secretion by the proton pump and the volume of gastric secretion. The PPI omeprazole binds directly to the proton pump and causes irreversible inhibition. Recovery of acid secretion requires regeneration of the proton pump by insertion of new H^+, K^+-ATPase enzyme molecules into the cell membrane, a process that takes 4–5 days (49). Unlike the H2 antagonists, the PPIs may not reduce the volume of gastric secretion (49).

Systematic overviews of the literature using meta-analysis have shown a clear hierarchy of effectiveness in the treatment of endoscopically proven GERD (20) (Table 1).

Sucralfate is a complex formed from sucrose octasulfate and polyaluminum hydroxide. It adheres strongly to ulcerated epithelium such as the base of ulcer craters and therefore confers protection from gastric acidity. It may have the additional benefit of binding bile acids, which may be

Table 1 Meta-Analysis of Studies Evaluating Medical Therapy for Gastroesophageal Reflux Disease

	Symptomatic relief (%) (20)	Healing of esophagitis (%) (20)	Remission after 6 months (%) (58)
Placebo	35	28.2 ± 15.6 (19.2–37.2)	10.6 (5.0–16.3)
Sucralfate	47	39.2 ± 22.4 (3.6–74.8)	
Cisapride		37.9 ± 4.5	
H2 receptor antagonists	47.6 ± 15.5	51.9 ± 17.1 (46.9–56.9)	52.3 (44.6–60.1)
PPI	77.4 ± 10.4	83.6 ± 11.4 (79.1–88.1)	82.4 (78.2–86.6)

important in nonacid (bile) reflux (49). Meta-analysis has shown a small but significant benefit of sucralfate in esophagitis (20)—see Table 1.

Cisapride was an effective agent for the healing of esophagitis (20) but is no longer available because of cardiac complications. Other prokinetic agents include bethanechol (50,51) and the dopamine antagonists metoclopramide (52,53) and domperidone (54). All these drugs have proven to be somewhat effective (less than cisapride) but side effects tend to limit the use of bethanechol and metoclopramide and domperidone is not available in the United States.

As Table 1 shows, the H2 antagonists are effective agents for both symptomatic relief and healing of esophagitis but the PPIs have a more rapid onset of effect and are overall much more effective in symptom relief and healing of esophagitis. Not all patients respond to PPIs and there is evidence of nocturnal acid breakthrough with PPI treatment even when given twice a day (55,56). Nighttime gastric acid secretion tends to be histamine-driven and a bedtime dose of H2 antagonist may be successful in reducing the nocturnal acid breakthrough (57).

A meta-analysis of long-term trials has shown that long-term continuous maintenance therapy with omeprazole achieves significantly better results than maintenance with ranitidine and that relief of heartburn with omeprazole is highly predictive of healing (58). More recent studies have shown that using a PPI on demand is an effective alternative to regular daily dosing (3). Again, as with healing of esophagitis, not all patients continue in remission with a PPI.

Helicobacter pylori is strongly implicated in the pathogenesis of peptic ulcer disease in the stomach and duodenum but most people with reflux disease are Helicobacter negative (59). Therefore opinion is that eradication of *H. pylori* is not part of the therapy of reflux (3).

NERD or Symptomatic Reflux

This condition (see preceding text in the discussion of symptoms) has been defined as "the presence of typical symptoms of GERD caused by intraesophageal gastric content reflux in the absence of esophageal mucosal breaks" (7). The following generalizations reflect the current views expressed in recent literature (7).

1. Likely to be the predominant variant of GERD in primary care and the population at large.
2. Symptomatically indistinguishable from classical erosive GERD with esophagitis and with a similar impairment of quality of life.
3. Higher proportion of women and lower incidence of smokers.
4. The LES resting tone may be normal so the predominant physiological mechanism is inappropriate LES relaxation. The 24 hr pH acid exposure tends to be lower and may be normal in up

to 50% of patients compared to about 25% in patients with erosive GERD.

5. Less responsive to therapy. The response to PPI is less predictable—10–30% may not respond to PPI and if response is achieved it may take longer to achieve.
6. Few develop erosive esophagitis or complications.
7. May have 24 hr pH in the normal range but symptoms are triggered by esophageal acid, and perhaps nonacid gastric juice.
8. There may be underlying esophageal sensitivity.

Treatment of Gastroesophageal Reflux in Patients with Chronic Cough

The Irwin diagnostic protocol is the standard for the systematic evaluation of patients presenting with chronic cough (60) and forms the basis of the recommendations of a consensus group (1).

The original protocol description (61) was published in 1981, and updated in 1990 (60) and 1998 (1). It can be summarized as follows:

1. An initial history and physical and chest x-ray (CXR).
2. If the patient is taking an angiotensin converting enzyme (ACE) inhibitor this medication is stopped (or changed to an appropriate alternative) and the patient reassessed in 1 month.
3. For smokers and those exposed to environmental irritants the irritant is eliminated and the patient reassessed in a month.
4. If initial evaluation did not suggest an etiology pulmonary function testing and a methacholine inhalation test are performed.

   • If history and exam suggest postnasal drip syndrome, sinus x-rays and an allergy evaluation are done.
   • If the CXR is abnormal and consistent with either cancer or infection sputum evaluation and/or bronchoscopy are arranged.

5. If still no cause is identified for the chronic cough the following tests for gastroesophageal reflux (even in the absence of upper gastrointestinal symptoms) are arranged: a barium swallow and if the barium swallow is negative, 24 hr pH monitoring.
6. If still no cause is identified, the patient undergoes fiberoptic bronchoscopy and cardiac evaluation.

A cause for the chronic cough was determined if specific therapy was deemed successful "patients no longer complained of cough because it had markedly improved, was controlled on treatment, or disappeared" (60). Many studies have endorsed the clinical utility and validity of this approach (60, 62–78). The results of these studies regarding reflux are summarized in Table 2.

(*text continues on pg. 282*)

Table 2   Evaluation and Treatment of Gastroesophageal Reflux in Patients
with Chronic Cough Using the Anatomical Diagnostic Protocol

Author(s)	*N*	Symptoms	Investigations
Irwin et al. (61)	49	Heartburn or sour taste in the mouth	1. Barium swallow showed reflux 2. Esophagoscopy with biopsy esophagitis 3. pH monitoring demonstrated reflux
Irwin et al. (60)	102	Heartburn or sour taste in the mouth more often than once every 3 weeks	1. Barium swallow showed reflux 2. Esophageal biopsy esophagitis 3. Abnormal 24 hr pH in the absence of upper GI symptoms
Smyrnios et al. (67)	71	Same as Irwin (1990)	Same as Irwin (1990)
Mello et al. (68)	88	Same as Irwin (1990)	Same as Irwin (1990)
Smyrnios et al. (73)	30	Same as Irwin (1990)	1. Barium esophagogram showed reflux of barium to the middle of the esophagus or higher

Treatment protocol	Definition of success	Resolution/ improvement (%)	N GERD
1. Diet modification 2. Bed elevation 6–8 in. 3. Antacids 30 mL (aluminum hydroxide 400 mg, magnesium hydroxide 400 mg, simethicone 30 mg) immediately after meal 4. Cimetidine 300 mg at bedtime and avoidance of bedtime snack 5. Encouragement to lose weight	Patients no longer complained of cough because it had markedly improved, was controlled on treatment, or disappeared	90	5
1. High protein, low fat antireflux diet 2. H2 blocker and/or metoclopramide 3. Elevation head of the bed 4. Three meals a day with nil for 2–3 hr before bed	Same as Irwin (1981)	98	28
Same as Irwin (1990)	Same as Irwin (1981)	97	20
Same as Irwin (1990). With the addition of 5. Dietary consult with weight monitoring	Same as Irwin (1981)	97	63
Same as Irwin (1990)	Same as Irwin (1981)	100	8

(Continued)

Table 2 Evaluation and Treatment of Gastroesophageal Reflux in Patients
with Chronic Cough Using the Anatomical Diagnostic Protocol (*Continued*)

Author(s)	*N*	Symptoms	Investigations
			2. 24 hr pH monitoring showed abnormality in the absence or upper GI complaints or if barium swallow was nondiagnostic
French et al. (72)	154	Same as Irwin (1990)	Same as Irwin (1990)
Hoffstein (66)	198	Heartburn, acid taste in the mouth, or nocturnal cough	Spontaneous or induced reflux on barium swallow
Wongtim et al. (69)	122	Heartburn and sour taste	Reflux during barium swallow
Marchesani et al. (71)	87	No patients with cough and GERD had any GERD symptoms	1. Esophagoscopy and biopsy (9 positive) 2. 24 hr pH monitoring with antimony electrode 10 cm above pH transition between gastric and esoph pH. DeMeester normals (5 positive)
McGarvey et al. (70)	43	Cough associated with dyspepsia. occurring after meals, when stooping, or when	24 hr pH monitoring

Treatment protocol	Definition of success	Resolution/ improvement (%)	N GERD
Same as Irwin (1990)	Same as Irwin (1981)	100	111
1. Avoidance of food for 3 hr before bed 2. 6 in. bed blocks 3. Metoclopramide or domperidone 15 min before evening meal 4. Ranitidine or famotidine	Patient reported that the cough was no longer a problem	88	47
1. Avoidance of caffeine, alcohol, chocolate, and other known dietary triggers 2. Ranitidine 3. Metoclopramide	Not specified	96	3
1. Prokinetic 2. Ranitidine 150 mg twice daily 3. Bed elevation 4. Three meals a day without snacking 5. Nothing to eat or drink for 2–3 hr before lying down	Disappearance of the cough with specific therapy	91	10
1. Dietary advice (weight loss, low-fat low-calorie foods, avoidance	Patient reported that cough had subsided to the extent that it was no longer		

(*Continued*)

Table 2 Evaluation and Treatment of Gastroesophageal Reflux in Patients with Chronic Cough Using the Anatomical Diagnostic Protocol (*Continued*)

Author(s)	N	Symptoms	Investigations
		supine	
Brightling et al. (74)	91	Heartburn, flatulence, waterbrash	In selected cases: 1. **Barium swallow** 2. **Endoscopy** 3. **Esophageal manometry and 24 hr pH monitoring**
Palombini et al. (76)	78	Heartburn, burning, and/or sour taste in the mouth	1. **Reflux of barium to the middle of the esophagus or higher** 2. **24 hr pH monitoring if no GERD symptoms**
Pratter et al. (75)	36	Symptoms of reflux	1. **2-week trial with omeprazole** 2. **If no clear response to step 1 or no symptoms of GERD 24 hr pH study** 3. **If pH study positive PPI**
Al-Mobeireek et al. (77)	100	Heartburn and/or sour taste in the mouth	1. **Endoscopy suggestive of reflux** **OR** 2. **2 Positive 24 hr pH monitoring**Avoidance of

Treatment protocol	Definition of success	Resolution/ improvement (%)	N GERD
of late night snacks)	troublesome		
2. Postural advice (avoidance of stooping, elevation of head of bed)			
3. 20 mg omeprazole for 8 weeks. If symptoms persisted increased to twice a day			
1. Weight reduction	Patients asked if their cough had improved		
2. Elevation head of the bed			
3. Nothing to eat for 2 hr before bed			
4. Acid suppression			
5. Prokinetic agent in selected cases			
1. Bed blocks, weight loss, avoidance of alcohol chocolate, and caffeine	Cough was controlled and/or disappeared after treatment		
2. H2 blockers (unspecified) for 90–160 days			
Prolonged treatment with PPI (drug, dose, and duration not specified)	Cough resolution		
1. Dietary precautions	Response assessed on a scale from 0 (no improvement) to 100% (complete resolution). Success		
2. H2 receptor antagonist or PPI			

(*Continued*)

Table 2 Evaluation and Treatment of Gastroesophageal Reflux in Patients with Chronic Cough Using the Anatomical Diagnostic Protocol (*Continued*)

Author(s)	N	Symptoms	Investigations
			food for 3 hr before bed 6 in. bed blocks
Poe and Kallay (78)	183	Symptomatic criteria for diagnosis not given	Diagnosis of GERD based on either response to an antireflux treatment trial or positive 24 hr pH test

Treatment protocol	Definition of success	Resolution/ improvement (%)	*N* GERD
	defined as > 75%		
1. Weight reduction, high protein antireflux diet, elevation of head of bed; avoidance of caffeine and smoking	Resolution of cough		
2. 40 mg omeprazole, 30 mg lansoprazole, or 20 mg rabeprazole			
3. If limited response to PPI alone, or dysphagia, prokinetic added			
4. 24 hr pH test if no response to above			
5. If no response to medical therapy, 24 hr pH positive, and no other cause, fundoplication			

There are six studies reporting prospective case series using the anatomic diagnostic protocol in which Irwin was an author (60,61,67,68,73,79). The incidence of reflux as a cause of chronic cough changed markedly in two of the more recent studies. In the Mello et al. (68) and French et al. (79) papers 72% of patients had reflux as a cause of their cough. In the remainder of the papers (60,61,67,73) between 10% and 28% of patients had reflux as a cause of their cough. If we pool the results of these four papers there were a total of 61 patients with reflux-related cough out of a total of 252 reported patients—24%. It is not possible to determine the specific response to antireflux therapy in these patients but the cough resolved in 96% (range 90–100%) of the patients studied.

There are nine other papers that use the "Irwin protocol" and report the data in a similar way (66,69–71,74–78). In these studies the proportion of patients with reflux-related cough varied from 8% to 41% and the overall success rate for the protocol ranged from 82% to 99%. Because these studies all used a similar systematic protocol it is again reasonable to pool the results which identify 187 patients with reflux-related cough out of a total of 938 reported patients (20%) which is consistent with the earlier Irwin data. Pooling the overall success rate of the protocol in the same way gives an overall success rate in these patients of 93% which again is similar to the reported Irwin experience.

Based on these and other studies up to 1998, Irwin and his colleagues concluded that reflux was the sole or a contributing cause of chronic cough in about 21% of patients (1) and a profile of patients with probable reflux related chronic cough was proposed (80). "Such patients have normal or near normal chest radiographs, are not smoking or taking an angiotensin-converting enzyme inhibitor, and their cough has not disappeared with specific therapy for postnasal drip syndrome and/or asthma" (80).

Did the patients with cough that responded to antireflux therapy have reflux? Unfortunately, this fundamental question is hard to answer. The Irwin studies usually define reflux symptoms as "heartburn or sour taste in the mouth more often than once every 3 weeks" (60). However, there is no clear definition of what is meant by heartburn, this definition is not in accordance with that proposed by the Genval conference (3), and 36% of the healthy adult population complain of heartburn on a monthly or more frequent basis (81). In the presence of typical reflux symptoms a response to specific therapy (usually a PPI) is considered diagnostic of GERD and unless there are worrying symptoms such as dysphagia, weight loss or hematemesis, further investigation may not be necessary (3). However, up to 75% of the Irwin patients do not have symptoms. The diagnosis of reflux in these atypical patients depends on specific investigations. Most of the studies rely on the barium swallow but this is known to have poor sensitivity and specificity for the diagnosis of reflux, especially in the absence of significant esophagitis. Many of the studies use "high reflux"—that is, reflux

of barium above either the carina or the thoracic inlet—to identify significant reflux but, as discussed earlier, this has not been evaluated against
objective reflux studies.

Twenty-four-hour pH studies were used in patients whose cough did
not respond to antireflux therapy. The methodology used by the Irwin
group (80) is not the standardized approach recommended by the American
Gastroenterology Association (82) in which the pH electrode is placed 5 m
above the manometrically determined LES. This group positioned the
catheters fluoroscopically (80). These studies were being used predominantly to determine whether or not there was an association between cough
and acid in the esophagus rather than to diagnose reflux by the usual criteria based on the overall duration of lower esophageal acid exposure (82).

The final difficulty with these studies is that, by today's standards, the
treatment is fairly "low level" and in all reported reflux treatment trials in
patients with esophagitis 20–30% of patients respond to placebo
(Table 1). In patients with endoscopic esophagitis, the healing rate with
H2 antagonists is 52% (20), the heartburn free rate 48% (20), and the
relapse rate 47% (58). The cough patients may be more analogous to the
NERD patients with their esophageal sensitivity. The published treatment
data in these patient is less well developed than in the GERD patients
but from the GI symptom perspective they are less (not more) responsive
to treatment (7).

Despite these criticisms, what is striking is that the Irwin data has
been reproduced by others. These criticisms apply to the other studies
but these results appear consistent. Of particular interest is the McGarvey
et al. study (70). In this study all patients underwent 24 hour pH monitoring
(standard procedure with laboratory controls) and all the patients with a
positive study were treated with omeprazole in doses consistent with current guidelines for the treatment of reflux disease. The final outcome used
to evaluate treatment was very similar to that used in the Irwin protocol:
"Patient reported that the cough had subsided to the extent that it was
no longer troublesome." Forty-three nonsmoking patients with a negative
CXR and who were not taking an ACE inhibitor were studied. Nineteen
of the 43 patients (44%) had a positive pH study. Of these 19 patients 13
(68%) responded to omeprazole (27% of all patients who presented with
chronic cough).

There are two small randomized controlled trials of omeprazole in
patients with chronic cough and a positive 24 hr pH study (83,84). In the
first study (83) 48 patients were studied. All these patients were nonsmokers
with a normal CXR, had a negative methacholine test, and were not using
an ACE inhibitor. Postnasal drip was excluded by absence of symptoms
suggestive of post-nasal drip, normal upper airway examination, and
negative sinus x-rays. Patients did not receive an empirical trial of therapy
for postnasal drip. All these 48 patients underwent 24 hr pH monitoring and

it was abnormal (pH $< 4.5\%$ of the total recording time or DeMeester score >14.5) in 29 (60% of patients studied). These 29 patients were randomized to receive either placebo for 8 weeks followed by a 2-week washout and cross-over omeprazole 40 mg daily for 8 weeks or omeprazole first followed by placebo. Unfortunately, there was carry-over from the omeprazole period to the placebo period so this group of patients could not be analyzed according to the original experimental design. There were 12 patients who received placebo first. There was a fall in the median daytime cough score in these 12 patients from a baseline of 8.0 (on a 21 point scale) to a median of 6.5. This small change was statistically significant ($p < 0.05$). Part of the reason why this change was modest was that there were only six patients who showed a greater than one point improvement (that is, six did not appear to respond to the intervention). There was no change in the night-time cough score.

The second study (84) was equally controversial. Seventy-one patients with chronic cough were screened and excluded if they were a current or ex-smoker, had an abnormal CXR, a positive methacholine test, were receiving ACE inhibitors, or had a history of any respiratory condition. Patients then received a two-week trial with a second generation antihistamine, oral decongestant, and nasal corticosteroid. They were enrolled in the study if their cough score was greater than 3 on an 8-point scale after a treatment trial for postnasal drip. Twenty-three patients were enrolled and underwent 24 hr pH monitoring. Seventeen of these 23 patients (74%) had an abnormal duration of reflux, eight were randomized to receive omeprazole 40 mg twice a day and nine to receive placebo for 12 weeks. At the end of the 12-week study period the nine placebo-treated patients received 1 month of omeprazole. Response was defined as a cough score of ≤ 1 on the 8-point scale. By these criteria, a total of six (36%) of the patients responded. None of the patients with a negative 24 hr pH test responded to open label omeprazole.

From these two small randomized studies the following conclusions can be drawn.

1. In patients with chronic cough and a clinical profile suggesting that reflux was the cause (80), 24 hr pH tests were positive in 60–74% of patients.
2. In patients with chronic cough and a positive 24 hr pH test according to the "usual" criteria, 35–50% experienced improvement in cough after at least 2 months treatment with omeprazole.
3. No patient with a negative pH test improved.
4. The total number of patients studied was only 52.

Why were the results of the randomized studies so disappointing when compared to the remarkably consistent results obtained with the anatomic diagnostic protocol? There are a number of possibilities. In randomized studies it is important to use objective outcomes with known measurement properties so that the study is adequately powered to answer the question posed. Neither study used such outcomes and they were both underpowered. It may also be unrealistic to expect complete elimination of cough which was the response criterion of the Ours et al. study (83). Most studies define response according to the Irwin protocol—"patients no longer complained of cough because it had markedly improved, was controlled on treatment, or disappeared" (60).

There may have been causes of cough other than GERD which were unrecognized. The patients in Kiljander et al.'s study (84) did not receive an empirical trial with a first generation antihistamine as recommended by the consensus conference (1) and in the Ours et al. study (83) Irwin and Zawacki contended that the empirical treatment for postnasal drip was inadequate (85). No patients were evaluated for eosinophilic bronchitis (86), either by treatment trial or sputum analysis. In one study (83) the dose of omeprazole may have been inadequate.

There may have been a problem with the selection of patients. The association of cough with an abnormal lower esophageal acid exposure in a 24 hr pH study does not prove causality. The relationship is more likely to be significant if there is association of cough with reflux episodes and may be Irwin and Zawacki are right when they say that association of cough with fall in pH is more important than the total duration of the acid exposure (87).

Perhaps in cough due to GERD, and other GERD-related upper airway disorders, regurgitation is more important than in reflux esophagitis where the importance of acid is unequivocal. The PPIs are extremely effective in suppressing gastric acid secretion but have little effect on the volume of gastric secretion (49). The H2 antagonists may be less effective in reducing acid secretion but do reduce the volume of gastric secretion (49). The other antireflux measures that have been used in the successful cough management protocols include dietary measures, elevation of the head of the bed, and prokinetics, all of which may reduce regurgitation and promote gastric emptying.

Nighttime reflux may be of particular importance to the development of cough and other upper airway disorders. Recent studies have identified that nocturnal acid secretion may continue in patients on twice daily PPI (55,56) and that H2 antagonists may successfully control this nocturnal acid breakthrough (57). Nonacid refluxate may contain bile which can be very corrosive to the airway (88,89) and increasing importance is being attached to the possibility of nonacid reflux as a cause of symptoms in patients with effective acid suppression from PPIs (90).

However one interprets the results of the randomized studies, it is clear that not all patients with the Irwin profile suggestive of reflux-related cough have reflux and not all those with reflux respond to optimal modern antireflux therapy. For these patients antireflux surgery can be considered.

Antireflux Surgery

Guidelines published by the Society of Gastrointestinal Endoscopic Surgeons (SAGES) give the following recommendations for antireflux surgery (91).

There should be documented GERD with evidence of mucosal injury (esophagitis) and/or excessive reflux during a 24 hr pH monitoring and in addition the patients should:

1. Have failed medical management

OR

2. Opt for surgery despite successful medical management (due to lifestyle considerations including age, time, expense of medications, etc.)

OR

3. Have complications of GERD (e.g., Barrett's/stricture, grade 3 or 4 esophagitis)

OR

4. Have "atypical" symptoms (asthma, hoarseness, cough, chest pain, aspiration) and reflux documented on 24 hr pH monitoring.

Most surgeons would also want an assessment of esophageal motility with esophageal manometry. Additionally, it is desirable to demonstrate the association of cough with esophageal acid exposure (18).

In patients with normal esophageal motility, the most widely accepted procedure is the Nissen complete or 360° fundoplication (92). This was first described by Nissen as an open procedure and since 1991 the laparoscopic Nissen fundoplication has been introduced (93). The tension in the fundoplication can be varied according to esophageal motility and clinical need by varying the size of the bougie around which the surgeon constructs the repair (94). If there is poor motility some surgeons recommend a partial fundoplication such as the Toupet (posterior 180–270°) or Belsey Mark IV (anterior 270°) (95). The latter Belsey operation requires the transthoracic approach.

In general, postoperative complications are likely to be more severe after an open, particularly transthoracic, procedure and the hospital stay is substantially longer. Laparoscopic fundoplication is associated with a much more rapid recovery, a hospital stay of 2–4 days, and a lower mortality (96). Some surgeons have reported doing laparoscopic fundoplications as day cases (97). The immediate respiratory complications can be related to the impairment in ventilatory capacity resulting from inhibition of the diaphragm and underlying lung disease (such as that due to chronic aspiration). The pulmonary function changes after laparoscopic fundoplication have been described (98) and provided the FEV_1 is greater than 1.5 L or 50% of predicted clinically significant ventilatory impairment or respiratory failure are unlikely (98). Other immediate respiratory complications include pneumothorax and pneumomediastinum related to the pneumoperitoneum necessary for laparoscopic fundoplication. The pneumoperitoneum is created with carbon dioxide and after release of the pneumoperitoneum at the end of the procedure the carbon dioxide is usually rapidly eliminated by ventilation and the pneumothorax or pneumomediastinum rapidly reabsorb (96).

Surgical complications in the immediate postoperative period include gastroparesis if there is bilateral vagal injury, dysphagia, bloating, esophageal leak, and trans-hiatal herniation of stomach (95,96). Vagal injury is uncommon with an experienced laparoscopic esophageal surgeon particularly as there is such good visualization of the surgical field with the laparoscopic approach and if there is minimal dissection (94). Trans-hiatal herniation is minimized by tethering the wrap to the right crus of the diaphragm (94) together with good control of coughing and retching in the immediate perioperative and postoperative periods. It is our practice (94) to give the patient an intravenous (IV) bolus of lidocaine immediately before extubation and use IV ondansetron in the first 36 hr. Patients undergoing surgery for cough may pose a particular problem. While most patients who are properly selected experience almost immediate improvement in their cough after surgery some patients will need expert respiratory medicine involvement to manage any associated reactive airways disease, control airway inflammation, and use effective antitussive therapy while minimizing respiratory depression. The most effective antitussive agents are probably codeine and morphine. If there is concern about respiratory depression, nebulized morphine may be helpful (99) and if necessary nebulized lidocaine (100).

All patients have a gastrograffin swallow on the first postoperative day to rule out esophageal leak and if negative begin oral fluids (94). After a few days on a fluid diet the patients will be on a soft diet for about 6 weeks. Weight loss is common during this period. Some dysphagia is to be expected in the first few months after surgery but in the majority of patients this will improve (101). A few patients may require esophageal dilatation, but it is extremely uncommon for the surgery to have to be revised if it was performed by an experienced esophageal surgeon. Bloating is reduced by appropriate dietary counseling and avoidance of carbonated beverages, and it too will improve with time (102). In general, if a patient has a motility disorder such as dysphagia, bloating, constipation, nausea, or diarrhea before surgery, and they have been properly selected for surgery, these symptoms will improve after surgery. In contrast, patients who did not complain of these symptoms before surgery may experience them to a mild or moderate degree after surgery but will improve over time.

Some patients may experience return of esophageal symptoms after surgery. This does not necessarily mean that reflux has returned and may reflect underlying esophageal mucosal sensitivity. It is now recognized that some patients will resume therapy with a PPI after successful antireflux surgery but these patients usually continue to experience greatly improved quality of life compared to their preoperative state (94,103).

The long-term success of open fundoplication is well described with up to 20 years follow-up (104) but as laparoscopic fundoplication has only been available since 1991 there is still limited long-term follow-up data. The 5-year follow-up data for laparoscopic fundoplication demonstrate that > 90% of patients will continue to experience excellent symptom control if the procedure was performed by an experienced laparoscopic esophageal surgeon (94,103).

Results of Surgery for Patients with Cough

There are no prospective controlled trials comparing medical and surgical antireflux therapy in patients with chronic cough. In a study evaluating our reflux symptom score, which includes cough, there are data comparing the change in cough in patients who underwent surgery with similar patients who did not have surgery and continued on medical therapy (105). The groups were similar but not prospectively randomized. The data shown in Figure 1 demonstrate that surgical therapy was superior to continuing medical therapy.

The literature with regard to surgery in patients with cough is summarized in Table 3 (106–117). Many of the studies are small and include patients who underwent open fundoplication. In most of the studies the outcomes regarding cough were subjective and did not use an objective cough score. However, it is evident that at least 80% of appropriately selected

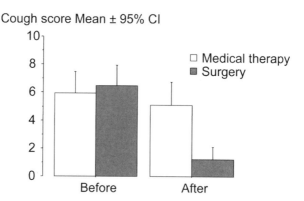

Figure 1   Mean cough score before and 6 months after laparoscopic Nissen fundoplication compared with patients who continued on medical therapy for 6–12 months. Data from Allen et al. (105).

Table 3 Surgical Treatment of Patients with Chronic Cough or Unspecified Respiratory Symptoms

Author(s)	Study	Surgery	Number (followed-up)	Percent improved (cough)		Follow-up
Johnson et al. (106)	Respiratory symptoms	Open	115 (50)	76%		3 years (median)
Allen and Anvari (107)	Total 195, 133 with cough, 62 primarily respiratory 178 complete preoperative data	LNF	178 (154)	Improved No cough	6 mos 82% 51%	Validated cough score. Success of surgery documented with postop pH and motility testing. Hunter et al. only other study with pH and motility post op
Allen and Anvari (108)	5 year follow up data. 905 patients, 523 with cough	LNF	6 months, 878 (715); 2 years, 740 (538); 5 years 487 (289)	Improved No cough	6 mos 5 yrs 84% 71% 52% 36%	One of two studies with 5-year follow-up. Validated cough symptom score. Postop motility and pH monitoring
Ekstrom and Johansson (109)	Chronic cough	Mainly open	11	47% daytime 80% nighttime 45% no cough		1 year
Chen and Thomas (110)		LF	90 (83)	13% no cough 41% improved 46% no change		1–5 years

(Continued)

Table 3 Surgical Treatment of Patients with Chronic Cough or Unspecified Respiratory Symptoms (*Continued*)

Author(s)	Study	Surgery	Number (followed-up)	Percent improved (cough)	Follow-up
Novitsky et al. (111)	Cough	LNF 18, open 3	21 (21)	18 (86%) improved 13 (62%) no cough 3 (14%) moderately improved 2 (10%) mild to moderate improvement 3 (14%) not improved	1 year (but improvement data reported 6–12 weeks after surgery)
DeMeeester et al. (112)	Cough wheeze or recurrent pneumonia. 77 patients evaluated and 17 underwent open fundo. No separate cough data	Open (Belsey IV)	17	14 (82%) improved—resp. not specified 9 (53% complete relief from resp. symptoms)	63 months (median) range 36 to 103
Wetscher et al. (113)	Respiratory symptoms	LNF	21 (21)	86%	6 months
So et al. (114)	35 with pulmonary symptoms from 150	LF	35	58% (pulmonary symptoms)	1 year
Patti et al. (115)	39 with respiratory symptoms from 340	LF	39	73% cough resolved	28 months (median)
Gadenstatter et al. (116)	62 with respiratory symptoms from 80	LNF	62	86% (respiratory symptoms)	6 months
Hunter et al. (117)	57 with respiratory from 300	LNF	300 (126)	Atypical symptoms with included cough improved or cured in 86%	17 months (median)

Abbreviations: LNF, laparoscopic Nissen fundoplication; LF, laparoscopic fundoplication using a variety of techniques.

patients should experience improvement in cough 6 months after surgery. Data with longer-term follow-up are limited. Cough will return in some patients but overall 70% of patients continue to experience improvement in their cough (108,111). In patients whose cough returns it is important to carefully re-evaluate the patients in a systematic manner because return in cough does not necessarily mean that the antireflux procedure has failed. The return of cough after surgery may be due to other causes such as cough-variant asthma, postnasal drip syndrome, and eosinophilic bronchitis. This point is illustrated in Figure 2, which compares the change in cough scores in the patients who presented primarily with cough and those who presented with reflux symptoms in whom cough was an incidental finding. Six months after surgery the absolute improvement in cough was identical in the two groups suggesting a similar mechanism for the cough. The improvement in cough was maintained in most of the GI patients in whom multiple causes for the cough were unlikely, but in the respiratory patients, the tendency for the scores to rise reflected the causes other than reflux. Note also that although the aggregate data showed a rise in cough score the majority of patients remained improved compared to their baseline status, quality of life was improved, and the patients were satisfied (108,118).

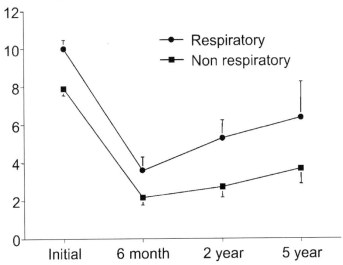

Figure 2   Mean cough score before surgery, 6 months, 2 years, and 5 years after surgery. The respiratory patients are those who presented primarily with cough and the nonrespiratory patients are those who presented with typical reflux symptoms.

Summary: Approach to the Management of Patients with Cough Due to Gastroesophageal Reflux

The approach that we recommend, based on the available literature and our own clinical experience, is summarized in Figure 3. Specific issues or controversies are discussed in the following text.

All patients are prescreened in a standard way in accordance with the current guidelines (1). All patients entering the protocol are nonsmokers (or are sustained quitters for at least a month), are no longer exposed to environmental irritants, have a normal (or stable) CXR, and are not on an ACE inhibitor.

The evaluation of GERD symptoms will depend on the clinical situation and the expertise that is available locally. If patients have alarm symptoms such as dysphagia, weight loss, hematemesis, or melena, they should be immediately referred to a gastroenterologist (3). Some writers believe that patients with chronic reflux symptoms should have an endoscopy to rule out Barrett's esophagus (5), but in general, current opinion is that it is reasonable to embark on a trial of antireflux therapy with a PPI in patients with typical reflux symptoms (3). In patients with cough and GERD our experience, and that of others (4), is that higher starting doses of PPI are necessary so we begin a trial of therapy with diet and lifestyle measures, PPI before breakfast and supper in a dose of 40 mg twice a day (omeprazole, esomeprazole, pantoprazole), 30 mg twice a day for lansoprazole, or 20 mg twice a day for rabeprazole, an H2 antagonist at bedtime, and in many patients a prokinetic. Where domperidone is available this prokinetic agent is preferred but in the United States domperidone is not available so metoclopramide is used. Many patients, however, cannot tolerate metoclopramide because of side effects.

If the patient has no other cause for chronic cough, there are no typical reflux symptoms, but reflux is suspected, a 24 hr pH test is recommended. A positive pH test will include an abnormal duration of acid exposure (based on local laboratory normal values) and/or association between episodes of acid reflux and cough.

A treatment trial should be continued for up to 6 months. If patients respond to antireflux therapy, this should be continued for a further 6 months and then reassessed. Patients are kept on their diet and lifestyle measures and the dose of PPI is gradually tapered over at least 2 weeks (ideally longer). Sudden cessation will lead to a surge of gastric acid over the next 5 days which may lead to immediate relapse whereas slow tapering may be successful. If patients can be weaned off PPI they should still have it available to be used on demand if symptoms recur. This on-demand approach to maintenance reflux therapy has been shown to be satisfactory in patients with GERD but has not been formally studied in patients with reflux and cough. If patients are well controlled on PPI but cannot be

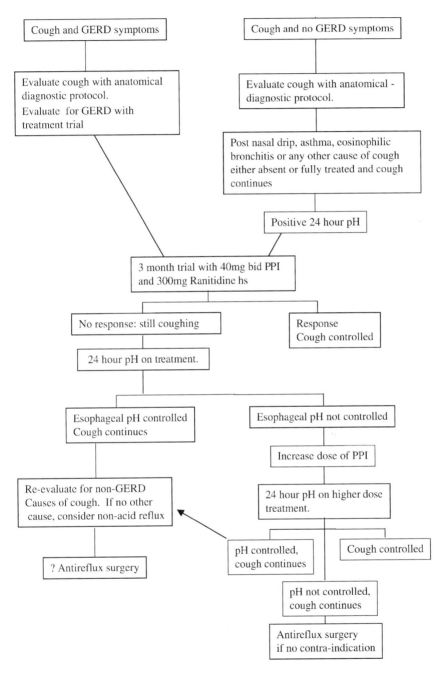

Figure 3 Recommended algorithm for the evaluation and treatment of gastroesophageal reflux in patients with chronic cough.

weaned they are likely to need long-term therapy with PPI. Some of these patients may opt for laparoscopic fundoplication (119).

If the patient does not respond to antireflux therapy the best approach is to perform a 24 hr pH study on treatment. If there is effective acid suppression (we strive for a pH <1% of the total 24 hr recording time) but the patient continues to cough, there are two possibilities: either the patient has another cause for their cough, or nonacid (bile) reflux is the cause. Establishing nonacid reflux as a cause of chronic cough is currently difficult in most centers. Irwin and Madison (120) suggest a barium swallow on medication and if there is spontaneous reflux above the thoracic inlet assuming that the patient has nonacid reflux. Esophageal impedance monitoring has now been developed (121) and is entering clinical practice with the commercial availability of 24 hr ambulatory combined pH and esophageal impedance monitoring (122,123). Esophageal impedance changes occur with the passage of gas or liquid boluses and the simultaneous measurement of pH will identify whether the liquid bolus is acid or non-acid. If nonacid reflux can be shown to occur in patients with effective acid suppression, and there is evidence that episodes of non-acid reflux are associated with cough, these patients can be considered for fundoplication.

Some patients do not respond to PPI even in high dosage. These non-responders will be identified by pH monitoring on medication and can be considered for fundoplication.

A systematic approach to patients with cough and reflux should lead to control of the cough in most patients. The majority will respond to a trial of intensive medical therapy (80), but some will require fundoplication. This surgery can be done laparoscopically with low morbidity and mortality and good long-term results. Greater than 90% of patients will experience control of reflux symptoms 5 or more years after surgery and 70% of patients with cough and reflux unresponsive to medical therapy will experience long-term control of their cough (108,111,118).

References

1. Irwin RS, Boulet L-P, Cloutier MM, Fuller RPMG, Hoffstein V, Ing AI, McCool D, O'Byrne P, Poe RH, Prakash UBS, Pratter MR, Rubin BK. Managing cough as a defense mechanism and as a symptom. A consensus panel of the American College of Chest Physicians. Chest 1998; 114:133s–181s.
2. Irwin RS, Madison JM. The diagnosis and treatment of cough. N Engl J Med 2000; 343:1715–1721.
3. Dent J, Brun J, Fendrick AM, Fennerty MB, Janssens J, Kahrilas PK, Lauritsen K, Reynolds JC, Shaw M, Talley NJ. on behalf of the Genval Workshop Group. An evidence-based appraisal of reflux disease management—the Genval Workshop Report. Gut 1999; 44(suppl 2):S1–S16.

4. DeVault KR, Castell DO. Updated guidelines for the diagnosis and treatment of gastroesophageal reflux disease. The Practice Parameters Committee of the American College of Gastroenterology. Am J Gastroenterol 1999; 94: 1434–1442.

5. Beck IT, Champion MC, Lemire S, Thomson AB, et al. The Second Canadian Consensus Conference on the Management of Patients with Gastroesophageal Reflux Disease. Can J Gastroenterol 1997; 11(suppl B):7B–20B..

6. Katz PO, Castell DO. Diagnosis of Gastroesophageal Reflux Disease. In: Stein MR, ed. Gastroesophageal Reflux Disease and Airway Disease. New York: Marcel Dekker Inc., 1999:55–68.

7. Fass R. Epidemiology and pathophysiology of symptomatic gastroesophageal reflux disease. Am J Gastroenterol 2003; 98:S2–S7.

8. Ott DJ. Barium Esophagogram. In: Castell DO, Wu WC, Ott DJ, eds. Gastroesophageal Reflux Disease. Pathogenesis, Diagnosis, Therapy. Mount Kisco, New York: Futura Publishing Company Inc., 1985:109–118.

9. Ott DJ, Wu WC, Gelfand DW. Reflux esophagitis revisited: prospective analysis of radiological accuracy. Gastrointest Radiol 1981; 6:1–7.

10. Richter JE, Castell DO. Gastroesophageal reflux. Pathogenesis, diagnosis, and therapy. Ann Intern Med 1982; 97:93–103.

11. Johnston BT, Troshinsky MB, Castell JA, Castell DO. Comparison of Barium radiology with esophageal pH monitoring in the diagnosis of gastroesophageal reflux disease. Am J Gastroenterol 1996; 91:1181–1185.

12. Linsman JF. Gastroesophageal reflux elicited while drinking water (water siphonage test). Am J Roent Radium Ther 1965; 94:325–332.

13. Paterson WG, Murat BW. Combined ambulatory esophageal manometry and dual-probe pH-metry in evaluation of patients with chronic unexplained cough. Dig Dis Sci 1994; 39:1117–1125.

14. Katzka DA, Paoletti V, Leite L, Castell DO. Prolonged ambulatory pH monitoring in patients with persistent gastroesophageal reflux disease symptoms: testing while on therapy identifies the need for more aggressive anti-reflux therapy. Am J Gastroenterol 1996; 91:2110–2113.

15. Bernstein LM, Baker LA. A clinical test for esophagitis. Gastroenterology 1958; 34:760–781.

16. Mansfield LE, Stein MR. Gastroesophageal reflux and asthma: a possible reflex mechanism. Ann Allergy 1978; 41:224–226.

17. Ing AJ, Ngu MC, Breslin AB. Pathogenesis of chronic persistent cough associated with gastroesophageal reflux. Am J Respir Crit Care Med 1994; 149:160–167.

18. Allen CJ, Anvari M. Preoperative symptom evaluation and esophageal acid infusion predict response to laparoscopic Nissen fundoplication in gastroesophageal reflux patients who present with cough. Surg Endosc 2002; 16: 1037–1041.

19. Kitchin LI, Castell DO. Rationale and efficacy of conservative therapy for gastroesophageal reflux. Arch Intern Med 1991; 151:448–454.

20. Chiba N, De Gara CJ, Wilkinson JM, Hunt RH. Speed of healing and symptom relief in grade II to IV gastroesophageal reflux disease: a meta-analysis. Gastroenterology 1997; 112:1798–1810.

21. Robertson D, Aldersley M, Shepherd H, Smith LS. Patterns of reflux in complicated oesophagitis. Gut 1987; 28:1484–1488.

22. Gudmundsson K, Johnsson F, Joelsson B. The time pattern of gastroesophageal reflux. Scand J Gastroenterol 1988; 23:75–79.

23. Meyers WF, Herbst JJ. Effectiveness of positioning therapy for gastroesophageal reflux. Pediatrics 1982; 69:768–772.

24. Stanciu C, Bennett JR. Effects of posture on gastro-oesophageal reflux. Digestion 1977; 15:104–109.

25. Becker DJ, Sinclair J, Castell DO, Wu WC. A comparison of high and low fat meals on postprandial esophageal acid exposure. Am J Gastroenterol 1989; 84:782–786.

26. Murphy DW, Castell DO. Chocolate and heartburn: evidence of increased esophageal acid exposure after chocolate ingestion. Am J Gastroenterol 1988; 83:633–636.

27. Sigmund CJ, McNally EF. The action of a carminative on the lower esophageal sphincter. Gastroenterology 1969; 56:13–18.

28. Wendl B, Pfeiffer A, Pehl C, Schmidt T, Kaess H. Effect of decaffeination of coffee or tea on gastro-oesophageal reflux. Aliment Pharmacol Ther 1994; 8:283–287.

29. Allen ML, Mellow MH, Robinson MG, Orr WC. The effect of raw onions on acid reflux and reflux symptoms. Am J Gastroenterol 1990; 85:377–380.

30. Pehl C, Wendl B, Pfeiffer A, Schmidt T, Kaess H. Low-proof alcoholic beverages and gastroesophageal reflux. Dig Dis Sci 1993; 38:93–96.

31. Waring JP, Eastwood TF, Austin JM, Sanowski RA. The immediate effects of cessation of cigarette smoking on gastroesophageal reflux. Am J Gastroenterol 1989; 84:1076–1078.

32. Kahrilas PJ. Cigarette smoking and gastroesophageal reflux disease. Dig Dis 1992; 10:61–71.

33. Stanciu C, Bennett JR. Smoking and gastro-esophageal reflux. Br Med J 1972; 3:793–795.

34. Beauchamp G. Gastroesophageal reflux and obesity. Surg Clin North Am 1983; 63:869–876.

35. Harvey RF, Gordon PC, Hadley N, Long DE, Gill TR, MacPherson RI, Beats BC, Tottle AJ. Effects of sleeping with the bed-head raised and of ranitidine in patients with severe peptic oesophagitis. Lancet 1987; 2:1200–1203.

36. van Herwaarden MA, Katzka DA, Smout AJ, Samsom M, Gideon M, Castell DO. Effect of different recumbent positions on postprandial gastroesophageal reflux in normal subjects. Am J Gastroenterol 2000; 95:2731–2736.

37. Galmiche JP, Letessier E, Scarpignato C. Treatment of gastro-oesophageal reflux disease in adults. Br Med J 1998; 316:1720–1723.

38. Stanciu C, Bennett JR. Alginate/antacid in reduction of gastroesophageal reflux. Lancet 1974; 1:109–111.

39. Washington N, Greaves JL, Iftikhar SY. A comparison of gastro-oesophageal reflux in volunteers assessed by ambulatory pH and gamma monitoring after treatment with either liquid Gaviscon or Algicon suspension. Aliment Pharmacol Ther 1992; 6:579–588.

40. Barnardo DE, Lancaster-Smith M, Strickland ID, Wright JT. A double-blind controlled trial of "Gaviscon" in patients with symptomatic gastro-oesophageal reflux. Curr Med Res Opin 1975; 3:388–391.
41. Buts JP, Leclercq V. Gaviscon and gastroesophageal reflux in children [letter]. J Pediatr Gastroenterol Nutr 1987; 6:482–483.
42. Buts JP, Barudi C, Otte JB. Double-blind controlled study on the efficacy of sodium alginate (Gaviscon) in reducing gastroesophageal reflux assessed by 24 h continuous pH monitoring in infants and children. Eur J Pediatr 1987; 146:156–158.
43. Chevrel B. A comparitive crossover study on the treatment of heartburn and epigastric pain: liquid Gaviscon and a magnesium–aluminium antacid gel. J Int Med Res 1980; 8:300–302.
44. McHardy GA. A multicentric, randomized clinical trial of Gaviscon in reflux esophagitis. South Med J 1978; 71(suppl 1):16–21.
45. Smart HL, Atkinson M. Comparison of a dimethicone/antacid (Asilone gel) with an alginate/antacid (Gaviscon liquid) in the management of reflux oesophagitis. J R Soc Med 1990; 83:554–556.
46. Ward AE. Comparative study of Algicon versus Gaviscon in symptomatic gastro-oesophageal reflux. Br J Clin Pract Symp Suppl 1989; 66:52–55.
47. Graham DY, Smith JL, Patterson DJ. Why do apparently healthy people use antacid tablets? Am J Gastroenterol 1983; 78:257–260.
48. Poynard T. Relapse rate of patients after healing of oesophagitis - a prospective study of alginate as self-care treatment for 6 months. French Co-operative Study Group. Aliment Pharmacol Ther 1993; 7:385–392.
49. Brunton LL. Control of gastric acidity and treatment of peptic ulcers. In: Hardman JG, Limbird LE, Goodman Gilman A, eds. Goodman and Gilman's The Pharmacological Basis of Therapeutics. New York: McGraw-Hill, 1996.
50. Euler AR. Use of bethanechol for the treatment of gastroesophageal reflux. J Pediatr 1980; 96:321–324.
51. McCallum RW, Kline MM, Curry N, Sturdevant RA. Comparative effects of metoclopramide and bethanechol on lower esophageal sphincter pressure in reflux patients. Gastroenterology 1975; 68:1114–1118.
52. McCallum RW, Ippoliti AF, Cooney C, Sturdevant RA. A controlled trial of metoclopramide in symptomatic gastroesophageal reflux. N Engl J Med 1977; 296:354–357.
53. McCallum RW, Fink SM, Winnan GR, Avella J, Callachan C. Metoclopramide in gastroesophageal reflux disease: rationale for its use and results of a double-blind trial. Am J Gastroenterol 1984; 79:165–172.
54. Maddern GJ, Kiroff GK, Leppard PI, Jamieson GG. Domperidone, metoclopramide, and placebo. All give symptomatic improvement in gastroesophageal reflux. J Clin Gastroenterol 1986; 8:135–140.
55. Peghini PL, Katz PO, Bracy NA, Castell DO. Nocturnal recovery of gastric acid secretion with twice-daily dosing of proton pump inhibitors. Am J Gastroenterol 1998; 93:763–767.
56. Klinkenberg-Knol EC, Meuwissen SG. Combined gastric and oesophageal 24 hour pH monitoring and oesophageal manometry in patients with reflux

disease, resistant to treatment with omeprazole. Aliment Pharmacol Ther 1990; 4:485–495.

57. Peghini PL, Katz PO, Castell DO. Ranitidine controls nocturnal gastric acid breakthrough on omeprazole: a controlled study in normal subjects. Gastroenterology 1998; 115:1335–1339.

58. Carlsson R, Galmiche JP, Dent J, Lundell L, Frison L. Prognostic factors influencing relapse of oesophagitis during maintenance therapy with antisecretory drugs: a meta-analysis of long-term omeprazole trials. Aliment Pharmacol Ther 1997; 11:473–482.

59. Csendes A, Smok G, Cerda G, Burdiles P, Mazza D, Csendes P. Prevalence of Helicobacter pylori infection in 190 control subjects and in 236 patients with gastroesophageal reflux, erosive esophagitis or Barrett's esophagus. Dis Esophagus 1997; 10:38–42.

60. Irwin RS, Curley FJ, French CL. Chronic cough. The spectrum and frequency of causes, key components of the diagnostic evaluation, and outcome of specific therapy. Am Rev Respir Dis 1990; 141:640–647.

61. Irwin RS, Corrao WM, Pratter MR. Chronic persistent cough in the adult: the spectrum and frequency of causes and successful outcome of specific therapy. Am Rev Respir Dis 1981; 123:413–417.

62. Irwin RS, Pratter MR, Hamolsky MW. Chronic persistent cough: an uncommon presenting complaint of thyroiditis. Chest 1982; 81:386–388.

63. Poe RH, Israel RH, Utell MJ, Hall WJ. Chronic cough: bronchoscopy or pulmonary function testing? Am Rev Respir Dis 1982; 126:160–162.

64. Poe RH, Harder RV, Israel RH, Kallay MC. Chronic persistent cough. Experience in diagnosis and outcome using an anatomic diagnostic protocol. Chest 1989; 95:723–728.

65. Pratter MR, Bartter T, Akers S, DuBois J. An algorithmic approach to chronic cough. Ann Intern Med 1993; 119:977–983.

66. Hoffstein V. Persistent cough in nonsmokers. Can Respir J 1994; 1:40–47.

67. Smyrnios NA, Irwin RS, Curley FJ. Chronic cough with a history of excessive sputum production. The spectrum and frequency of causes, key components of the diagnostic evaluation, and outcome of specific therapy. Chest 1995; 108:991–997.

68. Mello CJ, Irwin RS, Curley FJ. Predictive values of the character, timing, and complications of chronic cough in diagnosing its cause. Arch Intern Med 1996; 156:997–1003.

69. Wongtim S, Mogmeud S, Limthongkul S, Chareonlap P, Udompanich V, Nuchprayoon C, Chochaipanichnont L. The role of the methacholine inhalation challenge in adult patients presenting with chronic cough. Asian Pac J Allergy Immunol 1997; 15:9–14.

70. McGarvey LP, Heaney LG, Lawson JT, Johnston BT, Scally CM, Ennis M, Shepherd DR, MacMahon J. Evaluation and outcome of patients with chronic non-productive cough using a comprehensive diagnostic protocol. Thorax 1998; 53:738–743.

71. Marchesani F, Cecarini L, Pela R, Sanguinetti CM. Causes of chronic persistent cough in adult patients: the results of a systematic management protocol. Monaldi Arch Chest Dis 1998; 53:510–514.

72. French CL, Irwin RS, Curley FJ, Krikorian CJ. Impact of chronic cough on quality of life. Arch Intern Med 1998; 158:1657–1661.

73. Smyrnios NA, Irwin RS, Curley FJ, French CL. From a prospective study of chronic cough: diagnostic and therapeutic aspects in older adults. Arch Intern Med 1998; 158:1222–1228.

74. Brightling CE, Ward R, Goh KL, Wardlaw AJ, Pavord ID. Eosinophilic bronchitis is an important cause of chronic cough. Am J Respir Crit Care Med 1999; 160:406–410.

75. Pratter MR, Bartter T, Lotano R. The role of sinus imaging in the treatment of chronic cough in adults. Chest 1999; 116:1287–1291.

76. Palombini BC, Villanova CA, Araújo E, Gastal OL, Alt DC, Stolz DP, Palombini CO. A pathogenic triad in chronic cough: asthma, postnasal drip syndrome, and gastroesophageal reflux disease. Chest 1999; 116:279–284.

77. Al-Mobeireek AF, Al-Sarhani A, Al-Amri S, Bamgboye E, Ahmed S. Chronic cough at a non-teaching hospital: are extrapulmonary causes overlooked? Respirology 2002; 7:141–146.

78. Poe RH, Kallay MC. Chronic cough and gastroesophageal reflux disease: experience with specific therapy for diagnosis and treatment. Chest 2003; 123: 679–684.

79. French CT, Irwin RS, Fletcher KE, Adams TM. Evaluation of a cough-specific quality-of-life questionnaire. Chest 2002; 121:1123–1131.

80. Irwin RS, French CL, Curley FJ, Zawacki JK, Bennett FM. Chronic cough due to gastroesophageal reflux. Clinical, diagnostic, and pathogenetic aspects. Chest 1993; 104:1511–1517.

81. Nebel OT, Fornes MF, Castell DO. Symptomatic gastroesophageal reflux: incidence and precipitating factors. Dig Dis 1976; 21:953–956.

82. Kahrilas PJ, Quigley EM. Clinical esophageal pH recording: a technical review for practice guideline development. Gastroenterology 1996; 110: 1982–1996.

83. Ours TM, Kavuru MS, Schilz RJ, Richter JE. A prospective evaluation of esophageal testing and a double-blind, randomized study of omeprazole in a diagnostic and therapeutic algorithm for chronic cough. Am J Gastroenterol 1999; 94:3131–3138.

84. Kiljander TO, Salomaa ER, Hietanen EK, Terho EO. Chronic cough and gastro-oesophageal reflux: a double-blind placebo-controlled study with omeprazole. Eur Respir J 2000; 16:633–638.

85. Irwin RS, Zawacki JK. Accurately diagnosing and successfully treating chronic cough due to gastroesophageal reflux disease can be difficult. Am J Gastroenterol 1999; 94:3095–3098.

86. Gibson PG, Dolovich J, Denburg J, Ramsdale EH, Hargreave FE. Chronic cough: eosinophilic bronchitis without asthma. Lancet 1989; 1:1346–1348.

87. Irwin RS, Zawacki JK. Response to Drs Ours and Richter. Am J Gastroenterol 2000; 95:1834–1836.

88. Schwartz DJ, Wynne JW, Gibbs CP, Hood CI, Kuck EJ. The pulmonary consequences of aspiration of gastric contents at pH values > 2.5. Am Rev Resp Dis 1980; 121:119–126.

89. Wynne JW, Ramphal R, Hood CI. Tracheal mucosal damage after aspiration. A scanning electron microscope study. Am Rev Respir Dis 1981; 124: 728–732.
90. Katz PO. Review article: the role of non-acid reflux in gastro-oesophageal reflux disease. Aliment Pharmacol Ther 2000; 14:1539–1551.
91. Guidelines for surgical treatment of gastroesophageal reflux disease (GERD). Society of American Gastrointestinal Endoscopic Surgeons (SAGES). Surg Endosc 1998; 12:186–188.
92. Nissen R. Gastroplexy and fundoplication in surgical treatment of hiatal hernia. Am J Dig Dis 1961; 6:954–961.
93. Dallemagne B, Weerts JM, Jehaes C, Markiewicz S, Lombard R. Laparoscopic Nissen fundoplication: preliminary report. Surg Laparosc Endosc 1991; 1:138–143.
94. Anvari M, Allen CJ. Laparoscopic Nissen fundoplication. Two year comprehensive follow-up of a technique of minimal paraesophageal dissection. Ann Surg 1998; 227:25–32.
95. DeMeester SR, DeMeester TR. Surgical treatment of gastroesophageal reflux disease with emphasis on respiratory symptoms. In: Stein MR, ed. Gastroesophageal Disease and Airway Disease. New York: Marcel Dekker, 1999: 209–236.
96. Anvari M. Complications of laparoscopic Nissen fundoplication. Semin Laparosc Surg 1997; 4:154–161.
97. Milford MA, Paluch TA. Ambulatory laparoscopic fundoplication. Surg Endosc 1997; 11:1150–1152.
98. Anvari M, Allen C, Moran LA. Immediate and delayed effects of laparoscopic Nissen fundoplication on pulmonary function. Surg Endosc 1996; 10: 1171–1175.
99. Rutherford RM, Azher T, Gilmartin JJ. Dramatic response to nebulized morphine in an asthmatic patient with severe chronic cough. Ir Med J 2002; 95: 113–114.
100. Udezue E. Lidocaine inhalation for cough suppression. Am J Emerg Med 2001; 19:206–207.
101. Anvari M, Allen CJ. Prospective evaluation of dysphagia before and after laparoscopic Nissen fundoplication without routine division of short gastrics. Surg Laparosc Endosc 1996; 6:424–429.
102. Anvari M, Allen C. Postprandial bloating after laparoscopic Nissen fundoplication. Can J Surg 2001; 44:440–444.
103. Anvari M, Allen C. Five-year comprehensive outcomes evaluation in 181 patients after laparoscopic Nissen fundoplication. J Am Coll Surg 2003; 196:51–57.
104. DeMeester TR, Bonavina L, Albertucci M. Nissen fundoplication for gastroesophageal reflux disease. Evaluation of primary repair in 100 consecutive patients. Ann Surg 1986; 204:9–20.
105. Allen CJ, Parameswaran K, Belda J, Anvari M. Reproducibility, validity, and responsiveness of a disease-specific symptom questionnaire for gastroesophageal reflux disease. Dis Esophagus 2000; 13:265–270.

106. Johnson WE, Hagen JA, DeMeester TR, Kauer WK, Ritter MP, Peters JH, Bremner CG. Outcome of respiratory symptoms after antireflux surgery on patients with gastroesophageal reflux disease. Arch Surg 1996; 131: 489–492.
107. Allen CJ, Anvari M. Gastro-oesophageal reflux related cough and its response to laparoscopic fundoplication. Thorax 1998; 53:963–968.
108. Allen CJ, Anvari M. Does laparoscopic fundoplication provide long-term control of gastroesophageal reflux related cough? Surg Endosc 2004; 18:633–637.
109. Ekstrom T, Johansson KE. Effects of anti-reflux surgery on chronic cough and asthma in patients with gastro-oesophageal reflux disease. Respir Med 2000; 94:1166–1170.
110. Chen RY, Thomas RJ. Results of laparoscopic fundoplication where atypical symptoms coexist with oesophageal reflux. Aust NZJ Surg 2000; 70:840–842.
111. Novitsky YW, Zawacki JK, Irwin RS, French CT, Hussey VM, Callery MP. Chronic cough due to gastroesophageal reflux disease: efficacy of antireflux surgery. Surg Endosc 2002; 16:567–571.
112. DeMeester TR, Bonavina L, Iascone C, Courtney JV, Skinner DB. Chronic respiratory symptoms and occult gastroesophageal reflux. A prospective clinical study and results of surgical therapy. Ann Surg 1990; 211:337–345.
113. Wetscher GJ, Glaser K, Hinder RA, Perdikis G, Klingler P, Bammer T, Wieschemeyer T, Schwab G, Klingler A, Pointner R. Respiratory symptoms in patients with gastroesophageal reflux disease following medical therapy and following antireflux surgery. Am J Surg 1997; 174:639–642; discussion 642–643.
114. So JB, Zeitels SM, Rattner DW. Outcomes of atypical symptoms attributed to gastroesophageal reflux treated by laparoscopic fundoplication. Surgery 1998; 124:28–32.
115. Patti MG, Arcerito M, Tamburini A, Diener U, Feo CV, Safadi B, Fisichella P, Way LW. Effect of laparoscopic fundoplication on gastroesophageal reflux disease-induced respiratory symptoms. J Gastrointest Surg 2000; 4:143–149.
116. Gadenstatter M, Wykypiel H, Schwab GP, Profanter C, Wetscher GJ. Respiratory symptoms and dysphagia in patients with gastroesophageal reflux disease: a comparison of medical and surgical therapy. Langenbecks Arch Surg 1999; 384:563–567.
117. Hunter JG, Trus TL, Branum GD, Waring JP, Wood WC. A physiologic approach to laparoscopic fundoplication for gastroesophageal reflux disease. Ann Surg 1996; 223:673–685.
118. Allen CJ, Anvari M. Chronic cough and gastroesophageal reflux—5 year follow up after laparoscopic Nissen fundoplication [abstr]. Am J Respir Crit Care Med 2000; 161:A60.
119. Anvari M, Allen CJ, Borm A. Laparoscopic Nissen fundoplication is a satisfactory alternative to long-term omeprazole therapy. Br J Surg 1995; 82: 938–942.
120. Irwin RS, Madison JM. The persistently troublesome cough. Am J Respir Crit Care Med 2002; 165:1469–1474.
121. Silny J. Intraluminal multiple electrical impedance procedure for measurement of gastrointestinal motility. J Gastrointest Motil 1991; 3:151–162.

122. Kahrilas PJ. Will impedance testing rewrite the book on GERD? Gastroenterology 2001; 120:1862–1864.
123. Vaezi MF, Shay SS. New techniques in measuring nonacidic esophageal reflux. Semin Thorac Cardiovasc Surg 2001; 13:255–264.

16

Cough-Variant Asthma

ANTHONY E. REDINGTON

Department of Respiratory Medicine, Hammersmith Hospital,
London, U.K.

Introduction

Several early case series drew attention to the fact that cough can be the principal or only presenting complaint in asthma. Glauser (1) first used the term "variant asthma" in 1972 in a description of five patients with an essentially nonproductive paroxysmal nocturnal cough that responded rapidly to short-term treatment with systemic corticosteroids. Spirometry was performed in three of the five cases and was consistent with mild airflow obstruction. In 1975, McFadden (2) described seven patients with a past history of intermittent wheezing who, at the time of study, complained only of intractable paroxysms of nonproductive cough. Plethysmography demonstrated a moderately severe obstructive pattern with abnormalities of airway resistance, specific conductance, maximum midexpiratory flow, and residual volume. There were marked improvements in all these aspects of pulmonary mechanics in response to bronchodilator treatment.

In a defining report in 1979, Corrao et al. (3) described six adults who complained of chronic persistent cough without any history of dyspnea or wheezing. Their baseline spirometric data were normal, in contrast to the above reports, but airway hyperresponsiveness was demonstrated in each case by methacholine challenge. The symptom of cough promptly disappeared in all six cases after starting maintenance therapy with either terbutaline or theophylline. Cough rapidly recurred when these agents were stopped but disappeared once again when they were reinstated.

Cough-variant asthma is the term now usually used to refer to those cases of asthma in which cough is the predominant or only symptom. Published guidelines on the diagnosis and management of asthma, such as those of the American Thoracic Society (4) and British Thoracic Society (5), acknowledge the existence of this variant form of the condition. However, cough-variant asthma is not currently assigned an individual code in the international classification of disease (ICD) system and cannot be searched separately as a Medline indexing term.

Cough-Variant Asthma in Adults

Surveys of adult patients presenting with chronic cough have established that asthma is in fact one of the most frequent underlying diagnoses. In an early case series of patients investigated according to an "anatomic diagnostic" protocol, Irwin et al. (6) identified asthma, either alone or in association with other pathology, as a cause of cough in 21 of 49 cases. Many subsequent surveys have confirmed that asthma is a major cause of chronic cough in adults (7–23) (Table 1). Despite the various differences in patient population and study design, these reports have been largely consistent in estimating that asthma is present in the region of 20–40% of cases and is usually one of the three most common diagnoses (Table 1). The patients described vary greatly in terms of age, with subjects up to 74 years (10). It is also apparent that the cough has sometimes remained undiagnosed for substantial periods, with cough durations as long as 20 years reported (10).

In some of these studies, a proportion of the cases in fact have had additional symptoms (such as breathlessness, wheeze, and chest tightness), wheeze on auscultation, or spirometric evidence of airflow obstruction. Such patients might more accurately be described as suffering from cough-predominant asthma. In other cases—the majority in some studies—cough is the only symptom that can be elicited, physical examination is entirely normal, and resting spirometry also shows no abnormality. In this situation, the diagnosis of cough-variant asthma rests primarily on the demonstration of airway hyperresponsiveness by inhalation challenge, most commonly with methacholine, together with a subsequent favorable response to a trial of antiasthma treatment . A positive methacholine test alone is regarded as insufficient, as false-positive results may be seen in a number of conditions (24). A detailed analysis of the shape of the methacholine

Table 1 Frequency of Asthma as a Diagnosis in Case Series of Adults with Chronic Cough

Study	Design	Number of patients studied[a]	Number (% total) with asthma	Number (% asthma) diagnosed with the aid of inhalation challenge
Irwin et al. (6)	Prospective, cough ≥3 wk, consecutive unselected	49	21 (43)	12 (57)
Poe et al. (7)	Retrospective, cough ≥8 wk, CXR normal or noncontributory	109	39 (36)	14 (36)
Poe et al. (8)	Retrospective, cough ≥8 wk, no other symptoms, CXR noncontributory, community hospital	139	46 (33)	38 (83)
Puolijoki and Lahdensuo (9)	Prospective, cough ≥8 wk and ≤2 years	198	46[b] (23)	14 (30)
Irwin et al. (10)	As Irwin et al. (6)	102	32 (31)	9 (28)
Pratter et al. (11)	Prospective, cough ≥3 wk, nonsmokers >1 year	45	14 (31)	N/A
Hoffstein (12)	Retrospective, cough >4 wk, CXR normal, lifelong nonsmokers	198	49 (25)	N/A
O'Connell et al. (13)	Prospective, cough ≥8 wk, CXR normal	87	9 (10)	N/A
Smyrnios et al. (14)	Excess sputum, otherwise as Irwin et al. (6)	71	31 (44)	2 (6.5)
Mello et al. (15)	As Irwin et al. (6)	88	21 (24)	N/A
	Cough ≥3 wk, CXR noncontributory, nonsmokers >1 year	122	49 (40)	N/A
Wongtim et al. (16)	Cough ≥4 wk, otherwise as Irwin et al. (6)	87	13 (15)	13 (100)
Marchesani et al. (17)	Retrospective, cough >3 wk	124	34 (27)	N/A

(Continued)

Table 1 Frequency of Asthma as a Diagnosis in Case Series of Adults with Chronic Cough (*Continued*)

Study	Design	Number of patients studied[a]	Number (% total) with asthma	Number (% asthma) diagnosed with the aid of inhalation challenge
McGarvey et al. (18)	Cough > 3 wk, lifetime nonsmokers	43	15 (35)	15 (100)
McGarvey et al. (19)	Normal CXR, normal spirometry, cough > 3 wk, CXR normal	91	16 (18)	N/A
Brightling et al. (20)	Induced sputum, prospective, cough ≥3 wk	78	46 (59)	34 (74)
Palombini et al. (21)	Nonsmokers, CXR normal, prospective, cough > 3 wk	100	26 (26)	0
Al-Mobeireek et al. (22)	Prospective, probability-based algorithm	131	32 (24)	19 (59)
Kastelik et al. (23)				

[a]Excluding patients lost to follow-up or not included in the analysis for other reasons.
[b]Includes 14 patients classified with "suspicion of asthma," i.e., without typical symptoms but with positive histamine challenge and positive response to antiasthma treatment.
Abbreviations: CXR, chest radiograph; N/A, not available.

dose–response curve has revealed no particular features that are more diagnostically helpful than the conventional parameters of the provocative concentration (or dose) required to produce a 20% fall in FEV_1, PC_{20} (or PD_{20}) (24).

In initial accounts of cough-variant asthma, the cough was described as nonproductive or minimally productive of sputum (1–3). However, in a study of adults with chronic cough and a self-reported history of excessive sputum production, Smyrnios et al. (14) found that the overall pattern of diagnoses reached was similar to that in unselected patients with chronic cough, with asthma representing 24% of all causes. Consistent with this, Mello et al. (15) studied unselected patients with chronic cough and found that the proportion diagnosed with asthma was similar among those with a dry cough and those with a productive cough. These authors also failed to identify any association between a diagnosis of asthma and various specific features of cough character and timing.

Most surveys of patients with chronic cough have identified an overall excess of female patients, but the sex distribution in relation to individual diagnoses has usually not been specified. In our own series (23), female patients outnumbered male patients with asthma by almost 2 to 1. We have also demonstrated heightened cough reflex sensitivity to both capsaicin and citric acid in female compared with male patients with asthma (and other causes of chronic cough), which may go some way to explain the female preponderance (25).

Cough-Variant Asthma in Children

Cough-variant asthma was first suggested as a pediatric diagnosis in several reports in the early 1980s. Cloutier and Loughlin (26) described 15 children aged 6–16 years with chronic nonproductive cough. Ten had normal pulmonary function studies at rest and five had only isolated minor abnormalities. Exercise challenge, however, produced changes in lung function consistent with mild airflow obstruction in all 15 cases and induced cough, but not wheeze, in 10 children. With theophylline treatment, all children became cough-free within 5 days and the exercise-induced decrease in flow rates was blocked. In the same year, König (27) described similar findings in a group of 11 children aged 3–12 years complaining of chronic cough. Routine spirometric testing was mostly normal but exercise challenge induced airflow obstruction and again there was a good response to anti-asthma treatment. The condition was referred to as "hidden asthma." Yahav et al. (28) described 15 children aged 3–14 years with a persistent mainly dry cough but no wheeze or dyspnea. Nine had a bronchodilator response to inhaled salbutamol, four of these also had exercise-induced bronchospasm, and all responded rapidly to treatment with either salbutamol or theophylline. The condition was considered a "forme-fruste" of asthma.

It was with the publication of the study of Hannaway and Hopper (29) in 1982 that cough-variant asthma became an established clinical diagnosis in children. These authors described 32 children, mostly younger than 10 years, who presented with chronic cough that was typically nonproductive, nocturnal, and worsened by exercise and cold air. Over half the children were atopic. Baseline pulmonary function tests, where these could be performed, showed no abnormalities. All responded to a trial of treatment with oral theophylline, often with dramatic cessation of the cough.

Surveys of chronic cough in pediatric populations have indicated a substantially different pattern of diagnoses from those in adults. Nevertheless, asthma represents an important diagnosis in all age groups. In a study of 72 infants and children with recalcitrant cough, Holinger and Sanders (30,31) found that cough-variant asthma was the single most common diagnosis, accounting for 25% of those younger than 18 months, 27% of children aged from 1.5 to 6 years, and 45% of children aged from 6 to 16 years. Pulmonary function tests were performed in only a minority, the diagnosis resting on response to a therapeutic trial in those too young to cooperate. Asthma was also the most common erroneous diagnosis made by the referring physician.

Pathophysiology

Cough Reflex Sensitivity

A number of studies have examined whether cough reflex sensitivity is altered in asthma. Doherty et al. (32) reported that capsaicin responsiveness was significantly greater in a group of asthmatic subjects, all of whom were receiving regular treatment with inhaled corticosteroids, than in healthy control subjects (where a C5 value could not be recorded in the majority of cases). Within the asthmatic group, capsaicin responsiveness was greater in those subjects who reported cough most days than those who did not, and there were inverse correlations between C5 values and subjective measures of cough frequency and severity. Consistent with this, Choudry and Fuller (33) found that responsiveness to capsaicin was increased only in those asthmatic subjects who described regular cough as a symptom.

Other studies, in contrast, have failed to demonstrate any change in the sensitivity of the cough reflex in asthma (34–38). Millqvist et al. (36) used a method based on prolonged inhalation of increasing concentrations of capsaicin and counting the total number of evoked coughs. These authors found no difference between a group of 10 subjects with well-controlled asthma and hyperresponsiveness to methacholine, half of whom were taking regular treatment with inhaled corticosteroids, and 23 healthy control subjects. Using an inhalation challenge protocol based on tidal breathing, Fujimura et al. reported no differences between asthmatic and healthy subjects in cough threshold to either inhaled tartaric acid (34,35) or capsaicin (37). The predominance of cough as a symptom of asthma was not specified in these reports.

These conflicting findings may perhaps relate to methodological differences in the challenge protocols, which are far from standardized, or to the choice of tussigenic stimulus. They may also reflect differences in the populations studied with regard, for example, to disease severity, symptom pattern, and treatment requirements. Few studies have focused specifically on cough-variant asthma. Dicpinigaitis et al. (39,40) reported that capsaicin responsiveness was greater in a group of eight adults with cough-variant asthma than in a group of eight adults with typical asthma. However, the former subjects had a form of the condition that was resistant to treatment with inhaled β-agonists and inhaled corticosteroids (but responsive to the leukotriene receptor antagonist zafirlukast—see below) and should probably therefore be regarded as having a relatively severe, and perhaps unusual, form of the condition. In children hospitalized with acute severe asthma exacerbations, Chang et al. (41) reported that cough reflex sensitivity was greater in those who reported cough as a regular symptom than those who did not. After clinical recovery capsaicin responsiveness was similar between these two groups.

On the basis of these studies, heightened cough reflex sensitivity appears to be a feature of both cough-variant asthma and other cases of asthma where cough is a major symptom.

Airway Responsiveness

Patients with asthma may have varying degrees of airway hyperresponsiveness and this feature can be used to classify them in terms of disease severity. Most reports of cough-variant asthma indicate airway responsiveness values in the mild to moderate range. Such patients, of course, usually also have mild disease in terms of other conventional parameters, for example, their normal or near-normal lung function. Many studies have confirmed the absence of any correlation between airway responsiveness and cough reflex sensitivity.

Wheezing Threshold

Koh et al. (42) examined the possibility that cough-variant asthma is associated with a high "wheezing threshold." These authors studied 32 children with classic asthma, some of whom were receiving treatment with an inhaled corticosteroid, and 12 children with cough-variant asthma. Inhalation challenge with methacholine was performed to calculate both a conventional PC_{20} and a "PCW," i.e., the provocative concentration when wheeze became audible by auscultation over the trachea. The baseline FEV_1 and PC_{20} did not differ between the two groups. However, the ratio of PCW to PC_{20} was significantly higher in cough-variant asthma. Wheezing was detected at a mean fall in FEV_1 of 47% in the cough-variant asthma group compared with 31% in classic asthma.

In an extension of this work, Koh et al. (43) prospectively examined longitudinal changes in wheezing threshold and methacholine responsiveness in 36 children with cough-variant asthma. Over a 4-year study period, cough persisted as the only symptom or resolved in 13 children, 29 developed clinical wheezing, and 7 were lost to follow-up. Airway responsiveness increased significantly in those children who developed wheezing but was unchanged in those who did not. There was no significant change in wheezing threshold in either group. In this study, the authors also confirmed their previous observation of a higher wheezing threshold in cough-variant asthma compared with classic asthma.

Although these studies suggest that a greater degree of airway narrowing may be required to produce an audible wheeze in cough-variant asthma, the significance of this observation is unclear. The site and mechanism of production of wheeze are not well defined and the relationship between wheeze and degree of airflow obstruction in asthma is complex and poorly understood (44).

Pathology

Airways inflammation and remodeling are both well established as characteristic features of classic asthma. Evidence derives from bronchoscopic studies involving bronchoalveolar lavage (BAL) fluid and/or endobronchial biopsy and, more recently, from the examination of induced sputum. Together, these reports have shown infiltration and activation of mast cells, eosinophils, and T-lymphocytes together with structural changes, the most characteristic of which is thickening of the reticular layer of the subepithelial basement membrane. Relatively few such studies, however, have focused specifically on cough-variant asthma.

McGarvey et al. (45) examined BAL fluid in a group of 12 adults with cough-variant asthma, five of whom had an additional pathology contributing to cough. Compared with a group of 10 healthy subjects, the proportion of BAL fluid eosinophils was significantly greater in cough-variant asthma and the proportion of mast cells also tended to be higher. However, interpretation of these findings is complicated by the fact that several of the patients with cough-variant asthma had coexistent gastroesophageal reflux disease, as BAL fluid eosinophilia was also present in subjects with gastroesophageal reflux disease alone. When the seven subjects with cough-variant asthma alone were considered separately, the difference in eosinophils no longer achieved statistical significance. Levels of histamine, tryptase, and eosinophil cationic protein (ECP) did not differ significantly between the cough-variant asthma and control groups. This study did not include subjects with classic asthma for comparison.

Niimi et al. (46) obtained BAL fluid and bronchial biopsy specimens from subjects with cough-variant asthma and subjects with classic asthma. A proportion of subjects in both groups received treatment with inhaled corticosteroids and theophylline. The numbers of eosinophils, but not of other leukocytes, in BAL fluid were significantly elevated in both cough-variant asthma and classic asthma compared with healthy control subjects. Similar findings were reported with regard to tissue eosinophil, but numbers of other inflammatory cells were not reported. No significant differences in these parameters were evident between the two asthmatic groups. Thickening of the subepithelial basement membrane was also described in cough-variant asthma, with measurements inter mediate between those of subjects with classic asthma and healthy control subjects (47).

In another bronchoscopy-based study, Lee et al. (48) obtained biopsy specimens from 25 subjects with chronic nonproductive cough and from five healthy control subjects. All of the patients with cough were considered to have evidence of inflammatory change, which was categorized as eosinophil-predominant in 21 cases and lymphocyte-predominant in the remaining four cases. Five of the 21 cases with eosinophilic inflammation had airway hyperresponsiveness to methacholine and were regarded on this basis to have cough-variant asthma. There are unfortunately several problems that significantly limit the interpretation of this study, for instance, (a) no therapeutic trials were performed so that the conventional criteria for a positive diagnosis of cough-variant asthma were not fulfilled; (b) the extent to which other diagnoses, particularly gastroesophageal reflux disease and postnasal drip syndrome, were excluded is unclear; (c) the method of quantitation and in particular the definition of abnormality was arbitrary and unvalidated; and (d) the number of subjects in the control group was very small for a study of this sort.

Examination of induced sputum provides a less invasive method to assess airway inflammation and has gained popularity in recent years. Fujimura et al. (49) reported that eosinophils were present in 100% of 25 induced sputum specimens from patients with classic asthma and 66% of 12 specimens from patients with cough-variant asthma, but less than 9% of 23 healthy control specimens. The mean percentage of eosinophilia was very similar in classic asthma (23%) and cough-variant asthma (27%), and was unrelated to either the degree of airway responsiveness or the capsaicin cough threshold. Comparable findings were reported by Okada et al. (50) who found 82% eosinophils in classic asthma and 67% in cough-variant asthma.

On the basis of these studies, it appears that airway inflammation is a feature of cough-variant asthma but the changes seen are both qualitatively and quantitatively similar to those in classic asthma. Interpretation is limited, however, by the fact that an inflammatory response appears also present in the airways of subjects with chronic cough due to etiologies other than asthma. As indicated earlier, McGarvey et al. (45) reported that chronic cough due to gastroesophageal reflux disease is associated with BAL fluid eosinophilia. Similarly, Boulet et al. (51) described airway inflammation in bronchial biopsy specimens and BAL fluid obtained from subjects with nonasthmatic cough of various etiologies. These observations may indicate that, at least in some cases, airway inflammation is a prerequisite for cough to be triggered by some other pathologic process. The alternative possibility that chronic cough might itself cause airway inflammation also cannot be discounted on the basis of these observational studies.

Neuropeptide Expression

Studies on the expression of neuropeptides in asthma have produced some inconsistent findings. Using quantitative immunohistochemistry, Ollerenshaw et al. (52) reported an increase in the number and length of substance P (SP)-immunoreactive nerves in the lamina propria of 3 mm-diameter airways of three subjects with fatal asthma compared with three nonasthmatic control subjects. All of the asthmatic subjects studied received corticosteroid treatment. In proximal airway biopsy samples obtained bronchoscopically from asthmatic subjects with disease of varying severity and from nonasthmatic control subjects, in contrast, nerves immunoreactive for SP and for calcitonin gene-related peptide (CGRP) were either sparse or absent (53–55). Elevated concentrations of SP in induced sputum (56) and BAL fluid (57) have been reported in asthma whereas, conversely, the total content of SP in tracheal tissue was reduced (58).

Only a single published study has specifically addressed airway neuropeptide expression in cough-variant asthma. Lee et al. (59) obtained endobronchial biopsy specimens from 6 subjects with cough-variant asthma, 14 subjects with classic asthma, and 5 healthy control subjects. They reported that the density of SP-immunoreactive nerves within the airway epithelium was increased in cough-variant asthma compared with the other two groups, which were similar to each other. Unfortunately, there are a number of design weaknesses that limit the interpretability of this study. These include the small sample size, the lack of detail regarding subject characterization, and the failure to match adequately for antiasthma treatments and smoking status. There are also uncertainties regarding the validity of bronchial biopsy specimens for the quantitation of nerves present at low density, such as those immunoreactive for SP (60).

In another bronchoscopy-based study, O'Connell et al. (54) found that the density of epithelial CGRP-immunoreactive nerves was increased in tissue from patients with idiopathic chronic cough, in whom asthma had been excluded by normal histamine bronchoprovocation, compared with tissue from healthy control subjects. The density of epithelial SP immunostaining was also greater, although this difference did not achieve statistical significance. These findings emphasize the importance of including a control population of patients with cough from other causes in studies of cough-variant asthma.

Natural History

Progression to Classic Asthma

In a proportion of cases, cough-variant asthma may be the precursor of classic asthma. In their original report in adult patients, Corrao et al. (3) found that two of the six developed wheezing within 1.5 years of completion of the study. More recently, Fujimura et al. (61) described the development of typical asthma symptoms in 4 of 20 subjects with cough-variant asthma over a 9-year follow-up period. The rate appeared to be lower among those subjects who were receiving long-term treatment with an inhaled corticosteroid (15%) than among those who were not (29%). Studies in pediatric populations have also suggested that many children with cough-variant asthma—up to 80% in some studies—eventually develop episodic wheeze and/or dyspnea (27,29,43,62,63).

Koh et al. (62) examined factors that may predict the development of wheeze. In a group of 48 children diagnosed with cough-variant asthma who were followed up for 4 years, 21 (44%) developed wheeze whereas the remainder either continued to experience persistent ($n = 12$) or intermittent ($n = 9$) cough as their only symptom or else became symptom free ($n = 6$). The two groups were not significantly different with regard to age, sex, prevalence of atopy, or spirometric values. High-dose methacholine challenges were performed at entry into the study. The PC_{20} did not differ significantly between the two groups but the degree of maximal airway narrowing and the proportion of cases where a plateau response could not be achieved were greater in those children who subsequently developed wheeze. Airway responsiveness is recognized to be a composite disorder and maximal attainable airway narrowing may be the most clinically relevant aspect, as this will determine the degree of airway obstruction except at low stimulus levels (64).

The degree of eosinophilic inflammation may also act as a marker for the subsequent development of classic asthma. Kim et al. (63) performed sputum induction in 62 children with cough-variant asthma who were then followed up regularly for a period of 4 years. The percentage of eosinophils was higher in those children who developed classic asthma (median 7.3%) than in those who did not (median 3.0%). There was also a trend toward higher levels of ECP. Neither airway responsiveness to methacholine nor peak expiratory flow variability was predictive of the development of classic asthma. As with maximal airway narrowing (62), this study suggests that those subjects with more severe disease initially are more likely to progress to developing classic asthma.

Development of Fixed Airflow Obstruction

The majority of studies in classic asthma have suggested that the condition is associated with accelerated loss of lung function in adult life (65–69). In a community-based longitudinal study in Copenhagen, Denmark, for example, Lange et al. (69) found that unadjusted FEV_1 declined by an average of 38 mL/year among adults with self-reported asthma and 22 mL/year in nonasthmatic control subjects (69). The negative influence of asthma on FEV_1 was seen in both smokers and nonsmokers. Some patients experience very steep rates of decline in lung function, leading to poorly reversible or irreversible airflow obstruction (70–72). Cross-sectional studies have also shown that lung function measurements are lower than predicted in adults with asthma (73–76). The degree of impairment appears related to both the duration and the severity of disease.

Information about longitudinal changes in pulmonary function in cough-variant asthma is limited. Fujimura et al. (61) measured FEV_1 annually in 20 adults with cough-variant asthma for a median follow-up period of almost 9 years. The slope of the regression line was 29 mL/year, which was not significantly different from the slope of 28 mL/year recorded in a group of 271 healthy control subjects. There are problems, however, with the interpretation of this study. Nearly two-thirds of the subjects with cough-variant asthma were receiving long-term inhaled corticosteroids and, at least in more typical asthma, there is evidence that such treatment may modulate the unfavorable impact of asthma on loss of FEV_1 (77,78). Additionally, the number of subjects with cough-variant asthma studied was small and several developed typical asthma symptoms or became lost to follow-up over the study period. Further work is needed, therefore, before a confident conclusion can be reached regarding the development of irreversible airflow obstruction in cough-variant asthma.

Treatment

The initial descriptions of cough-variant asthma emphasized the good therapeutic response to oral or inhaled bronchodilators. Indeed, such a positive response formed a necessary component of the diagnostic criteria in most studies. Subsequent transfer to inhaled corticosteroid treatment results in sustained symptom control for the majority of patients (79). Where there is diagnostic uncertainty, and particularly if facilities for methacholine challenge are not available, a short course of oral corticosteroids can be helpful as a diagnostic–therapeutic trial (80).

An initial case report drew attention to a possible role for antileukotriene therapy in cough-variant asthma (81). Dicpinigaitis et al. (40) performed a randomized controlled crossover study of the leukotriene receptor antagonist zafirlukast 20 mg twice daily for 14 days in eight patients with cough-variant or cough-predominant asthma that had proved refractory to treatment with inhaled β-agonists and, in five cases, also to inhaled corticosteroids. Compared with placebo, zafirlukast decreased cough severity and frequency, as assessed by a simple scoring system, and also reduced cough reflex sensitivity measured by capsaicin inhalation challenge. This contrasts with the results of a study of similar design in subjects with mild to moderate asthma without cough where zafirlukast had no influence on capsaicin responsiveness (39).

The compound azelastine, a histamine H1 receptor antagonist, in addition to its various other properties, has reported activity in cough-variant asthma. In a placebo-controlled study, Shioya et al. (82) found that azelastine reduced cough and increased cough threshold to inhaled capsaicin in a group of eight subjects with cough-variant asthma. Other histamine H1 receptor antagonists such as terfenadine have reported antitussive effects in classic asthma (83,84).

A small proportion of patients with cough-variant asthma have a form of the condition that is relatively severe and unresponsive to treatment. The term "malignant" has been proposed to describe such cases (85). Typically, cough disrupts sleep and other activities, leads to emergency room visits or hospitalizations, and requires prolonged treatment with high doses of prednisolone. In a minority of cases, continuous prednisolone treatment may be necessary (79).

Relationship of Cough-Variant Asthma to Eosinophilic Bronchitis and to "Atopic Cough"

The term eosinophilic bronchitis was introduced by Gibson et al. (86,87) to describe a condition characterized by chronic cough with sputum eosinophilia, but—in contrast to asthma including its cough-variant form—without variable airflow obstruction or airway hyperresponsiveness. The cough is responsive to treatment with inhaled corticosteroids, which also produce a decrease in capsaicin responsiveness and a reduction in sputum eosinophilia (88). The series reported by Brightling et al. (20) suggests that eosinophilic bronchitis may account for up to 10–15% of cases of chronic cough in some populations. As discussed more fully in Chapter 17, recent progress has been made in elucidating the mechanisms underlying this condition. Both asthma and eosinophilic bronchitis are characterized by a similar pattern of eosinophilic airway inflammation (89,90). However, concentrations of the mast-cell products histamine and prostaglandin D_2 in induced sputum are greater in eosinophilic bronchitis than in asthma (91). Furthermore, localization of mast cells to airway smooth muscle appears to occur in asthma but not in eosinophilic bronchitis (89). Together these findings might predict that cough-variant asthma is associated with a more superficial localization of mast cells than classic asthma, but this possibility has not been examined in detail.

In a series of reports, Fujimura et al. (49,92–94) have described a condition that they have termed atopic cough. This is characterized by chronic cough without other respiratory symptoms, normal airway responsiveness to methacholine, and an excess of eosinophils in induced sputum and bronchial biopsy specimens. These features suggest that atopic cough is distinct from cough-variant asthma but shares many similarities with, and may perhaps be identical to, eosinophilic bronchitis. Indeed, the validity of atopic cough as a distinct diagnostic entity has been the subject of recent debate (95).

Conclusions

Cough-variant asthma is now well established as a common cause of chronic cough in adults and children. However, the fundamental features that distinguish this form of the disease from more typical asthma are largely obscure. More work is needed to define the pathophysiology and pathology of cough-variant asthma in greater detail. Ultimately, it is hoped that such lines of investigation will lead to novel and better forms of treatment.

References

1. Glauser FL. Variant asthma. Ann Allergy 1972; 30:457–459.
2. McFadden ER. Exertional dyspnea and cough as preludes to acute attacks of bronchial asthma. N Engl J Med 1975; 292:555–559.
3. Corrao WM, Braman SS, Irwin RS. Chronic cough as the sole presenting manifestation of bronchial asthma. N Engl J Med 1979; 300:633–637.
4. American Thoracic Society. Standards for the diagnosis and care of patients with chronic obstructive pulmonary disease (COPD) and asthma. Am Rev Respir Dis 1987; 136:225–243.
5. British Thoracic Society, Scottish Intercollegiate Guidelines Network. British Guideline on the Management of Asthma. Thorax 2003; 58(suppl 1):i1–i94.

6. Irwin RS, Corrao WM, Pratter MR. Chronic persistent cough in the adult: the spectrum and frequency of causes and successful outcome of specific therapy. Am Rev Respir Dis 1981; 123:413–417.
7. Poe RH, Israel RH, Utell MJ, Hall WJ. Chronic cough: bronchoscopy or pulmonary function testing? Am Rev Respir Dis 1982; 126:160–162.
8. Poe RH, Harder RV, Israel RH, Kallay MC. Chronic persistent cough: experience in diagnosis and outcome using an anatomic diagnostic protocol. Chest 1989; 95:723–728.
9. Puolijoki H, Lahdensuo A. Causes of prolonged cough in patients referred to a chest clinic. Ann Med 1989; 21:425–427.
10. Irwin RS, Curley FJ, French CJ. Chronic cough: the spectrum and frequency of causes, key components of the diagnostic evaluation, and outcome of specific therapy. Am Rev Respir Dis 1990; 141:640–647.
11. Pratter MR, Bartter T, Akers S, DuBois J. An algorithmic approach to chronic cough. Ann Intern Med 1993; 119:977–983.
12. Hoffstein V. Persistent cough in nonsmokers. Can Respir J 1994; 1:40–47.
13. O'Connell F, Thomas VE, Pride NB, Fuller RW. Capsaicin cough sensitivity decreases with successful treatment of chronic cough. Am J Respir Crit Care Med 1994; 150:374–380.
14. Smyrnios NA, Irwin RS, Curley FJ. Chronic cough with a history of excessive sputum production: the spectrum and frequency of causes, key components of the diagnostic evaluation, and outcome of specific therapy. Chest 1995; 108:991–997.
15. Mello CJ, Irwin RS, Curley FJ. Predictive values of the character, timing, and complications of chronic cough in diagnosing its cause. Arch Intern Med 1996; 156:997–1003.
16. Wongtim S, Mogmeud S, Limthongkul S, Chareonlap P, Udompanich V, Nuchprayoon C, Chochaipanichnont L. The role of the methacholine inhalation challenge in adult patients presenting with chronic cough. Asian Pac J Allerg Immunol 1997; 15:9–14.
17. Marchesani F, Cecarini L, Pela R, Sanguinetti CM. Causes of chronic persistent cough in adult patients: the results of a systematic management protocol. Monaldi Arch Chest Dis 1998; 53:510–514.
18. McGarvey LPA, Heaney LG, MacMahon J. A retrospective survey of diagnosis and management of patients presenting with chronic cough to a general chest clinic. Int J Clin Pract 1998; 52:158–161.
19. McGarvey LPA, Heaney LG, Lawson JT, Johnston BT, Scally CM, Ennis M, Shepherd DRT, MacMahon J. Evaluation and outcome of patients with chronic non-productive cough using a comprehensive diagnostic protocol. Thorax 1998; 53:738–743.
20. Brightling CE, Ward R, Goh KL, Wardlaw AJ, Pavord ID. Eosinophilic bronchitis is an important cause of chronic cough. Am J Respir Crit Care Med 1999; 160:406–410.
21. Palombini BC, Villanova CAC, Araújo E, Gastal OL, Alt DC, Stolz DP, Palombini CO. A pathogenic triad in chronic cough: asthma, postnasal drip syndrome, and gastroesophageal reflux disease. Chest 1999; 116:279–284.

22. Al-Mobeireek AF, Al-Sarhani A, Al-Amri S, Bamgboye E, Ahmed SS. Chronic cough at a non-teaching hospital: are extrapulmonary causes overlooked? Respirology 2002; 7:141–146.
23. Kastelik JA, Aziz I, Ojoo JC, Thompson RH, Redington AE, Morice AH. Investigation and management of chronic cough using a probability-based algorithm. Eur Respir J 2005; 25:232–243.
24. Irwin RS, French CT, Smyrnios NA, Curley FJ. Interpretation of positive results of a methacholine inhalation challenge and 1 week of inhaled broncho-dilator use in diagnosing and treating cough-variant asthma. Arch Intern Med 1997; 157:1981–1987.
25. Kastelik JA, Thompson RH, Aziz I, Ojoo JC, Redington AE, Morice AH. Sex-related differences in cough reflex sensitivity in patients with chronic cough. Am J Respir Crit Care Med 2002; 166:961–964.
26. Cloutier MM, Loughlin GM. Chronic cough in children: a manifestation of air-way hyperreactivity. Pediatrics 1981; 67:6–11.
27. König P. Hidden asthma in childhood. Am J Dis Child 1981; 135:1053–1055.
28. Yahav Y, Katznelson D, Benzaray S. Persistent cough—a forme-fruste of asthma. Eur J Respir Dis 1982; 63:43–46.
29. Hannaway PJ, Hopper DK. Cough variant asthma in children. J Am Med Assoc 1982; 247:206–208.
30. Holinger LD. Chronic cough in infants and children. Laryngoscope 1986; 96:316–322.
31. Holinger LD, Sanders AD. Chronic cough in infants and children: an update. Laryngoscope 1991; 101:596–605.
32. Doherty MJ, Mister R, Pearson MG, Calverley PMA. Capsaicin responsive-ness and cough in asthma and chronic obstructive pulmonary disease. Thorax 2000; 55:643–649.
33. Choudry NB, Fuller RW. Sensitivity of the cough reflex in patients with chronic cough. Eur Respir J 1992; 5:296–300.
34. Fujimura M, Sakamoto S, Kamio Y, Matsuda T. Cough receptor sensitivity and bronchial responsiveness in normal and asthmatic subjects. Eur Respir J 1992; 5:291–295.
35. Fujimura M, Sakamoto S, Kamio Y, Saito M, Miyake Y, Yasui M, Matsuda T. Cough threshold to inhaled tartaric acid and bronchial responsiveness to methacholine in patients with asthma and sino-bronchial syndrome. Intern Med 1992; 31:17–21.
36. Millqvist E, Bende M, Löwhagen O. Sensory hyperreactivity—a possible mechanism underlying cough and asthma-like symptoms. Allergy 1998; 53:1208–1212.
37. Fujimura M, Kamio Y, Hashimoto T, Matsuda T. Airway cough sensitivity to inhaled capsaicin and bronchial responsiveness to methacholine in asthmatic and bronchitic subjects. Respirology 1998; 3:267–272.
38. Dicpinigaitis PV. Capsaicin responsiveness in asthma and COPD. Thorax 2001; 56:162.
39. Dicpinigaitis PV, Dobkin JB. Effect of zafirlukast on cough reflex sensitivity in asthmatics. J Asthma 1999; 36:265–270.

40. Dicpinigaitis PV, Dobkin JB, Reichel J. Antitussive effect of the leukotriene receptor antagonist zafirlukast in subjects with cough-variant asthma. J Asthma 2002; 39:291–297.
41. Chang AB, Phelan PD, Robertson CF. Cough receptor sensitivity in children with acute and non-acute asthma. Thorax 1997; 52:770–774.
42. Koh YY, Chae SA, Min KU. Cough variant asthma is associated with a higher wheezing threshold than classic asthma. Clin Exp Allergy 1993; 23:696–701.
43. Koh YY, Jeong JH, Park Y, Kim CK. Development of wheezing in patients with cough variant asthma during an increase in airway responsiveness. Eur Respir J 1999; 14:302–308.
44. Spence DPS, Graham DR, Jamieson G, Cheetham BMG, Calverley PMA, Earis JE. The relationship between wheezing and lung mechanics during methacholine-induced bronchoconstriction in asthmatic subjects. Am J Respir Crit Care Med 1996; 154:290–294.
45. McGarvey LPA, Forsythe P, Heaney LG, MacMahon J, Ennis M. Bronchoalveolar lavage findings in patients with nonproductive cough. Eur Respir J 1999; 13:59–65.
46. Niimi A, Amitani R, Suzuki K, Tanaka E, Murayama T, Kuze F. Eosinophilic inflammation in cough variant asthma. Eur Respir J 1998; 11:1064–1069.
47. Niimi A, Matsumoto H, Minakuchi M, Kitaichi M, Amitani R. Airway remodelling in cough-variant asthma. Lancet 2000; 356:564–565.
48. Lee SY, Cho JY, Shin JJ, Kim HK, Kang KH, Yoo SH, In KH. Airway inflammation as an assessment of chronic nonproductive cough. Chest 2001; 120:1114–1120.
49. Fujimura M, Songür N, Kamio Y, Matsuda T. Detection of eosinophils in hypertonic saline-induced sputum in patients with chronic nonproductive cough. J Asthma 1997; 34:119–126.
50. Okada C, Horiba M, Matsumoto H, Torigoe R, Mizuuchi H, Murao M, Soda R, Takahashi K, Kimura G, Tanimoto Y. A study of clinical features of cough variant asthma. Int Arch Allergy Immunol 2001; 125(suppl 1):51–54.
51. Boulet L-P, Milot J, Boutet M, St. Georges F, Laviolette M. Airway inflammation in nonasthmatic subjects with chronic cough. Am J Respir Crit Care Med 1994; 149:482–489.
52. Ollerenshaw SJ, Jarvis D, Sullivan CE, Woolcock AJ. Substance P immunoreactive nerves in airways from asthmatics and nonasthmatics. Eur Respir J 1991; 4:673–682.
53. Howarth PH, Springall DR, Redington AE, Djukanovic R, Holgate ST, Polak JM. Neuropeptide-containing nerves in endobronchial biopsies from asthmatic and nonasthmatic subjects. Am J Respir Cell Mol Biol 1995; 13:288–296.
54. O'Connell F, Springall DR, Moradoghli-Haftvani A, Krausz T, Price D, Fuller RW, Polak JM, Pride NB. Abnormal intraepithelial airway nerves in persistent unexplained cough? Am J Respir Crit Care Med 1995; 152:2068–2075.
55. Chanez P, Springall D, Vignola AM, Moradoghi-Haftvani A, Polak JM, Godard P, Bousquet J. Bronchial mucosal immunoreactivity of sensory neuropeptides in severe airway diseases. Am J Respir Crit Care Med 1998; 158:985–990.

56. Tomaki M, Ichinose M, Miura M, Hirayama Y, Yamauchi H, Nakajima N, Shirato K. Elevated substance P content in induced sputum from patients with asthma and patients with chronic bronchitis. Am J Respir Crit Care Med 1995; 151:613–617.

57. Nieber K, Baumgarten CR, Rathsack R, Furkert J, Oehme P, Kunkel G. Substance P and beta-endorphin-like immunoreactivity in lavage fluid of subjects with and without allergic asthma. J Allergy Clin Immunol 1992; 90:646–652.

58. Lilly CM, Bai TR, Shore SA, Hall AE, Drazen JM. Neuropeptide content of lungs from asthmatic and nonasthmatic patients. Am J Respir Crit Care Med 1995; 151:548–553.

59. Lee SY, Kim MK, Shin C, Shim JJ, Kim HK, Kang KH, Yoo SH. Substance P-immunoreactive nerves in endobronchial biopsies in cough-variant asthma and classic asthma. Respiration 2003; 70:49–53.

60. Jesenik F, Springall DR, Redington AE, Doré CJ, Abrams D-C, Holgate ST, Howarth PH, Polak JM. Validation of endobronchial biopsy specimens for nerve quantitation by computer-assisted image analysis. J Pathol 2000; 192: 545–548.

61. Fujimura M, Nishizawa Y, Nishitsuji M, Abo M, Kita T, Nomura S. Longitudinal decline in pulmonary function in atopic cough and cough variant asthma. Clin Exp Allergy 2003; 33:588–594.

62. Koh YY, Park Y, Kim CK. The importance of maximal airway response to methacholine in the prediction of wheezing development in patients with cough-variant asthma. Allergy 2002; 57:1165–1170.

63. Kim CK, Kim JT, Kang H, Yoo Y, Koh YY. Sputum eosinophilia in cough-variant asthma as a predictor of the subsequent development of classic asthma. Clin Exp Allergy 2003; 33:1409–1414.

64. Sterk PJ, Bel EH. Bronchial hyperresponsiveness: the need for a distinction between hypersensitivity and excessive airway narrowing. Eur Respir J 1989; 2: 267–274.

65. Schachter EN, Doyle CA, Beck GJ. A prospective study of asthma in a rural community. Chest 1984; 85:623–630.

66. Peat JK, Woolcock AJ, Cullen K. Rate of decline of lung function in subjects with asthma. Eur J Respir Dis 1987; 70:171–179.

67. Ulrik CS, Backer V, Dirksen A. A 10 year follow up of 180 adults with bronchial asthma: factors important for the decline in lung function. Thorax 1992; 47:14–18.

68. Ulrik CS, Lange P. Decline of lung function in adults with bronchial asthma. Am J Respir Crit Care Med 1994; 150:629–634.

69. Lange P, Parner J, Vestbo J, Schnohr P, Jensen G. A 15-year follow-up study of ventilatory function in adults with asthma. N Engl J Med 1998; 339: 1194–1200.

70. Backman KS, Greenberger PA, Patterson R. Airways obstruction in patients with long-term asthma consistent with "irreversible asthma." Chest 1997; 112:1234–1240

71. Hudon C, Turcotte H, Laviolette M, Carrier G, Boulet L-P. Characteristics of bronchial asthma with incomplete reversibility of airflow obstruction. Ann Allergy Asthma Immunol 1997; 78:195–202.

72. Ulrik CS, Backer V. Nonreversible airflow obstruction in life-long nonsmokers with moderate to severe asthma. Eur Respir J 1999; 14:892–896.
73. Brown PJ, Greville HW, Finucane KE. Asthma and irreversible airflow obstruction. Thorax 1984; 39:131–136.
74. Finucane KE, Greville HW, Brown PJE. Irreversible airflow obstruction: evolution in asthma. Med J Aust 1985; 142:602–604.
75. Connolly CK, Chan NS, Prescott RJ. The relationship between age and duration of asthma and the presence of persistent airflow obstruction in asthma. Postgrad Med J 1988; 64:422–425.
76. Braman SS, Kaemmerlen JT, Davis SM. Asthma in the elderly: a comparison between patients with recently acquired and long-standing disease. Am Rev Respir Dis 1991; 143:336–340.
77. van Schayck CP, Dompeling E, van Herwaarden CLA, Folgering H, Verbeek ALM, van der Hoogen HJM, van Weel C. Bronchodilator treatment in moderate asthma or chronic bronchitis: continuous or on demand? A randomised controlled study. Br Med J 1991; 303:1426–1430.
78. Dompeling E, van Schayck CP, van Grunsven PM, van Herwaardeen CLA, Akkermans R, Molema J, Folgering H, van Weel C. Slowing the deterioration of asthma and chronic obstructive pulmonary disease observed during bronchodilator therapy by adding inhaled corticosteroids: a 4-year prospective study. Ann Intern Med 1993; 118:770–778.
79. Cheriyan S, Greenberger PA, Patterson R. Outcome of cough variant asthma treated with inhaled steroids. Ann Allergy 1994; 73:478–480.
80. Doan T, Patterson R, Greenberger PA. Cough variant asthma: usefulness of a diagnostic-therapeutic trial with prednisone. Ann Allergy 1992; 69:505–509.
81. Nishi K, Watanabe K, Ooka T, Fujimura M, Matsuda T. Cough-variant asthma successfully treated with a peptide leukotriene receptor antagonist. Jpn J Thorac Dis 1997; 35:117–123.
82. Shioya T, Ito N, Sasaki M, Kagaya M, Sano M, Shindo T, Kashima M, Miura M. Cough threshold for capsaicin increases by azelastine in patients with cough-variant asthma. Pulm Pharmacol 1996; 9:59–62.
83. Taytard A, Beaumont D, Pujet JC, Sapene M, Lewis PJ. Treatment of bronchial asthma with terfenadine: a randomised controlled trial. Br J Clin Pharmacol 1987; 24:743–746.
84. Rafferty P, Jackson L, Smith R, Holgate ST. Terfenadine, a potent histamine H1-receptor antagonist in the treatment of grass pollen sensitive asthma. Br J Clin Pharmacol 1990; 30:229–235.
85. Millar MM, McGrath KG, Patterson R. Malignant cough equivalent asthma: definition and case reports. Ann Allergy Asthma Immunol 1998; 80:345–351.
86. Gibson PG, Dolovich J, Denburg J, Ramsdale EH, Hargreave FE. Chronic cough: eosinophilic bronchitis without asthma. Lancet 1989; i:1346–1348.
87. Gibson PG, Hargreave FE, Girgis-Gabardo A, Morris M, Denburg JA, Dolovich J. Chronic cough with eosinophilic bronchitis: examination for variable airflow obstruction and response to corticosteroid. Clin Exp Allergy 1995; 25:127–132.
88. Brightling CE, Ward R, Wardlaw AJ, Pavord ID. Airway inflammation, airway responsiveness and cough before and after inhaled budesonide in patients with eosinophilic bronchitis. Eur Respir J 2000; 15:682–686.

89. Brightling CE, Bradding P, Symon FA, Holgate ST, Wardlaw AJ, Pavord ID. Mast-cell infiltration of airway smooth muscle in asthma. N Engl J Med 2002; 346:1699–1705.
90. Brightling CE, Symon FA, Birring SS, Bradding P, Wardlaw AJ, Pavord ID. Comparison of airway immunopathology of eosinophilic bronchitis and asthma. Thorax 2003; 58:528–532.
91. Brightling CE, Ward R, Woltmann G, Bradding P, Sheller JR, Dworski R, Pavord ID. Induced sputum inflammatory mediator concentrations in eosino-philic bronchitis and asthma. Am J Respir Crit Care Med 2000; 162:878–882.
92. Fujimura M, Sakamoto S, Matsuda T. Bronchodilator-resistive cough in atopic patients: bronchial reversibility and hyperresponsiveness. Intern Med 1992; 31:447–452.
93. Fujimura M, Kamio Y, Hashimoto, Matsuda T. Cough receptor sensitivity and bronchial responsiveness in patients with only chronic nonproductive cough: in view of effect of bronchodilator therapy. J Asthma 1994; 31:463–472.
94. Fujimura M, Ogawa H, Yasui M, Matsuda T. Eosinophilic trachobronchitis and airway cough hypersensitivity in chronic non-productive cough. Clin Exp Allergy 2000; 30:41–47.
95. McGarvey LPA, Morice AH. Atopic cough: little evidence to support a new clinical entity. Thorax 2003; 58:736–737.

17

Eosinophilic Bronchitis

CHRISTOPHER E. BRIGHTLING, SURINDER S. BIRRING,
MIKE A. BERRY, and IAN D. PAVORD

Respiratory Medicine, University Hospitals of Leicester NHS Trust,
    Glenfield Hospitals,
Leicester, U.K.

Introduction

Gibson et al. (1) first identified eosinophilic bronchitis without asthma as a cause of chronic cough in 1989. They described a condition that manifests as a corticosteroid responsive chronic cough in nonsmokers without the abnormalities of airway function that characterize asthma. These patients had evidence of airway inflammation in the form of a sputum eosinophilia, hence the term eosinophilic bronchitis. The development of safe and non-invasive methods of assessing airway inflammation using induced sputum has allowed the further characterization of this condition. Studies where assessment of airway inflammation has been undertaken in chronic cough patients have shown that eosinophilic bronchitis without asthma may account for up to 10–15% of cases referred for specialist investigation (2,3), although the incidence is likely to depend on the extent to which therapeutic trials of corticosteroids are undertaken in primary care. This chapter addresses the clinical features and management of eosinophilic bronchitis without asthma as a cause of chronic cough. It also highlights recent advances in our understanding of the pathogenesis of this disorder, which have particularly informed our understanding of the relationship between eosinophilic airway inflammation and disordered airway function in asthma.

Clinical Features and Diagnosis

Chronic cough, traditionally defined as a cough lasting for more than 3 weeks with no overt clinical or radiological evidence of lung disease, is a common reason for referral to a specialist. Several series have shown that a cause of persistent cough can be identified relatively simply in 80–95% of cases by using an "anatomic diagnostic" protocol (2,4–6). Cough-variant asthma, gastroesophageal reflux, rhinitis with postnasal drip, and eosinophilic bronchitis are the most common causes of chronic cough (2). Often there are multiple causes for the chronic cough (2) and therefore eosinophilic bronchitis should always be considered even when a primary cause has been established, especially if there is no or partial treatment response.

Eosinophilic bronchitis is defined as a chronic cough in subjects with no symptoms or objective evidence of variable airflow obstruction, normal airway responsiveness (provocative concentration of methacholine producing a 20% decrease in FEV_1 [PC_{20}] > 16 mg/mL) and a sputum eosinophilia (2). A similar corticosteroid responsive cough syndrome has been reported by Fujimura et al. (7) and has been given the diagnostic label "atopic cough" (7). This condition has been defined as an isolated chronic cough, no variable airflow obstruction or airway hyperresponsiveness, and one or more objective indication of atopy as defined by: blood or sputum eosinophilia, elevated total or specific IgE, or positive skin tests. Whether eosinophilic bronchitis and atopic cough represent distinct clinical entities is unclear (8). The main features and differences between eosinophilic bronchitis, cough-variant asthma, classic asthma, and atopic cough are summarized in Table 1.

As with other causes of cough, details of the nature and timing of the cough are of limited help in establishing a diagnosis of eosinophilic bronchitis but in our experience it is a predominantly dry cough with small amounts of tenacious sputum in the mornings that typically responds to inhaled corticosteroids. Making a positive diagnosis of eosinophilic bronchitis therefore requires assessment of lower airway inflammation, ideally using induced sputum analysis after other causes of cough have been excluded by clinical, radiologic, and physiologic (spirometry and methacholine challenge test) assessment. We use a >3% sputum eosinophil count as indicative of eosinophilic bronchitis as this is well outside our normal range (<1.9%) and this level of sputum eosinophilia has been associated with a corticosteroid response in chronic obstructive pulmonary disease (COPD) and asthma (9,10). Induced sputum is a safe, valid, and repeatable measure

Table 1 Clinical and Pathological Features of Eosinophilic Bronchitis Compared with Classical Asthma and Cough-Variant Asthma

	Eosinophilic bronchitis	Classical asthma	Cough-variant asthma	Atopic cough
Symptoms	Cough, often associated with upper airway symptoms	Dyspnoea, cough, wheeze	Isolated cough	Isolated cough
Atopy	Same as general population	Common	Common	Common
Airway hyperresponsiveness	Absent	Present	Present	Absent
Cough reflex hypersensitivity	Increased	Normal or increased	Normal or increased	Increased
Response to bronchodilator	Absent	Good	Good	Absent
Response to corticosteroids	Good	Good	Good	Good
Sputum eosinophilia	Always	Usually	Usually	Usually
Bronchial biopsy eosinophilia	Very common	Common	Common	Common
Mast cells within airway smooth muscle bundles	No	Yes	Yes	Unknown

of airway inflammation (11) but does require same-day processing for eosinophil quantification and cell viability, unlike routine cytology. Exhaled nitric oxide, another noninvasive marker of airway inflammation has been proposed as a simpler but more expensive alternative to induced sputum tests. Exhaled nitric oxide levels are usually higher in eosinophilic bronchitis (12,13) but its role in the diagnosis of eosinophilic bronchitis has not been formally evaluated.

We have recently reported a 2-year prospective study of chronic cough (2), where induced sputum was performed in all subjects in whom the diagnosis remained unclear after simple clinical assessment and a methacholine inhalation test (Fig. 1). Ninety-one patients with chronic cough were identified among 856 referrals. A diagnosis leading to a successful treatment was reached in 85 (93%) of the cases (Table 2). Eosinophilic bronchitis using the aforementioned definition was identified in 12 (13.2%) patients, representing 30% of those who undertook sputum induction.

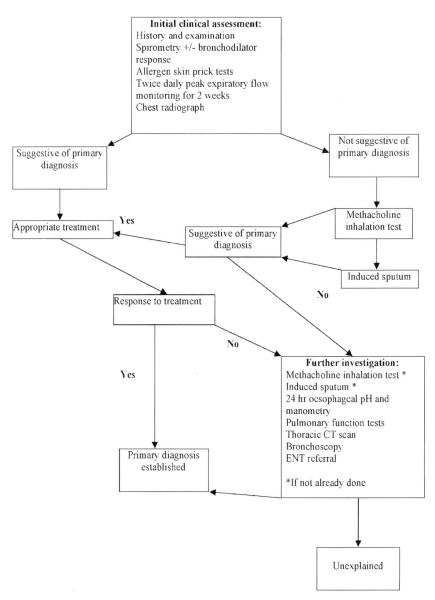

Figure 1 Diagnostic algorithm for investigating chronic cough including assessment of airway inflammation. (Adapted from Ref. 2.)

Table 2 Causes of Isolated Chronic Cough (*n* = 91)

Primary cause of cough	
Rhinitis	20 (24%)
Asthma	16 (17.6%)
Postviral	12 (13.2%)
Eosinophilic bronchitis	12 (13.2%)
Gastroesophageal reflux	7 (7.7%)
Unexplained	6 (6.6%)
COPD	6 (6.6%)
Bronchiectasis	5 (5.5%)
ACE inhibitor-induced cough	4 (4.4%)
Lung cancer	2 (2.2%)
Cryptogenic fibrosing alveolitis	1 (1.1%)

Abbreviations: ACE, angiotensin converting enzyme; COPD, chronic obstructive pulmonary disease. (Adapted from Ref. 2.)

Treatment

Anti-inflammatory treatment with inhaled corticosteroids is the mainstay of therapy for eosinophilic bronchitis. Patients improve symptomatically and have a significant fall in their sputum eosinophil count following inhaled corticosteroids (14,15). In one study, capsaicin cough sensitivity, which was moderately increased before treatment (15), improved towards normal following treatment with inhaled budesonide (400 µg twice daily) and there was a significant positive correlation between the treatment induced change in cough sensitivity and sputum eosinophil count. These findings suggest that heightened cough sensitivity contributes to the cough in eosinophilic bronchitis and that eosinophilic airway inflammation is causally associated with the increased cough sensitivity.

There are no data currently available to guide which inhaled corticosteroid should be used for eosinophilic bronchitis, at which dose, and for how long. The efficacy of inhaled corticosteroids remains to be determined in placebo controlled randomized trials. In our experience, improvement begins in 1–2 weeks. Very occasionally oral corticosteroids are required to control symptoms and eosinophilic inflammation. Although there may be basement membrane thickening and other changes to suggest airway remodeling (16), it remains unclear whether therapy for eosinophilic bronchitis should be discontinued when symptoms resolve. The role of other potential therapeutics agents such as antihistamines and antileuko-trienes needs to be explored (17).

Pathogenesis of Eosinophilic Bronchitis

One of the main interests is why an apparently similar pattern of airway inflammation is associated with different functional abnormalities in eosinophilic bronchitis and asthma. Conceivably this might reflect functionally important differences in site, state of activation, or regulation of inflammatory response. We have recently tested these hypotheses in a comparative immunopathological study of eosinophilic bronchitis and asthma.

We and others have found that both conditions were associated with a similar degree of sputum (13,17), bronchoalveolar lavage fluid (13,18), and biopsy eosinophilia and a similar degree of basement membrane thickening (13,16) in bronchial biopsy specimens suggesting that the site within the bronchial tree is similar. We assessed activation by measuring sputum supernatant concentration of various important effector mediators and found that eosinophilic bronchitis and asthma are both associated with increased levels of cysteinyl-leukotrienes and eosinophilic cationic protein (17). Interestingly, histamine and prostaglandin D_2 concentrations are only increased in eosinophilic bronchitis suggesting that activation of mast cells in superficial airway structures is a particular feature of this condition and raising the possibility that localization of activated mast cells might differ in asthma and eosinophilic bronchitis. In support of this, we have recently found that mast cell numbers in airway smooth muscle are increased in asthma, but not in eosinophilic bronchitis (16). Furthermore, airway smooth muscle mast cell numbers inversely correlated with airway hyperresponsiveness. Thus a key factor determining the different functional association of airway inflammation in eosinophilic bronchitis and asthma might be the microlocalization of mast cells with a predominant airway smooth muscle infiltration (Figs. 2a,b and 3), resulting in airway hyperre-

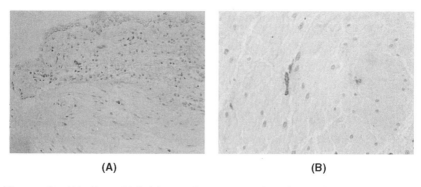

(A)   (B)

Figure 2 (**A**) Bronchial biopsy from an asthmatic subject demonstrating epithelium, submucosa, and smooth muscle with mast cells infiltrating the airway smooth muscle (×100). (**B**) Bronchial biopsy from another asthmatic illustrating mast cells within the airway smooth muscle (×400). (Adapted from Ref. 16.)

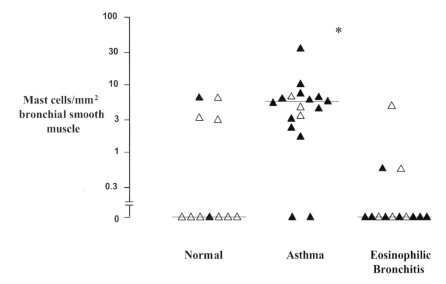

Figure 3 Mast cells (tryptase+) in airway smooth muscle/mm² in subjects with asthma, eosinophilic bronchitis, and normal controls (16). *, p < 0.0001 (Kruskal–Wallis test); closed triangles, atopic subjects; open triangles, nonatopic subjects.

sponsiveness and variable airflow obstruction, and an epithelial infiltration producing bronchitis and cough (Fig. 4). The specific role of the mast cell in the bronchial epithelium of patients with eosinophilic bronchitis and its interactions with cough sensory afferents needs further study.

Natural History of Eosinophilic Bronchitis

The natural history of eosinophilic bronchitis is unclear. A 10-year follow-up evaluation of the 12 patients from the original reports of eosinophilic bronchitis suggests that that this condition is generally benign and self-limiting (19). However, our experience is somewhat different. We have identified 52 patients from 1996 to 2003 with eosinophilic bronchitis and from 32 of these patients we have follow-up data of more than 1 year. Three (9%) of our patients developed asthma with typical symptoms and airway hyperresponsiveness. Twenty-one (66%) had persistent symptoms and or ongoing airway inflammation. Only one patient with eosinophilic bronchitis had complete resolution of symptoms and had no sputum eosinophilia whilst not on corticosteroid therapy. Five (16%) developed fixed airflow obstruction, although the decline in FEV_1 in the whole group of patients with eosinophilic bronchitis was not greater than in normal controls. Our findings are similar to that reported for atopic cough where there was no increased decline in lung function (20) and progression to asthma was rare (21).

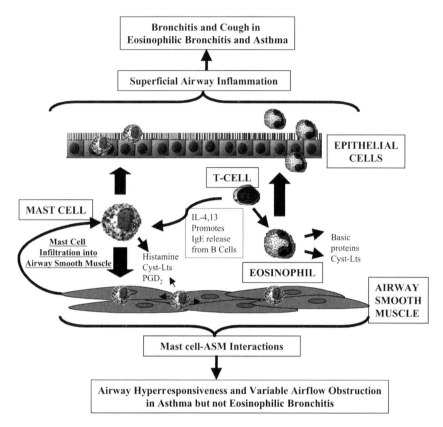

Figure 4   Schematic illustrating the importance of microlocalization of mast cells into the airway smooth muscle bundles in asthma in the development of disordered airway physiology and superficial mast cells and eosinophils in the development of cough in asthma and eosinophilic bronchitis.

We have reported one of the patients who over a 2-year period developed fixed airflow obstruction (22). The patient's cough improved with inhaled corticosteroids, but the sputum eosinophilia persisted. Several studies have observed that 30–40% of patients with COPD without a history of asthma and with no bronchodilator reversibility have sputum evidence of an airway eosinophilia (7,23). Our observation provides one possible explanation for the presence of eosinophilic airway inflammation in some patients with COPD without apparent pre-existing asthma in that eosinophilic bronchitis may in some circumstances be a prelude to COPD. Progressive irreversible airflow obstruction may occur due to remodeling of the airway secondary to the persistent eosinophilic airway inflammation in the presence of inadequate corticosteroid therapy. If this is true it has important implications in the early diagnosis and successful treatment of eosinophilic bronchitis. Further studies should be able to further define the natural history of this easily treatable condition.

Conclusions

Eosinophilic bronchitis is a common and treatable cause of chronic cough. The airway inflammation is similar to that seen in asthma although eosinophilic bronchitis is associated with quite different abnormalities of airway function. Recent findings support that these differences might be related to the site of mast cell infiltration of the airways. The main challenge for the future is for clinicians to consider eosinophilic bronchitis in their differential diagnosis of chronic cough and to develop noninvasive techniques to measure airway inflammation so that the condition can be positively identified. Future studies should look at the role of other noninvasive markers of airway inflammation in the chronic cough clinic, define the natural history of eosinophilic bronchitis and investigate the effects of other therapies.

References

1. Gibson PG, Dolovich J, Denburg J, Ramsdale EH, Hargreave FE. Chronic cough: eosinophilic bronchitis without asthma. Lancet 1989; I:1346–1348.
2. Brightling CE, Ward R, Goh KL, Wardlaw AJ, Pavord ID. Eosinophilic bronchitis is an important cause of cough. Am J Respir Crit Care 1999; 160:406–410.
3. Carney IK, Gibson PG, Murnee-Allen K, Saltos N, Olsen LG, Hensley MJ. A systematic evaluation of mechanisms in chronic cough. Am J Respir Crit Care 1997; 156:211–216.
4. Irwin RS, Corrao WM, Pratter MR. Chronic persistent cough in the adult: the spectrum and frequency of causes and successful outcome of specific therapy. Am Rev Respir Dis 1981; 123:413–417.
5. Irwin RS, Curley FJ, French CL. Chronic cough. The spectrum and frequency of causes, key components of the diagnostic evaluation, and outcome of specific therapy. Am Rev Respir Dis 1990; 141:640–647.
6. McGarvey LP, Heaney LG, Lawson JT, Johnston BT, Scally CM, Ennis M, Shepherd DR, MacMahon J. Evaluation and outcome of patients with chronic non-productive cough using a comprehensive diagnostic protocol. Thorax 1998; 53:738–743.
7. Fujimura M, Ogawa H, Yasui M, Matsuda T. Eosinophilic tracheobronchitis and airway cough hypersensitivity in chronic non-productive cough. Clin Exp Allergy 2000; 30:41–47.
8. Brightling CE, Pavord ID. Eosinophilic bronchitis—what is it and why is it important? Clin Exp Allergy 2000; 30:4–6.

9. Pizzichini E, Pizzichini MMM, Gibson P, Parameswaran K, Gleich GJ, Berman L, Dolovich J, Hargreave FE. Sputum eosinophilia predicts benefit from prednisolone in smokers with chronic obst.uctive bronchitis. Am J Respir Crit Care Med 1998; 158:1511–1517.
10. Pavord ID, Brightling CE, Woltmann G, Wardlaw AJ. Non-eosinophilic corticosteroid unresponsive asthma. Lancet 1999; 353:2213–2214.
11. Pavord ID, Pizzichini MMM, Pizzichini E, Hargreave FE. The use of induced sputum to investigate airway inflammation. Thorax 1997; 52:498–501.
12. Berlyne GS, Parameswaran K, Kamada D, Efthimiadis A, Hargreave FE. A comparison of exhaled nitric oxide and induced sputum markers of airway inflammation. J Allergy Clin Immunol 2000; 106:638–644.
13. Brightling CE, Symon FA, Birring SS, Bradding P, Wardlaw AJ, Pavord ID. Comparison of airway immunopathology of eosinophilic bronchitis and asthma. Thorax. 2003; 58:528–532.
14. Gibson PG, Hargreave FE, Girgis-Gbardo, Morris M, Denburg JA, Dolovich J. Chronic cough with eosinophilic bronchitis: examination for variable airflow obstruction and response to corticosteroid. Clin Exp Allergy 1995; 25: 127–132.
15. Brightling CE, Ward R, Wardlaw AJ, Pavord ID. Airway inflammation, airway responsiveness and cough before and after inhaled budesonide in patients with eosinophilic bronchitis. Eur Respir J 2000; 15:682–686.
16. Brightling CE, Bradding P, Symon FA, Holgate ST, Wardlaw AJ, Pavord ID. Mast cell infiltration of airway smooth muscle in asthma. N Engl J Med 2002; 346:1699–1705.
17. Brightling CE, Ward R, Woltmann G, Bradding P, Sheller JR, Dworski R, Pavord ID. Induced sputum inflammatory mediator concentrations in eosino-philic bronchitis and asthma. Am J Respir Crit Care Med 1999; 162:878–882.
18. Gibson PG, Zlatic K, Scott J, Sewell W, Woolley K, Saltos N. Chronic cough resembles asthma with IL-5 and granulocytes-macrophage colony-stimulating factor gene expression in bronchoalveolar cells. J Allergy Clin Immunol 1998; 101:320–326.
19. Hancox RJ, Leigh R, Kelly MM, Hargreave FE. Eosinophilic bronchitis. Lan-cet 2001; 358:1104.
20. Fujimura M, Nishizawa Y, Nishitsuji M, Abo M, Kita T, Nomura S. Longitu-dinal decline in pulmonary function in atopic cough and cough variant asthma. Clin Exp Allergy 2003; 33:588–594.
21. Fujimura M, Ogawa H, Nishizawa Y, Nishi K. Comparison of atopic cough with cough variant asthma: is atopic cough a precursor of asthma? Thorax 2003; 58:14–18.
22. Brightling CE, Woltmann G, Wardlaw AJ, Pavord ID. The development of irre-versible airflow obstruction in a patient with eosinophilic bronchitis without asthma. Eur Respir J 1999; 14:1228–1230.
23. Brightling CE, Monteiro W, Ward R, Morgan MDL, Wardlaw AJ, Pavord ID. Sputum eosinophilia and the short-term response to prednisolone in chronic obstructive pulmonary disease: a randomised controlled trial. Lancet 2000; 356:1480–1485.

18

Upper Airway Causes of Chronic Cough

**THADDEUS BARTTER, ZIAD C. BOUJAOUDE, and
MELVIN R. PRATTER**

Division of Pulmonary and Critical Care Medicine, Robert Wood Johnson Medical
   School at Camden,
Camden, New Jersey, U.S.A.

Introduction

Cough receptors have been documented to be present in the pharynx and
the larynx and have been inferred to be present in other locations in the
upper respiratory system (see Chapters 2 and 3) (1). Postnasal drip
(PND) is clearly the most common and dominant mechanism whereby disease of the upper airway causes cough. *Bordetella pertussis* causes acute
cough that may persist. *B. pertussis* may be a common upper airway cause
of chronic cough in some communities (2). There are several other disorders that can involve the upper airway and be associated with cough. At
times, these disorders may have cough as their sole or presenting manifestation. These causes will be listed but will not be considered further in this
chapter (Table 1) (1–6). The focus of this chapter will be on PND because
of its dominant role in cough due to upper airway disease.

   PND is not only the commonest upper airway cause of chronic cough
but also the commonest overall cause of chronic cough in most large studies
(7–9). There is presumably an interaction between the amount of material
dripping into the upper airway and the sensitivity of cough receptors; in

Table 1 Upper Airway Causes of Chronic Cough

Post-nasal drip (see text)
Swallowing disorders (e.g., neuromuscular disorders) (3)
Bordetella pertussis (2,6)
Thyroiditis (4)
Mediastinal masses (retrosternal goiter, lymphoma) (5)
Laryngeal or tracheal nodules or tumors
Foreign bodies or irritants in the ear (1)
Elongated uvula (1)
Vocal tics

some cases cough may be due to copious secretions, whereas in others very sensitive receptors may amplify the response to a relatively minor amount of PND.

PND is the act or sensation of secretions dripping into the posterior pharynx from the nose or sinuses. There is no clear-cut separation between normal and abnormal amounts of PND; PND is a physiologic clearance mechanism for irritant or particulate substances. It is therefore a normal process that only becomes "pathological" when it produces symptoms perceived as interfering with normal function. The major manifestations are excessive throat clearing and cough. Patients may also describe episodic gagging or choking, a tickle in the throat, dyspnea, or, occasionally, nausea and vomiting (10–13).

A negative physical examination of the upper airways is not a reliable method for ruling out PND as an etiology of cough (9). Several findings, however, are often associated with symptomatic PND. These include nasal edema, heavy nasal secretions, visible posterior pharyngeal secretions, and cobblestoning of the posterior pharynx (13,14).

There is no specific test that can document the quantity of PND and its impact on symptoms. The only way to definitively confirm PND as an etiology of cough is to document a response to specific treatment. PND does have a broad differential diagnosis, and specific etiologies may need to be evaluated to optimize therapy. The differential diagnosis is discussed below.

Differential Diagnosis of PND

Allergic Rhinitis

Allergic rhinitis is widely prevalent; it affects an estimated 20–40 million people in the United States alone. Allergic rhinitis can be seasonal (20% of cases), perennial (40% of cases), or mixed (40% of cases) (15). Allergic rhinitis is characterized clinically by one or more symptoms including sneezing, itching, nasal congestion, and rhinorrhea. Many causative agents have been linked to allergic rhinitis including pollens, molds, dust mites, and animal dander. Seasonal allergic rhinitis is fairly easy to identify because of the rapid and reproducible onset and offset of symptoms in association with pollen exposure (tree, grass, and weed) and outdoor mold spores during a defined season in which aeroallergens are abundant in the outdoor air. Perennial allergic rhinitis is defined as allergic rhinitis occurring during nine or more months of the year as a result of exposure to dust mites, cockroaches, indoor molds, or danders (including cat and dog) (15).

Careful history and physical examination are the most effective diagnostic maneuvers for the identification of allergic rhinitis. Laboratory confirmation of the presence of IgE antibodies to specific allergens, such as dust mites, pollens, or animal dander, is helpful in establishing a specific allergic diagnosis, especially if the history of specific allergen exposure is not clear-cut. The gold standard of allergen testing, however, remains dermal skin testing with specific allergens. In many cases, it is necessary to test for specific allergens to convince the family and patient of allergic diagnosis and to reinforce the importance of environmental control measures.

Vasomotor Rhinitis

Vasomotor rhinitis, or perennial nonallergic rhinitis, manifests with a spectrum of symptoms that range from predominantly obstructive to predominantly secretory. Nasal blockage is the most common symptom and, unlike allergic rhinitis, sneezing and nasal pruritus are less common (16).

Little is known about the pathophysiology of vasomotor rhinitis except that nonspecific nasal hyperreactivity occurs on exposure to nonimmunologic stimuli such as changes in temperature or relative humidity, alcohol ingestion, strong odors, and other airborne irritants. Vasomotor rhinitis is unrelated to allergy, infection, structural lesions, systemic disease, or drug abuse. Vasomotor rhinitis is therefore a diagnosis of exclusion (16).

Bacterial Sinusitis

Viral infections of the upper airway are a major cause of acute cough (17,18). Acute viral upper respiratory tract infection (URIs), do, however, sometimes produce chronic cough by causing a persistent, secondary bacterial sinusitis. (Persistent PND may at times be a chronic residuum of acute viral URI after the infection has resolved. This is discussed later.) The mechanism in bacterial sinusitis is obstruction of the sinus ostia and impairment of mucus clearance. Other listed causes of mucosal edema and obstruction can also lead to secondary sinus infection; the primary physiology is the conversion of the sinuses into a closed space. When caused by viral infection, bacterial sinusitis usually develops approximately 7 days after the acute infection (19). *Streptococcus pneumoniae* and *Haemophilus influenzae* are the most commonly isolated bacteria from infected maxillary sinuses followed by *Streptococcus pyogenes, Moraxella catarrhalis,* and anaerobic bacteria (19).

The clinical diagnosis of bacterial sinusitis is difficult and is generally overdone. The clinical characteristics lack specificity. Duration of illness of less than 7 days makes bacterial sinusitis unlikely, but duration of ≥ 7 days does not reliably distinguish prolonged viral infection from bacterial rhinosinusitis (17,20); purulent nasal discharge, tooth or facial pain (especially when unilateral), unilateral maxillary sinus tenderness, and worsening of symptoms after initial improvement seem to be helpful for predicting a higher likelihood of bacterial infection in patients with rhinosinusitis symptoms. Sinus radiography has limited value given the limited characteristics of the findings and the known high prevalence of abnormal findings in patients with viral rhinosinusitis. In a study using computed tomographic scanning, maxillary sinus abnormalities were present in 87% of acute viral URIs within 48 hr of onset (21). In another study, maxillary sinus radiographs of patients with typical viral URIs showed sinusitis in 39% of cases on the seventh day of illness (20).

Allergic Fungal Rhinosinusitis

Allergic fungal rhinosinusitis is generally recognized as an immunologically mediated disorder of the immunocompetent, distinct from other fungal forms of sinusitis. The pathophysiology is unclear, but allergic fungal rhinosinusitis is not an infection; it appears to be analogous to allergic bronchopulmonary aspergillosis in the lungs. At the present time, it is believed that exposure to specific fungal elements initiates an inflammatory cascade which involves IgE-mediated sensitivity (atopy), specific T-cell HLA receptor expression, and aberrancy of local mucosal defense mechanisms (22). Allergic fungal rhinosinusitis accounts for 5–10% of patients with chronic rhinosinusitis. It is most common among adolescents and young adults residing in temperate regions with relatively high humidity. It is associated with nasal polyposis and the presence of allergic fungal mucin. Atopy is characteristic of the disease: roughly two thirds of patients report a history of allergic rhinitis and 90% show elevated specific IgE to one or more fungal antigens (22).

The clinical presentation is usually subtle. Patients typically have gradual nasal airway obstruction and production of semisolid nasal crusts. Occasionally, the presentation may be dramatic, giving rise to acute visual loss, gross facial dysmorphia, or complete nasal obstruction. Pain is uncommon. Unresponsiveness to antihistamines, intranasal corticosteroids, and immunotherapy or recurrence after surgery are other clues suggestive of diagnosis.

Nonallergic Rhinitis with Eosinophilia Syndrome

Described first in 1981 (23), nonallergic rhinitis with eosinophilia syndrome (NARES) represents approximately 15–33% of adults with nonallergic rhinitis. NARES manifests with perennial symptoms of sneezing paroxysms, profuse watery rhinorrhea, and nasal pruritus; patients tend to have more intense nasal symptoms than patients with either vasomotor rhinitis or allergic rhinitis. Additionally, the presence of anosmia is common.

The pathophysiology of NARES syndrome is not understood. NARES usually occurs as an isolated disorder, but in some cases it is associated with the well-known triad of aspirin intolerance, non-IgE-mediated asthma, and nasal polyps. Nasal smears show marked eosinophilia, but allergic disease cannot be identified by skin testing or by RAST. Eosinophilia may contribute to nasal mucosal dysfunction. However, its presence in mild amounts is generally regarded as a good prognostic indicator for response to treatment with topical steroid therapy.

Anatomic Abnormalities

Anatomic abnormalities account for approximately 5–10% of chronic nasal disorders (16). Common anatomic causes of nasal obstruction include nasal polyps, deviated septum, enlarged turbinates, and dysfunctional nasal valve. Nasal polyps occur in approximately 1% of the general population. Nasal polyps are worthy of mention because of their association with chronic sinusitis, probably via the physiology of sinus osteal obstruction. Sinus polyps can occur alone or in association with a number of other entities. The triad of aspirin intolerance, nasal polyps, sinusitis, and asthma could be called a tetrad, with chronic sinusitis its fourth component (24). Other diseases associated with nasal polyps are Young syndrome, cystic fibrosis, Kartagener syndrome, Churg-Strauss syndrome, and allergic fungal sinusitis. Adenoid hypertrophy is a noncongenital abnormality that can engender rhinosinal disease. A number of tumors can be associated with sinus disease. These include chordoma, chemodectoma, neurofibroma, angiofibroma, inverting papilloma, squamous cell carcinoma, sarcoma, and encephaloceles or meningocele (16).

Rhinitis Medicamentosa

Many drugs can induce rhinitis in allergic and nonallergic individuals (16). The term "rhinitis medicamentosa" is most commonly used to describe the rebound nasal congestion that occurs with overuse of topical decongestants/ vasoconstrictor nasal preparations (oxymetazolone, phenylephrine) as well as from abuse of cocaine (16,25,26). This is important because the chronic use of topical decongestants can perpetuate the very symptoms that they are being used to treat. It is for this reason that topical decongestants, although very effective, can be recommended only for acute/short-term treatment of nasal congestion.

Atrophic Rhinitis

Atrophic rhinitis is a disease characterized by symptoms of epistaxis, severe crusting, and stuffiness associated with a foul or fetid odor and *Klebsiella ozaenae* colonization. In industrialized countries, atrophic rhinitis is usually seen only as a rare complication of nasal/septal surgery aimed to relieve obstruction. In underdeveloped countries, atrophic rhinitis can result from chronic undertreated infection and perhaps from nutritional deficiencies (27).

Physical/Chemical/Irritant-Induced Rhinitis

Physical triggers of rhinitis include cold and dry air, ingestion of spicy food, exposure to bright light, and outdoor air pollutants including dust, ozone, sulfur dioxide, formaldehyde, volatile organic compounds, wood smoke, and environmental tobacco smoke. Most of these triggers are nasal irritants causing reduced nasal airflow, rhinorrhea, and sneezing. The pathophysiology of this disorder may involve both mast cell degranulation and increased neuronal reflex mechanisms. Avoidance is effective. Prophylaxis with topical ipratropium prior to exposure to a known irritant may also be effective (16).

Occupational Rhinitis

Occupational rhinitis is defined as the episodic, work-related occurrence of sneezing, rhinorrhea, and nasal obstruction (28). Unlike the other entities discussed herein, occupational rhinitis is defined more by context than by pathophysiology; groupings of occurrences can be traced to a workplace exposure. Occupational rhinitis can be induced by exposure to strong odors, irritation from exposure to one or more known respiratory irritants at levels exceeding threshold limits, stimulation of immunologic pathways, or corrosive exposure from high concentrations of irritating and soluble chemical gases. A case of occupational rhinitis could therefore be allergic due to exposure to workplace aeroallergens, irritant, or it could represent aggravation of underlying allergic rhinitis by a separate workplace exposure. The greater the number of symptomatic workers, the more likely it is that the offending agent is nonimmunogenic. Environmental control is the mainstay of therapy, achieved by removing the etiologic agent, improving ventilation, wearing protective masks, or changing the work site. Nasal saline lavage can be used to remove accumulated particulates when particulate matter is responsible.

Miscellaneous

Rhinitis can be associated with metabolic conditions such as the hormonal changes of pregnancy and thyroid dysfunction. It can also be seen with systemic vasculitis and granulomatous diseases (16).

Postinfectious and Idiopathic PND

While different specific etiologies of PND have been discussed, it appears that some PND has no obvious or persistent underlying cause; it appears clinically as though some trigger initiated PND, which then persists as a vicious cycle and causes cough until interrupted. Poe and Israel used the term "postinfectious" after noting (as have others) that in some cases chronic cough appears to have been triggered by a URI (7). Others have noted this association but have included "postinfectious" with other causes of PND (9,13). It seems reasonable to label this as postinfectious PND when an upper respiratory infection was the historical precipitant and as idiopathic PND when no such initiating trigger can be identified.

Treatment of Cough Due to PND

As noted above, PND is the commonest cause of cough in large series. Its diagnosis and treatment are complicated by the fact (mentioned above) that there is no objective study that can demonstrate, in a given patient, that PND is the cause of cough. An algorithmic approach to chronic cough has demonstrated that a diagnostic/therapeutic approach to PND in the initial work-up of cough is very effective (9). Interestingly, this approach does not involve the classification of an etiology of PND prior to intervention. We recommend a diagnostic "testing" approach to PND only if PND persists despite an initial diagnostic/therapeutic trial. We recommend that evaluations for asthma and GERD be deferred until the issue of PND has been fully addressed unless initial history and physical are highly suggestive of one of these diagnoses. In recent years, the armamentarium of pharmacological options for treating PND has increased significantly. This gives the clinician a number of choices if initial approaches are not well tolerated.

Most of the etiologies of PND listed above may be suggested by history and physical but are unlikely to be proven. There are some exceptions. Anatomic abnormalities should be evident on initial physical examination. A diagnosis of atrophic rhinitis should be quite clear after history and physical. In many cases of chronic cough, the diagnosis after initial history and physical is not clear-cut; there is a potential for PND as an etiology of cough although the specific etiology of PND is not clear.

The two most universally effective and time-honored therapies for PND are antihistamine/decongestants (A/D) and topical nasal steroids.

A/D are usually well tolerated, although there may be excessive dryness, excessive stimulation, drowsiness, or (in men) urinary retention. They are of value in the diagnosis and treatment of cough; if there was some response after 7–10 days of A/D, then PND is almost certainly an etiology of cough (9). If there is no response, PND becomes much less likely. Note that the "nonsedating" antihistamines are not as universally effective as the more classical antihistamines. Nonsedating antihistamines are clearly less effective in vasomotor rhinitis (14,18). We therefore recommend that the initial diagnostic/therapeutic approach to chronic cough involve a "classical" antihistamine coupled with a decongestant.

Topical nasal steroids have nonspecific anti-inflammatory properties. They are well tolerated and easy to administer. They are effective across a broad spectrum of the diagnoses listed above (16,29–32). Topical nasal steroids are therefore a reasonable second medication if there is a persistence of PND symptoms and cough after initial A/D therapy or if A/D therapy is not tolerated. The addition of nasal steroids may allow successful treatment with a lower dose of A/D.

Four other classes of topical preparations are available; topical anticholinergics, topical antihistamines, topical vasoconstrictors, and cromolyn. Ipratropium is an anticholinergic with direct antisecretory action which can be effective in some hypersecretory states, particularly vasomotor rhinitis (33–36). Azelastine is a topical antihistamine shown to have some efficacy in allergic and vasomotor rhinitis (16,37,38). Both drugs are potential alternatives or adjuncts to an A/D approach to PND. Topical vasoconstrictors are useful to help open the nasal passageways and promote drainage when sinusitis is present. It is recommended that they generally should not be used for more than 3–5 days to avoid rebound effects (25,26). Intranasal cromolyn can be helpful in managing allergic rhinitis, although the need to use it several times a day in many patients limits compliance and its effectiveness compared to other modalities for allergic rhinitis (39,40).

Leukotriene inhibitors have also recently been documented to have efficacy similar to nonsedating antihistamines in the treatment of allergic rhinitis (41). They may be less effective than topical steroids (42), but they have appeal, particularly in cases of allergic rhinitis coupled with asthma and cough.

If an initial nonspecific diagnostic/therapeutic trial fails to achieve resolution of both PND symptoms and cough, evaluation of the specific etiologies listed is reasonable. Radiographic imaging of the sinuses is definitely indicated, as occult chronic sinusitis can have cough as its only manifestation (43). If sinusitis is present, then a therapy of combined short-term topical alpha adrenergic blockers, nasal steroids, and antibiotics is often effective. Chronic sinusitis may require courses of antibiotics significantly longer than those used for acute infections. Other investigations relevant in the face of nonresponsive PND would include allergy testing, antifungal allergen assays, nasal smears, and, at times, nasal biopsy/drainage. A more extensive search for occupational and/or irritant exposures would also be advised.

If further diagnostic modalities yield a diagnosis of allergic fungal rhinosinusitis, systemic steroids may produce some relief of symptoms, but definitive management depends on removal of all fungal mucin from the nasosinal passages. The availability of oral antifungals such as itraconazole may increase the likelihood of success with medical therapy, although this remains to be confirmed (22).

If the ultimate diagnosis is NARES, then topical steroid therapy is often effective. Systemic steroid therapy may be required intermittently for exacerbations (23).

Atrophic rhinitis is relatively resistant to treatment and usually not cured. The standard modality is antibiotic treatment of bacterial overgrowth coupled with aggressive nasal saline irrigation. Intermittent surgical intervention may be required (27).

There are several experimental approaches to different diagnoses. In vasomotor rhinitis, local capsaicin treatment of the nasal mucosa has been shown to reduce symptoms in one study (44). Another study demonstrates efficacy of local application of different concentrations of silver nitrate (45). There are also surgical approaches to vasomotor rhinitis, which include endoscopic vidian nerve section and/or electrocoagulation of the anterior ethmoidal nerve (46). While these therapies may have some efficacy, the established armamentarium is usually effective, and they should need to be used extremely rarely.

A final issue in the treatment of upper airway causes of chronic cough is the question of when to look for additional etiologies of cough. Many patients have two or three major causes of cough. Effective treatment of PND would, in those cases, only be expected to effect partial resolution of cough. How aggressively to pursue the differential diagnosis of PND in any individual is in part clinical judgment. A general guideline is that the persistence of symptomatic PND would warrant further work-up of PND before addressing asthma and GERD. Conversely, if there are no symptoms of PND in a patient who continues to cough after initial diagnostic/therapeutic interventions for PND, it is probably advisable to look at other etiologies of cough prior to an extensive evaluation for occult PND that did not respond to that initial therapy.

Conclusion

The upper airway is a major cause of chronic cough. The most common mechanism whereby upper airway disease causes cough is through PND. The differential diagnosis of PND is broad. In the clinical approach to

common cough, it makes sense to treat PND with an empiric diagnostic/
therapeutic trial prior to embarking on a search for a specific upper airway
cause of PND.

References

1. Irwin RS, Rosen MJ, Braman SS. Cough. A comprehensive review. Arch Intern Med 1977; 137(9):1186–1191.
2. Birkebaek NH, Kristiansen M, Seefeldt T, Degn J, Moller A, Heron I, et al. *Bordetella pertussis* and chronic cough in adults. Clin Infect Dis 1999; 29: 1239–1242.
3. Buckler RA, Pratter MR, Chad DA, Smith TW. Chronic cough as the presenting symptom of oculopharyngeal muscular dystrophy. Chest 1989; 95:921–922.
4. Irwin RS, Pratter MR, Hamolsky MW. Chronic persistent cough: an uncommon presenting complaint of thyroiditis. Chest 1982; 81:386–388.
5. Akers SM, Bartter TC, Pratter MR. Chronic cough as the sole manifestation of Hodgkin's disease. Chest 1992; 101:853–854.
6. Birkebaek NH. *Bordetella pertussis* in the aetiology of chronic cough in adults. Diagnostic methods and clinic. Dan Med Bull 2001; 48:77–80.
7. Poe RH, Harder RV, Israel RH, Kallay MC. Chronic persistent cough. Experience in diagnosis and outcome using an anatomic diagnostic protocol. Chest 1989; 95:723–728.
8. Irwin RS, Curley FJ, French CL. Chronic cough. The spectrum and frequency of causes, key components of the diagnostic evaluation, and outcome of specific therapy. Am Rev Respir Dis 1990; 141:640–647.
9. Pratter MR, Bartter T, Akers S, DuBois J. An algorithmic approach to chronic cough. Ann Intern Med 1993; 119:977–983.
10. Pratter MR, Curley FJ, DuBois J, Irwin RS. Cause and evaluation of chronic dyspnea in a pulmonary disease clinic. Arch Intern Med 1989; 149:2277–2282.
11. Irwin RS, Pratter MR, Holland PS, Corwin RW, Hughes JP. Postnasal drip causes cough and is associated with reversible upper airway obstruction. Chest 1984; 85:346–352.
12. Irwin RS, Pratter MR. Postnasal drip and cough. Clin Notes Respir Dis 1980; 18:11–12.
13. Irwin RS, Corrao WM, Pratter MR. Chronic persistent cough in the adult: the spectrum and frequency of causes and successful outcome of specific therapy. Am Rev Respir Dis 1981; 123:413–417.
14. Irwin RS, Boulet LP, Cloutier MM, Fuller R, Gold PM, Hoffstein V, et al. Managing cough as a defense mechanism and as a symptom. A consensus panel report of the American College of Chest Physicians. Chest 1998; 114(suppl 2): 133S–181S.
15. Skoner DP. Allergic rhinitis: definition, epidemiology, pathophysiology, detection, and diagnosis. J Allergy Clin Immunol 2001; 108(suppl 1):S2–S8.
16. Settipane RA, Lieberman P. Update on nonallergic rhinitis. Ann Allergy Asthma Immunol 2001; 86:494–507.

17. Curley FJ, Irwin RS, Pratter MR, Stivers DH, Doern GV, Vernaglia PA, et al. Cough and the common cold. Am Rev Respir Dis 1988; 138:305–311.
18. Irwin RS, Madison JM. The diagnosis and treatment of cough. N Engl J Med 2000; 343:1715–1721.
19. Gwaltney JM Jr. Acute community-acquired sinusitis. Clin Infect Dis 1996; 23:1209–1223.
20. Puhakka T, Makela MJ, Alanen A, Kallio T, Korsoff L, Arstila P, et al. Sinusitis in the common cold. J Allergy Clin Immunol 1998; 102:403–408.
21. Gwaltney JM Jr, Phillips CD, Miller RD, Riker DK. Computed tomographic study of the common cold. N Engl J Med 1994; 330:25–30.
22. Marple BF. Allergic fungal rhinosinusitis: current theories and management strategies. Laryngoscope 2001; 111:1006–1019.
23. Jacobs RL, Freedman PM, Boswell RN. Nonallergic rhinitis with eosinophilia (NARES syndrome). Clinical and immunologic presentation. J Allergy Clin Immunol 1981; 67:253–262.
24. Szczeklik A, Nizankowska E, Sanak M, Swierczynska M. Aspirin-induced rhinitis and asthma. Curr Opin Allergy Clin Immunol 2001; 1:27–33.
25. Scadding GK. Rhinitis medicamentosa. Clin Exp Allergy 1995; 25:391–394.
26. Graf P, Hallen H, Juto JE. The pathophysiology and treatment of rhinitis medicamentosa. Clin Otolaryngol 1995; 20:224–229.
27. Chand MS, MacArthur CJ. Primary atrophic rhinitis: a summary of four cases and review of the literature. Otolaryngol Head Neck Surg 1997; 116:554–558.
28. Slavin RG. Occupational rhinitis. Ann Allergy Asthma Immunol 2003; 90 (5 suppl 2):2–6.
29. Orgel HA, Meltzer EO, Bierman CW, Bronsky E, Connell JT, Lieberman PL, et al. Intranasal fluocortin butyl in patients with perennial rhinitis: a 12-month efficacy and safety study including nasal biopsy. J Allergy Clin Immunol 1991; 88:257–264.
30. Ratner PH, Howland WC III, Jacobs RL, Reed KD, Goode-Sellers ST, Prillaman BA, et al. Relief of sinus pain and pressure with fluticasone propionate aqueous nasal spray: a placebo-controlled trial in patients with allergic rhinitis. Allergy Asthma Proc 2002; 23:259–263.
31. Gross G, Jacobs RL, Woodworth TH, Georges GC, Lim JC. Comparative efficacy, safety, and effect on quality of life of triamcinolone acetonide and fluticasone propionate aqueous nasal sprays in patients with fall seasonal allergic rhinitis. Ann Allergy Asthma Immunol 2002; 89:56–62.
32. Scadding GK, Lund VJ, Jacques LA, Richards DH. A placebo-controlled study of fluticasone propionate aqueous nasal spray and beclomethasone dipropionate in perennial rhinitis: efficacy in allergic and non-allergic perennial rhinitis. Clin Exp Allergy 1995; 25:737–743.
33. Meltzer EO, Orgel HA, Bronsky EA, Findlay SR, Georgitis JW, Grossman J, et al. Ipratropium bromide aqueous nasal spray for patients with perennial allergic rhinitis: a study of its effect on their symptoms, quality of life, and nasal cytology. J Allergy Clin Immunol 1992; 90:242–249.
34. Dockhorn R, Aaronson D, Bronsky E, Chervinsky P, Cohen R, Ehtessabian R, et al. Ipratropium bromide nasal spray 0.03% and beclomethasone nasal spray

alone and in combination for the treatment of rhinorrhea in perennial rhinitis. Ann Allergy Asthma Immunol 1999; 82:349–359.

35. Grossman J, Banov C, Boggs P, Bronsky EA, Dockhorn RJ, Druce H, et al. Use of ipratropium bromide nasal spray in chronic treatment of nonallergic perennial rhinitis, alone and in combination with other perennial rhinitis medications. J Allergy Clin Immunol 1995; 95:1123–1127.

36. Druce HM, Spector SL, Fireman P, Kaiser H, Meltzer EO, Boggs P, et al. Double-blind study of intranasal ipratropium bromide in nonallergic perennial rhinitis. Ann Allergy 1992; 69:53–60.

37. LaForce C, Dockhorn RJ, Prenner BM, Chu TJ, Kraemer MJ, Widlitz MD, et al. Safety and efficacy of azelastine nasal spray (Astelin NS) for seasonal allergic rhinitis: a 4-week comparative multicenter trial. Ann Allergy Asthma Immunol 1996; 76:181–188.

38. Banov CH, Lieberman P. Efficacy of azelastine nasal spray in the treatment of vasomotor (perennial nonallergic) rhinitis. Ann Allergy Asthma Immunol 2001; 86:28–35.

39. Cohan RH, Bloom FL, Rhoades RB, Wittig HJ, Haugh LD. Treatment of perennial allergic rhinitis with cromolyn sodium. Double-blind study on 34 adult patients. J Allergy Clin Immunol 1976; 58:121–128.

40. Orgel HA, Meltzer EO, Kemp JP, Ostrom NK, Welch MJ. Comparison of intranasal cromolyn sodium, 4%, and oral terfenadine for allergic rhinitis: symptoms, nasal cytology, nasal ciliary clearance, and rhinomanometry. Ann Allergy 1991; 66:237–244.

41. Philip G, Malmstrom K, Hampel FC, Weinstein SF, LaForce CF, Ratner PH, et al. Montelukast for treating seasonal allergic rhinitis: a randomized, double-blind, placebo-controlled trial performed in the spring. Clin Exp Allergy 2002; 32:1020–1028.

42. Nathan RA. Pharmacotherapy for allergic rhinitis: a critical review of leukotriene receptor antagonists compared with other treatments. Ann Allergy Asthma Immunol 2003; 90:182–190.

43. Pratter MR, Bartter T, Lotano R. The role of sinus imaging in the treatment of chronic cough in adults. Chest 1999; 116:1287–1291.

44. Stjarne P, Rinder J, Heden-Blomquist E, Cardell LO, Lundberg J, Zetterstrom O, et al. Capsaicin desensitization of the nasal mucosa reduces symptoms upon allergen challenge in patients with allergic rhinitis. Acta Otolaryngol 1998; 118:235–239.

45. Bhargava KB, Shirali GN, Abhyankar US, Gadre KC. Treatment of allergic and vasomotor rhinitis by the local application of different concentrations of silver nitrate. J Laryngol Otol 1992; 106:699–701.

46. el Guindy A. Endoscopic transseptal vidian neurectomy. Arch Otolaryngol Head Neck Surg 1994; 120:1347–1351.

19

Psychogenic Cough

PAUL A. GREENBERGER

Department of Medicine, Northwestern University Feinberg School of Medicine,
Chicago, Illinois, U.S.A.

Introduction

Psychogenic cough or "habit cough" is a nonorganic cough that typically occurs in children or adolescents (1–7) but has been reported in adults (4,8,9). It is thought that there may not be underlying psychopathology although children may have school phobia or use the cough for attention getting (3,5,10). The cough may increase in intensity or frequency in the presence of medical personnel and be nonexistent during sleep or distraction. Most reports of psychogenic cough note that the subjects are not particularly troubled by the repetitive coughing in the setting of frustration on the part of teachers or parents. Some adults may be depressed, however (9). Antitussives and antiasthma medications including courses of prednisone are ineffective in suppressing the cough. The workup for common causes of cough such as postnasal drip from rhinitis, sinusitis, gastroesophageal reflux, and asthma will be normal or there will be a limited to absent response to pharmacotherapy . There may be a poor effort on inspiration during spirometry such that the flow-volume tracing will be consistent with extrathoracic obstruction.

International Classification of Diseases—9th Revision (11)

Chronic cough (not psychogenic) or bronchial cough is identified by the code 786.2, whereas psychogenic cough is coded for with 306.1. Functional "arising from mental factors" cough also is identified by 306.1. Stridor, which is not congenital in etiology, and which is not part of psychogenic cough, is coded for by 786.1. Psychogenic asthma is identified by 493.9.

Diagnosis

The diagnosis may be suspected when there is a nonproductive cough of over 8 weeks duration, consistent with a chronic cough (12), that has been resistant to pharmacologic therapy for cough, gastroesophageal reflux, and asthma with radiologic or bronchoscopic tests being within normal limits. Concomitantly, the patient appears not to be ill or bothered by the cough (9). The cough has several characteristics that are listed in Table 1. Although there are many causes of chronic cough, patients who present to specialists such as a pulmonologist or allergist-immunologist may be evaluated for rhinitis (allergic, nonallergic, or mixed), sinusitis, asthma specifically cough-variant asthma, and gastroesophageal reflux disease (12–15). Many adult patients with chronic cough will have more than one cause of chronic cough (12,14–16). In a study of 78 nonsmoking patients aged 15–81 years, one explanation for cough was found in 30 (38.5%) patients whereas the remaining 48 (61.5%) patients had more than one cause identified (16). Indeed, gastroesophageal reflux may be present in 25–50% of patients with asthma (14) and may persist in the absence of acid, suggesting that nonacid reflux may be present (13). The diagnosis of psychogenic cough may be overlooked in some situations while a careful diagnostic and therapeutic trial has been performed. Certainly, one would not want to label a patient with a psychogenic cough when there is bronchiectasis present or external compression of the tracheal from a mediastinal mass.

Differential Diagnosis

In the absence of an organic cause of chronic nonproductive cough in a patient who is not bothered excessively by the cough, psychogenic cough may be considered. Thus, often the diagnosis is made by exclusion of other causes, some of which are presented for contrast.

Cough-Variant Asthma

Ten patients were described who had debilitating cough for from 2 months to 20 years (17). Chest radiographs, expiratory flow rates, and otolaryngologic examinations were normal. The chest examination by auscultation did not reveal wheezing or crackles but patients would be coughing or would

Table 1 Some Characteristics of Psychogenic Cough

Clinical features
The cough is non-productive and has lasted at least 3 weeks
The cough may be "honking," "staccato," or "honking" that may begin suddenly
The cough is not associated with swallowing, eating or drinking
The patient does not seem appropriately troubled by the repetitive coughing (*la belle indifference*)
The cough has failed to respond to therapy for common causes of chronic cough such as asthma, gastroesophageal reflux disease, and post-nasal drip from rhinitis or sinusitis
A thoughtful diagnostic evaluation has not identified a cause
The cough may cease when the patient is distracted
Nonpharmacologic treatments such as lozenges may "control" the cough

Psychologic issues
Secondary gain is present (What situation or persons would the patient lose control of if the cough were to be "cured?")
The cough interferes with social activities but not sleep
The cough increases in intensity or frequency in the presence of family, medical professionals, teachers, or telephone use
Emotional distress will increase the cough, including during visits to physicians
Anxiety, depression, conversion disorder, or somatoform illness may be identified more frequently in adults than children
Psychologic or psychiatric evaluation may be refused by the patient
Pulmonary function tests
Expiratory flow rates (FEV$_1$, FVC, and FEF$_{25-75}$) are normal
Methacholine challenge tests are negative
The flow-volume loop may resemble extrathoracic obstruction consistent with vocal cord dysfunction
Poor effort may be present especially on inspiration

(From Ref. 11.)

report coughing spasms. By history, some patients had coughing spasms that had interfered with work, sleep, or social functions. Indeed, some patients had experienced fecal or urinary incontinence because of severe coughing. Because beta agonists, theophylline, nasal corticosteroids, and antitussives and in some cases orally inhaled corticosteroids were unsuccessful in diminishing the cough, prednisone at a minimum of 30 mg daily for 7–14 days was administered (17). This diagnostic–therapeutic trial was successful in all patients, some patients responding within 3 days. The patients then can be treated with inhaled corticosteroids for persistent asthma if needed. However, inhaled corticosteroids alone may not be sufficient initially for control of cough-variant asthma. Prednisone-dependent cough variant asthma may be recognized when it is not possible to control the coughing with high dose inhaled corticosteroids and other medications.

In 1975, E. R. McFadden, Jr. reported seven patients with mean age of 27 years who had "intractable paroxysms of coughing that tended to be nonproductive of sputum" (18). It was possible to induce wheezing in three of the patients. The FEV_1 was just 53.2% of predicted and the residual volume was 152% consistent with gas trapping. Additional measures of airways resistance demonstrated substantial increased values which would be expected with moderately severe airways obstruction. After a week of bronchodilator treatment, the FEV_1 had increased remarkably to 110% and the residual volume decreased to 105.9% (18). The findings were consistent with reversible large airways obstruction in patients with cough-variant asthma. There was some degree of small airways obstruction in that the maximum mid-expiratory flow (similar to FEF_{25-75}) initially was just 29% but increased to 98% after treatment (18). This group of patients did not have the chief complaint of wheezing but rather intractable cough. The site of airways obstruction primarily was large (and small) airways. In summary, both descriptions of patients with asthma who had cough as a primary symptom (17,18) required either oral bronchodilators or prednisone to improve symptoms and respiratory status. These patients are more common than patients with psychogenic cough and at times a diagnostic–therapeutic trial of inhaled corticosteroids and prednisone will be necessary to confirm or refute that the cough is consistent with cough-variant asthma.

The Irritable Larynx and Laryngeal Dysfunction Syndromes

The irritable larynx designation may include various terms such as vocal cord dysfunction, laryngeal dyskinesia, episodic paroxysmal laryngospasm, and irritable larynx syndrome (19). The symptoms that patients report vary but typically patients have chronic throat clearing and its resulting cough or other symptoms such as paroxysmal inspiratory stridor, intermittent dyspnea, dysphonia, intractable asthma that does not respond to antiasthma therapy. Some patients will have been intubated during acute respiratory distress when stridor is present. In a series of 39 patients with the irritable larynx syndrome, symptoms had included "episodic laryngospasm and or dysphonia with or without globus or chronic cough (20). There typically is a trigger such as a viral upper respiratory tract illness. However, gastroesophageal reflux was identified in over 90% of patients and a third had some psychologic factors that served as stimuli (20).

It is thought that either gastroesophageal acid reflux (12,13) or nonacid (pepsin) reflux (21) that causes posterior laryngitis (22) or better designated as laryngopharyngeal reflux (21) may irritate the vocal cords and arytenoids resulting in cough and various symptoms classified under the irritable larynx syndrome. Coughing can intensify gastroesophageal reflux (23) which can potentiate the process. Patients with laryngopharyngeal reflux often report cough, hoarseness, postnasal drainage, "asthma" or a globus sensation. The latter is the feeling of a lump in the throat or a choking sensation (24). The reflux can contribute to the intermittent but difficult to control cough. Antireflux therapy is recommended; however, when psychologic factors are present, the ideal approach would be to have the patient receive therapy by a psychologist or psychiatrist. However, patients do not seek such care and may not return for medical advice when they have been told to seek psychologic or psychiatric evaluation. Some patients with vocal cord dysfunction who present with difficult to treat asthma may respond to voice therapy.

Factitious Cough Conditions

Factitious cough was one of five conditions that were produced by a 37-year-old woman (25). She had been admitted to a hospital for 3 weeks' of cough associated with wheezing. She also reported shortness of breath. The cough was loud and "seal barking" in quality. The patient had stated that her asthma had been present for 7 years, and it was worsened by exposure to cleaning solutions, molds, and dust. She had recently been hospitalized for 5 weeks because of violent coughing and wheezing dyspnea. Her examination by this author was within normal limits except for anterior sternal-costal tenderness to palpation. When she produced a "seal barking" cough, she reported the sensation to produce mucus. She coughed so frequently that it was difficult to be certain that breath sounds were normal. The coughing episodes would last 15 min before stopping. There was no evidence of airflow obstruction and she had mild restrictive findings that improved after albuterol inhalation. An arterial blood gas on room air had pH of 7.43, pO_2 of 54 mmHg, and pCO_2 of 34 mmHg (25). The pulse oxygen saturation was 91%. The patient did not appear to be ill during this time, and it was concluded that these results were attributable to breath holding. It was determined that this patient had produced five factitious allergic conditions including (a) factitious severe coughing, (b) factitious fever with normal rectal temperature, (c) positive immediate skin tests which were negative skin tests for the first 20 min but "positive" results produced by linear scratching of the test sites, (d) factitious systemic allergic reactions to vaccine immunotherapy, and (e) factitious hypoxemia caused by breath holding (25). A psychiatrist concluded that there was agitated depression in that the patient's son had Down's syndrome. The patient refused to pursue psychiatric care and chose to receive counseling from a pastor-psychologist.

Direct laryngosopy can be useful when patients are suspected of having nonorganic upper airway obstruction during which cough is a major manifestation (26). A 61-year-old woman presented with coughing, a sensation of throat closure, dyspnea, and loss of voice attributable to inhalation of nail polish remover and perfumes (26). During an emergency department visit, it was noted that her uvula was not edematous and there was no rash or erythema that would help confirm an allergic mechanism. Her arterial pCO_2 was 25 mmHg and pH was 7.55 with pO_2 of 94 mmHg. These findings were consistent with acute respiratory alkalosis from hyperventilation, not airways obstruction from asthma or upper airway obstruction. Further-more, the flow-volume loop tracing was normal and not consistent with vocal cord dysfunction. At a time when she was asymptomatic, direct laryn-goscopy was performed which demonstrated absence of vocal cord or pha-ryngeal edema. When she was then challenged with exposure to an open bottle of nail polish, symptoms of coughing and choking occurred within seconds. The vocal cords did not swell and moved appropriately (26). Her voice sounded hoarse in the absence of objectively proved angioedema. It was concluded that she had hyperfunctioning vocal and laryngeal muscles consistent with a nonorganic etiology. In this case, speech therapy was helpful in preventing future episodes.

Definition of a Factitious Disorder

There are three requirements for a factitious disorder. First, the disorder is one in which the subject produces symptoms to assume the "sick" role. In other words, the symptoms are produced by the patient intentionally and may result in objectively confirmed findings. The second requirement is that there is motivation to be "ill." Third, the subject does not produce these symptoms or signs for a defined strategic reason such as avoiding jail or military service or to receive disability payments. For example, a medical resident was referred for severe asthma and on examination had unilateral crepitus in the right supraclavicular fossa. She did not appear to be ill and was not dyspneic. Her chest examination only revealed mild rhonchi and expiratory flow rates demonstrated mild airways obstruction only. A chest radiograph did not reveal a pneumomediastinum or pneumothorax. It was felt that she had used a 26.5 gauge needle to inject air into the supra-clavicular fossa so as to support her diagnosis of severe asthma with pneu-momediastinum. In contrast, malingering, which also results in production of objectively present findings, relates to a specific purpose such as receiv-ing continued disability payments. The factitious patient receives no appar-ent economic benefits as occurs with malingering. The subject is unaware of the motivating factors and the symptoms or signs may be physical, psycho-logic, or both.

Munchausen's Syndrome

Munchausen's syndrome refers to a chronic condition that is the most severe form of factitious disorder. In Munchausen's syndrome, there are (a) repeated hospitalizations, (b) fantastic and compelling stories about the subject's medical or surgical history that is a fabrication, and (c) traveling from hospital to hospital. Subjects knowingly can injure themselves for subconscious reasons. As opposed to severe coughing, some subjects emit loud stridorous sounds. There is no wheezing on auscultation of the chest and the patient is not cyanotic (27). Furthermore, the patient is not alarmed or frightened by the stridorous sounds. With distraction or sleep, the "stridor" and cough cease. In such a situation, Munchausen's stridor would not result in injury to the patient. However, if cough accompanies an acute anaphylactic reaction such that results from the deliberate ingestion of aspirin in a Munchausen's patient who has aspirin-intolerant asthma, the risk of severe, true airways obstruction is moderate to high because the bronchoconstriction is real. The Munchausen patient is able to generate sympathy, having assumed the "sick" role. Perhaps the motivating factor involves gratification from the attention that health care providers give to the patient; alternatively, there may be deep-seated anger and the Munchausen's patient seeks to control others.

Cough may be a component of Munchausen's anaphylaxis, which is true anaphylaxis. The patient, who is allergic to Brazil nuts, will ingest the particular nut to induce an anaphylactic reaction. Immediate skin testing with a Brazil nut extract will demonstrate the anti-Brazil nut IgE antibodies. One such patient, after producing a series of "idiopathic" ana-phylactic episodes erred when he presented with unilateral conjunctival injection and chemosis after he had inserted Brazil nut dust in his conjunctival sac. An astute allergist-immunologist determined that the previous attacks had been self-induced by ingestion of Brazil nut.

Some clinical tools to consider in the diagnosis of factitious asthma are presented in Table 2.

Factitious Sneezing

A 13-year-old adolescent female was described who had reported sneezing up to 2000 times a day (28). Intranasal beclomethasone dipropionate and oral brompheniramine helped reduce the number of sneezes in part;

Table 2 Some Clinical Issues When Considering Factitious Cough or Asthma

How ill does the patient appear compared to the reported symptoms?
Does the cough, wheeze, or emitted stridorous sounds cease with distraction, a deep breath, anxiolytic treatment (midazolam), or during sleep?
Is the wheeze heard loudest over the neck?
Does asking the patient to cough stop the wheeze or cough on the next inspiration?
Is there stridor or cough without auscultatory wheezing in lung fields?
Are the FEV_1 and FEF_{25-75} within normal limits or is effort unsatisfactory during expiratory or inspiratory efforts?

however, sneezing could last an hour straight. She had been sent to an emergency department for the sneezing and treated with subcutaneous epinephrine on one occasion. Subsequent treatments with flunisolide and triamcinolone acetonide were not of help. Manipulation of her vertebral column by a chiropractor was considered to be of "some benefit." During her examination at Northwestern University, there was not a single sneeze in 3 hr. Immediate skin tests for allergens were negative. The nasal examination was normal. The adolescent had missed 21 days of school over a 3-month period (28). One week later, the mother was called to ascertain the status of her daughter. She reported that the sneezing had decreased but she did not "hold with this psychologic stuff" (28). The patient had continued to be treated by a chiropractor who had located and treated the patient's "sneeze point" in the spine. In this case, the diagnosis was suspected when there was a history of a remarkable number and duration of sneezes, lack of anti-allergen IgE antibodies, absence of sneezing during sleep or during a 3-hr period of physician and nurse evaluation, poor to absent response to various nasal corticosteroids and a normal nasal exam.

Vocal Cord Dysfunction

Vocal cord dysfunction (29,30) may or may not coexist with asthma. It may present as intractable asthma of which cough is a major component. Vocal cord dysfunction may be overlooked by experienced physicians and result in intubations if stridor is a major component. Alternatively, the physician may be unwilling to accept the notion that the patient has stridor that is not caused by airway obstruction of an organic cause. In that case, the patient continues to receive treatment for asthma. Cough, associated with vocal cord dysfunction, may be difficult to suppress, and pulmonary function tests may show a truncated inspiratory loop or poor effort (Fig. 1). It is important to verify that the inspiratory and expiratory efforts are not suppressed by the patient. Some features of vocal cord dysfunction are presented in Table 3. The difference between a partial effort on spirometry and a correct maximal effort is illustrated in Figure 2A,B. A physician should be certain that the patient truly produces a full inspiratory and expiratory maneuver; otherwise, "asthma" may be suspected improperly.

Globus Sensation

The globus sensation is defined as the feeling of a lump in the throat that may be more pronounced during swallowing of saliva and clearing if there is drinking of liquids or eating solids (31). The literature describes the presence of neurotic behavior along with depression, phobias, anxiety, and obsessionality (31). In contrast, many structural causes may be identified including postcricoidal web, goiters, thyroid tumors, cervical osteophytes, increased tension of the pharyngeal musculature, and collapse of muscles

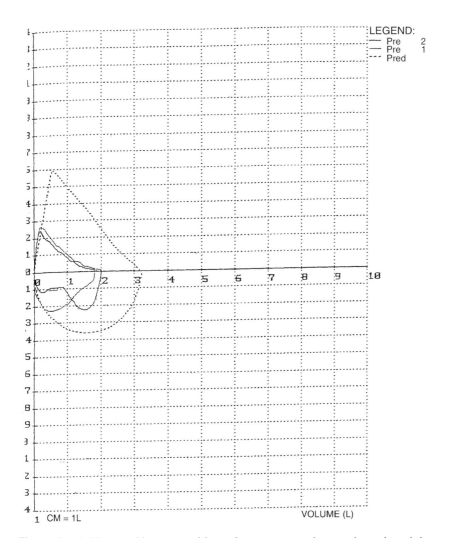

Figure 1 A 49-year-old woman with persistent severe asthma and vocal cord dysfunction. She has GERD as well. The FVC is 2.1 L (66%), FEV_1 1.3 L (49%), FEV% 62, FEF_{25-75} 0.7 L/sec (23%). The PEF is 3 L/sec (49%). The tracing shows reductions in both the inspiratory and expiratory loops compared to the predicted, which is the dotted line. Note the different inspiratory tracings.

of mastication (summarized in Ref. 31). In a series of 27 patients who had the globus sensation reported as persistent and 61 patients who had intermittent symptoms, 25/88 patients had described the onset of the globus sensation when there was intense fear, tension, or mental stress (31). The globus sensation was less pronounced during times of relaxation or distraction and

Table 3 Some Features of Vocal Cord Dysfunction

It may or may not coexist with asthma.

It may cause "severe steroid dependent" asthma.

It may be associated with gastroesophageal reflux disease, chronic sinusitis, and postnasal drainage.

The patient may or may not be aware of the vocal cord dysfunction.

Midazolam blocks vocal cord apposition so the bronchoscopic exam may be normal.

The inspiratory loop on a flow volume tracing is truncated and the expiratory loop may show obstruction if asthma is present or if the effort is poor.

Pulmonary function tests may be deemed "unsatisfactory."

The patient refuses to inspire to total lung capacity and will not phonate an "e" sound for 10 sec. The patient may expire no more than 3–6 sec.

during eating or drinking. It was noted that in some patients, burping or throat clearing cleared the sensation (31). When psychometric testing was carried out and compared with 80 patients in a gastroenterology clinic, the extent of depression was similar between the two groups (31). Some 24/58 globus patients were found to meet criteria for major depression ($n = 6$), generalized anxiety ($n = 6$), hypochondriasis ($n = 3$), agoraphobia ($n = 5$), and panic disorder ($n = 4$). However, after extensive evaluations, some 67/88 patients were found to have organic causes such as gastroesophageal reflux ($n = 13$), achalasia ($n = 24$), chronic pharyngitis ($n = 4$), n = 4), thyroid adenoma ($n = 3$), "nutcracker" esophagus ($n = 3$), and diffuse esophageal spasms ($n = 1$) (31). Thus, although the globus sensation may suggest anxiety or depression because patients do not report dysphagia, there should be an aggressive investigation for structural or mechanical causes.

Bronchomalacia

Bronchomalacia can result in cough, wheezing, stridor, and dyspnea. Sputum may or may not be produced. It may occur on an idiopathic basis, but many cases in the pediatric literature have been described in association with congenital heart disease or tracheoesophageal fistula (32). In adults, there may be bronchomalacia that occurs after lung transplantation, at the site of the anastomosis (33). However, when a patient, typically an adult, has persisting nonproductive coughing and louder ronchi over the neck and upper chest, while asthma may be suspected, a rare explanation is bronchomalacia. Indeed, patients may have been treated for asthma for years but the high resolution computerized tomographic examination will reveal areas of bronchomalacia. Bronchoscopic examination can confirm the diagnosis and stent placement (single or multiple) can provide relief of some symptoms for the patient. A possible clue is that the patient may report that flexing the cervical spine resulted in a sensation of transient dyspnea or

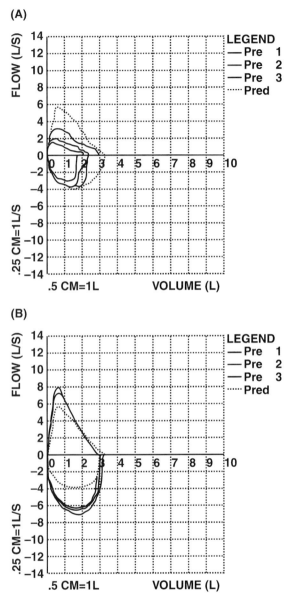

Figure 2 (**A**) A 45-year-old woman performed inspiratory and expiratory efforts with a good but only about a "half maximal effort." The PEF is 3.3 L/sec (52%). The FEV$_1$ is 2.2 L (77%) consistent with mild reduction. The FEV$_1$% is 65 consistent with airways obstruction. (**B**) The same patient who then performed in a true maximal fashion. The PEF is 8.2 L/sec (131%). The FEV$_1$ is 2.8 L (101%) and FEV$_1$% is 81. The dotted line is the predicted one. The subject has no respiratory condition.

throat constriction. This diagnosis suggests that although psychogenic cough implies an absence of organic cause, the differential diagnosis for cough is broad. While the common causes of cough account for over 90% of most cases, a physician may overlook structural or physiologic causes for a nonproductive cough (34). If there is a poor response to pharmacotherapy, there should be a reassessment of the working diagnoses regarding the patient's cough.

Clinical Management

The diagnosis of psychogenic cough may be suspected in children and adolescents (1–8) although less commonly, an adult presents with this condition (4,9,35,36). In an episode of mass psychogenic illness among 1000 military recruits in San Diego, cough was the most prevalent symptom and occurred in 275 (27.5%) of subjects (36). In that situation, the temperature had been very hot (33–42°C) and because of brush fires, there was poor air quality (36). Some 375 subjects required ambulance transportation to the hospital where little objective disease was present and hyperventilation was found. Some subjects had fainted. The symptoms resolved within 12 hr. It has been reported that psychogenic cough in adults may last for months or years (9) whereas in children, the cough may not have been present for as long. Furthermore, the cough may persist in adults whereas, in children, some behavioral interventions can stop or reduce the coughing within a few days (10,35,37).

Management of Children and Adolescents

Behavorial management has been successful (10) when an explanation or suggestion has not been effective. One approach has been to attempt to convince the child that the cough has weakened the chest muscles such that the cough cannot be contained and that a tight bedsheet is needed to support the chest and stop the cough (10,37). The cough is made much more difficult as the sheet is placed tightly for 1–2 days. Other approaches have included positive rewards for less or no coughing, instruction in mouth breathing, prevention of mouth breathing by having the child hold a button between the lips so as to prove that the cough does not occur, hypnosis, and psychologic counseling (35). When the characteristics of a psychogenic cough are present, one should assume that there is some aspect of secondary gain involved. Thus, an issue to consider is what would happen if the cough were to end? What situation or person would no longer be controlled? Nebulized lidocaine has been reported to be successful as a diagnostic and transient pharmacologic approach (38).

Management of Adults

As in children or adolescents, the features of psychogenic cough include the triad of (a) receipt of secondary gain from the cough, (b) la belle indifference, and (c) absence of organic abnormalities to explain the cough. Some adults have been referred for speech therapy, breathing exercises, relaxation strategies, self-hypnosis, psychologic counseling, or psychotherapy. When patients develop somatic type symptoms such as cough as a response to emotional triggers, a solution may be difficult to achieve. Indeed, some patients may refuse to seek psychologic or psychiatric advice. A remarkable approach was described in a 41-year-old patient with depression and a 7-year history of an intractable cough (35). It was determined that the patient sensed an urge to cough upon pressure to the right side of her neck and specifically over the sternocleidomastoid muscle (35). It was concluded that the patient had a trigger point on that muscle that resulted in afferent stimulation resulting in an intractable cough. In addition to stress management and diaphragmatic breathing exercises, she was treated by attaching electrodes to three areas of the skin over the sternocleidomastoid muscle for the purpose of active pacing of the muscle. It was concluded that this form of biofeedback was helpful in stopping the cough (35). Afferent impulses travel to the cough center in the medulla primarily not only via the vagus nerve but also by the trigeminal, glossopharyngeal, and phrenic nerves. The sternocleidomastoid, innervated by C2 and C3, is considered an efferent muscle for respiration. However, there appeared to be afferent fibers in the sternocleidomastoid that participated in the cough and were amenable to biofeedback! Another patient with psychogenic cough of 13-year duration and which never awakened her from sleep, found relief with throat lozenges (9). Indeed, a single lozenge suppressed the cough, and she used at least 20 per day (9). Her cough began after her husband's death from leukemia. As with other patients with psychogenic cough, she reported that the cough disrupted telephone conversations and limited her attending public activities such as theater and the symphony. Nevertheless, she was rather indifferent to the effects of the chronic cough. She was advised to seek psychiatric consultation, but she refused. When contacted 7 months later, the cough had continued; the patient had sought care from a homeopathic physician. However, that physician had not been able to stop the cough either.

Practical Issues

When the difficult-to-control or intractable cough persists, one should reconsider the working hypotheses as to what the cause or causes are of cough. Many patients examined by an allergist-immunologist or pulmonologist may well have asthma, gastroesophageal reflux disease (GERD), and postnasal drainage from rhinitis or sinusitis (14). For practical purposes, a

2-week course of prednisone 1–2 mg/kg in children and 40–60 mg daily in adults resolves or improves nearly all coughing from asthma. Less common causes of troublesome cough should be considered and excluded. When psychogenic cough appears to be present, one should discontinue many of the antitussive and antiasthma medications. Primarily, oral corticosteroids should be discontinued and then inhaled corticosteroids. There should be no deterioration in the patient's condition. A patient with psychogenic cough also may have GERD so appropriate treatment should be utilized in that case. Approaches to psychogenic cough may include distraction interventions initially to attempt to verify the nonorganic nature of the cough. Continued invasive procedures and polypharmacy should be avoided.

Summary

Psychogenic cough may be diagnosed in a patient who coughs excessively, has *la belle indifference*, derives secondary gain from the cough, and for which the diagnostic workup and therapeutic measures have proven ineffective. The diagnosis is one of exclusion. The patient may or may not accept the physician's judgment that the cough is not organic. In any event, the patient may be helped by measures aimed at stress management, distraction, biofeedback, voice therapy, psychologic or psychiatric consultation. Children may respond to aversive interventions which stops the cough in a few days. The physician or other health care specialists should attempt to identify reasons for why the patient seeks secondary gain from the persisting cough. One should avoid overtreating the patients with therapies that are of little to no value. The physician also can discourage other physicians from continuing the attempts to identify an organic basis for the persisting cough when none exists!

Acknowledgments

The study was supported by the Ernest S. Bazley Grant to Northwestern Memorial Hospital and Northwestern University.

References

1. Holinger LD. Chronic cough in infants and children. Laryngoscope 1996; 96:316–322.
2. Holinger LD, Sanders AD. Chronic cough in infants and children: an update. Laryngoscope 1991; 101:596–605.
3. Berman BA. Habit cough in adolescent children. Ann Allergy 1966; 24:43–46.

4. Gay M, Blager F, Bartsch K, Emery CF, Rosenstiel-Gross AK, Spears J. Psychogenic habit cough: review and case reports. J Clin Psychiatry 1987; 48:483–486.

5. Butani L, O'Connell EJ. Functional respiratory disorders. Ann Allergy Asthma Immunol 1997; 79:91–99.

6. McGarvey LP, Warke TJ, McNiff C, Heaney LG, MacMahon J. Psychogenic cough in a schoolboy: evaluation using an ambulatory cough recorder. Pediatr Pulmonol 2003; 36:73–75.

7. Bhatia MS, Chandra R, Vaid L. Psychogenic cough: a profile of 32 cases. Int J Psychiatry Med 2002; 32:353–360.

8. Blager F, Gay M, Wood R. Voice therapy techniques adapted to treatment of habit cough: a pilot study. J Commun Disord 1988; 21:393–400.

9. Mastrovich JD, Greenberger PA. Psychogenic cough in adults: a report of two cases and review of the literature. Allergy Asthma Proc 2002; 23:27–33.

10. Lavigne JV, Davis T, Fauber R. Behavioral management of psychogenic cough: alternative to the "bedsheet" and other aversive techniques. Pediatrics 1991; 87:532–537.

11. Hart AC, Hopkins CA. ICD 9 CM: Expert for Physicians. International Classification of Diseases. 9th Revision, Clinical Modification. St. Anthony Publishing Salt Lake City 2002; 67–71.

12. Irwin RS, Madison JM. The diagnosis and treatment of cough. N Engl J Med 2000; 343:1715–1721.

13. Irwin RS, Zawacki JK, Wilson MM, French CT, Callergy MP. Chronic cough due to gastroesophageal reflux disease: failure to resolve despite total/near-total elimination of esophageal acid. Chest 2002; 121:1132–1140.

14. Greenberger PA. Therapy in the management of the rhinitis/asthma complex. Allergy Asthma Proc 2003; 24:403–407.

15. Schaefer OP, Irwin RS. Unsuspected bacterial suppurative disease of the airways presenting as chronic cough. Am J Med 2003; 114:602–606.

16. Palombini BC, Castilhos Villanova CA, Araujo E, Gastal OL, Carneiro Alt D, Prestes Stolz D, Oliveira Palombini C. A pathogenic triad of chronic cough: asthma, postnasal drip syndrome, and gastroesophageal reflux disease. Chest 1999; 116:279–84.

17. Cheriyan S, Greenberger PA, Patterson R. Outcome of cough variant asthma treated with inhaled steroids. Ann Allergy 1994; 73:478–480.

18. McFadden ER Jr. Exertional dyspnea and cough as preludes to acute attacks of bronchial asthma. N Engl J Med 1975; 292:555–559.

19. Andrianopoulos MV, Gallivan GJ, Gallivan KH. PVCD, EPL, and the iritable larynx syndrome: what are we talking about and how do we treat it? J Voice 1999; 13:447–455.

20. Morrison M, Rammage L, Emami AJ. The irritable larynx syndrome. J Voice 1999; 13:447–455.

21. Balafsky PC. Abnormal endoscopic pharyngeal and laryngeal findings attribu-table to reflux. Am J Med 2003; 115:90S–96S.

22. Kamel PL, Hanson D, Kahrilas PJ. Omeprazole for the treatment of posterior laryngitis. Am J Med 1994; 96:321–326.

23. Kiljander TO. The role of proton pump inhibitors in the management of gastroesophageal reflux disease-related asthma and chronic cough. Am J Med 2003; 115:65S–71S.
24. Vaezi MF. Sensitivity and specificity of reflux-attributed laryngeal lesions: experimental and clinical evidence. Am J Med 2003; 115:97S–104S.
25. McGrath KG, Greenberger PA, Zeiss CR, Patterson R. Facilitious allergic disease: multiple factitious illness and familial Munchausen's stridor. Immunol Allergy Pract 1984; VI:41–49.
26. Ditto AM, Grammer LC, Kern RC. Direct laryngoscopy with provocation: a useful method to distinguish acute laryngeal edema from nonorganic disease. Ann Allergy Asthma Immunol 1995; 75:25–28.
27. Patterson R, Schatz M, Horton M. Munchausen's stridor: non-organic laryngeal obstruction. Clin Allergy 1974; 4:307–310.
28. Wiener D, McGrath K, Patterson R. Factitious sneezing. J Allergy Clin Immunol 1985; 75:741–742.
29. Beckman DB, Greenberger PA. Diagnostic dilemma. Vocal cord dysfunction. Am J Med 2001; 110:731–741.
30. Newman KB, Mason UB III, Schamling KB. Clinical features of vocal cord dysfunction. Am J Respir Crit Care Med 1983; 152:1382–1386.
31. Moser G, Wenzel-Abatzi T-A, Stelzeneder M, Wenzel T, Weber U, Wiesnagrotzki S, Schnieder C, Schima W, Stacher-Janotta G, Vacariu-Granser GV, Pokieser P, Bergmann H, Stacher G. Globus sensation: pharyngoesophageal function, psychometric and psychiatric findings, and follow-up in 88 patients. Arch Intern Med 1998; 158:1365–1373.
32. Masters IB, Chang AB, Patterson L, Wainwright C, Buntain H, Dean BW, Francis PW. Series of laryngomalacia, tracheomalacia, and bronchomalacia disorders and their associations with other conditions in children. Pediatr Pulmonol 2002; 34:189–195.
33. Gotway MB, Golden JA, LaBerge JM, Webb WR, Reddy GP, Wilson MW, Kerlan RK Jr, Gordon RL. Benign tracheobronchial stenoses: changes in short-term and long-term pulmonary function testing after expandable metallic stent placement. J Comput Assist Tomogr 2002; 26:564–572.
34. Irwin RS, Boulet L-P, Cloutier MM, Fuller R, Gold PM, Hoffstein V, Ing AJ, McCool FD, O'Byrne P, Poe RH, Prakash UB, Pratter MR, Rubin BK. Managing cough as a defense mechanism and as a symptom. A consensus panel report of the American College of Chest Physicians. Chest 1998; 114:133S–181S.
35. Riegel B, Warmoth JE, Middaugh SJ, Kee WG, Nicholson LC, Melton DM, Parikh DK, Rosenberg JC. Psychogenic cough treated with biofeedback and psychotherapy. A review and case report. Am J Phys Med Rehabil 1995; 74:155–158.
36. Struewing JP, Gray GC. An epidemic of respiratory complaints exacerbated by mass psychogenic illness in a military recruit population. Am J Epidemiol 1990; 132:1120–1129.
37. Cholan SQ, Stone SM. The cough and the bedsheet. Pediatrics 1984; 74:11–15.
38. Sherman JM. Breaking the cycle: lidocaine therapy for habit cough. J Fla Med Assoc 1997; 84:308–309.

20

Cough Reflex Sensitivity in Health and Disease

ALYN H. MORICE

Division of Academic Medicine, University of Hull, Hull, U.K.

Introduction

Central to our understanding of cough is the modulation of the cough reflex. We have all experienced cough as a useful phenomenon protecting the airways from accidental but potentially harmful aspiration. What is striking, however, is the transformation of the cough reflex into the debilitating and detrimental hypersensitivity seen in disease. We cough uncontrollably during viral upper respiratory tract infections to minor tussive stimuli such as a change in atmospheric conditions. Patients with chronic cough usually describe paroxysms precipitated by nonspecific irritants such as perfume or cigarette smoke. How this dramatic transformation of the cough reflex is regulated is largely unknown but important clues can be garnered from clinical observation, the effect of drugs, animal models, and, more recently, the expression and molecular pharmacology of the putative cough receptors themselves in vitro.

There are several possible mechanisms whereby a normally tuned reflex may be made hypersensitive. These are best considered by the anatomical location of those factors influencing the reflex. While no morphologically

distinct cough receptor has been unequivocally described (Undem has
recently described a branching structure lying beneath the airways epithelium which responds to mechanical but not chemical stimuli), it is clear that
those sensory receptors located within the airway, esophagus, and even the
ear can be modulated by local factors to cause reflex hypersensitivity. At
the relay stations of the jugular and nodose ganglia a further opportunity
for regulation occurs by cross-talk with adjacent neurones. Finally, and perhaps most importantly, central modulation of the reflex in the relay from the
nucleus tractus solitarius through the "cough centres" to the efferent pathway provides for both conscious and involuntary regulation. It is here that
most antitussives in current use have their activity and it is key to our understanding of the major difference between cough in man and the cough
response of animals. It should be emphasized that our knowledge is rudimen-
tary at best and certainly a synthesis of this knowledge is yet to be achieved.

Cough Reflex Sensitivity in Normal Subjects

Given a sufficient stimulus, all normal subjects cough. However, the individual degree of cough sensitivity varies enormously within the population
such that it is difficult to describe a normal range. Mechanical stimulation
is perhaps the most consistent: even insensitive individuals will cough in
response to laryngeal irritation with say a pretzel, to give a presidential
example. This reflects the primary protective role of the cough reflex—the
prevention of foreign body inhalation—and may suggest, as electrophysiological studies do, that cough is not a single hardwired reflex with a single
input but a complex polymodal phenomenon with its different facets differentially regulated. There is no doubt, however, that protection against
aspiration is the most important function. The diminished cough reflex sensitivity in disease states such as Parkinsonism (1) and stroke (2) leads to
inhalation pneumonia, bronchial sepsis, and ultimately death.

Where the greatest variation in cough reflex sensitivity is seen is in
cough in response to chemical stimulation. Others in this volume have
described in detail methods of cough induction using vanilloids, organic
acids, and distilled water. Each of these three individual methodologies
shows enormous variation both in their normal range and in an individual's
sensitivity to each challenge methodology (3). This variation is an individual
characteristic since within-subject cough challenge is highly reproducible
(4). We have previously shown (5) that different organic acids and indeed
highly protonated inorganic acids, such as phosphoric acid, have similar
sensitivities within subjects indicating a common mechanism (Fig. 1).
However, there is no correlation between the response to citric acid and that
to capsaicin within a population of normal subjects. This differential sensitivity suggests that acid challenge and capsaicin work through different

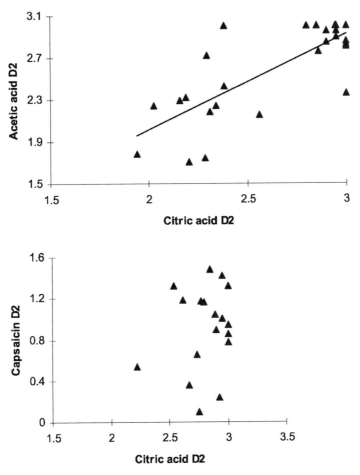

Figure 1 Correlation between citric acid- and acetic acid-induced cough but lack of correlation with capsaicin-induced cough in normal subjects. (Redrawn from Ref. 5.)

mechanisms and indeed an acid-sensitive putative cough receptor has been described in afferent neurones. Against this hypothesis there is cross-tachyphylaxis between the different modalities (6) and the observation that the vanilloid antagonist capsazepine inhibited both citric acid- and capsaicin-induced cough in guinea pigs seems to imply a common mode of action (7). Help in differentiating these two possibilities has been provided by recent investigation of the molecular pharmacology of the TRPV1 (VR1) capsaicin receptor. In this model protons and capsaicin act allosterically (Fig. 2) Protons bind to an extracellular domain of the TRPV1, whereas

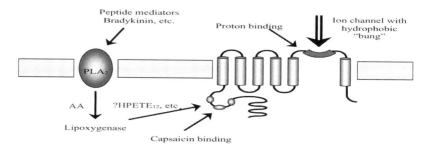

Figure 2 The TRPV1 or VR1 vanilloid receptor. Protons and capsaicin bind at different allosteric sites to independently modulate this putative cough receptor. (From Ref. 7a.)

the capsaicin-binding site is located on the intracellular loop. Thus, the lack of competitive interaction may reflect on independent alterations in the opening probability of the ion channel rather than direct steric competition. Both agonists, however, enhance the cough reflex through the capsazepine-sensitive TRPV1.

Sex Differences in the Cough Reflex

Perhaps the largest observable difference in cough receptor sensitivity in normal subjects lies in the effect of sex. A number of studies have shown that in healthy female volunteers inhalation of a variety of tussive substances produces either a greater number of coughs for a given stimulus or a leftward shift in the cough dose–response curve (8–12). This is unlikely to be due to anatomical differences producing an artifactual augmentation of deposition of tussive stimuli in female subjects since a higher frequency of ACE inhibitor-induced cough is also found in women (13). A hormonal influence is implied by the observation that cough reflex sensitivity is similar in boys and girls (14) but the reason for the marked gender difference in adults remains obscure. This relationship between sex and the cough reflex remains true despite the influence of underlying pathology enhancing the reflex. Women with chronic cough have a heightened cough reflex compared with men (15).

One interesting observation that may shed light on this difference is the demonstration of estrogen receptors on mast cells (16). In eosinophilic bronchitis it has been shown that the distribution of mast cells within the airways differs from that in classic asthma (17). If mast cell activation, which is clearly an important component of the cough reflex in disease, also modulates cough reflex sensitivity in normal subjects then sex hormones may work through the well-described mast cell/neuronal cross-talk.

Higher Influences

In man the cough reflex is under a marked degree of cortical control . Thus, if subjects are asked to inhibit cough using a traffic light system of instruction a highly significant reduction in cough frequency is seen in viral cough (18). Some subjects are able to completely suppress cough whereas others "break" the cough suppression after a few minutes. Similarly, capsaicin-induced cough, albeit at low concentrations, can be suppressed by the majority of normal subjects (19). A further illustration of the profound effect of the cortex on cough is given by anesthesia. As each level of sedation is passed, cough becomes more and more difficult to provoke (20).

These illustrations of cortical influences have important consequences in the pharmacology of antitussives. There appears to be a large component of activity that resides in what is commonly called the placebo effect. Indeed, the pharmacokinetics of this response can be modeled (21). Cough suppression with placebo is maximal at 4 hr postdose. Not only must an allowance be made for this placebo effect, which in some studies using cough challenge methodology is as large as that seen with the active agent, but it may also underlie the activity of some of the branded antitussives currently on the market. The contrary difficulty arises in that translating antitussive effects seen in animal models into clinically important cough suppression in man can be fraught with difficulty. A number of compounds (neurokinin antagonists, peripheral sensory nerve blockers) have shown good activity in guinea pigs but have proven to be without significant activity in man.

To suggest, however, that cough is "all in the mind" is clearly incorrect. The uncontrolled paroxysms of cough referred to in the opening of this chapter produce profound psychosocial morbidity. Indeed quality of life assessments have demonstrated that the heightened cough reflex of chronic cough produces a similar decrement in quality of life to that seen in disabling illness such as chronic obstructive pulmonary disease (22). While cortical influences alter cough reflex sensitivity, the clinical entity of psychogenic cough of central origin is vanishingly rare, the one exception being the isolated cough tic of childhood (23).

The Cough Reflex and Irritant Exposure

The relationship of irritant exposure with cough reflex sensitivity is not simple. It might be expected that heightened cough sensitivity would be seen, and indeed in a number of occupational lung diseases, particularly asthma, cough is a prominent feature. Cough as an isolated finding may occur following chronic exposure to low-molecular weight irritants. In glass bottle factory workers exposed to hydrochloric acid and organic oils a chronic cough develops without airways hypersensitivity to methacholine (24). Cough reflex hypersensitivity was demonstrated by inhalation challenge with capsaicin and citric acid (25). In contrast, cigarette smoking has been shown to be associated with a reduction in cough reflex sensitivity (26).

Cough Reflex Sensitivity Is Enhanced in Disease

In acute viral cough, capsaicin sensitivity increases whereas methacholine responsiveness does not change (27). This observation illustrates the separation of cough and reflex bronchoconstriction and implies that there are specific stimuli for cough, which are subtended by a different reflex pathway or more likely pathways. The physiology and pharmacology of these pathways are dealt with in other chapters in this volume. Here, I have concentrated on the factors regulating sensitivity rather than the factors causing cough.

One of the most important concepts in understanding the cough reflex in disease is the global nature of cough reflex hypersensitivity . It does not appear to matter whether the irritant stimulus leading to cough is a particular anatomical area or another. The whole of the cough reflex is upregulated. Thus, in gastroesophageal reflux-induced cough there is an increase in sensitivity to inhaled capsaicin (28–30). There are several possible mechanisms to explain this observation. Reflux may be leading to aspiration, which causes localized hypersensitivity of airway receptors. However, Ing et al. (31) have shown that reflux cough may occur commonly in the absence of aspiration and that local instillation of acid (and indeed saline) in the distal esophagus leads to cough. The hypothesis of vagal hypersensitivity suggests that noxious stimuli lead to upregulation of the gate controlling cough reflex sensitivity, a situation analogous to the gate theory of pain. Where this regulation occurs—at a receptor, ganglion or central level—is currently the subject of much debate since modulation of the hypersensitivity is the holy grail of antitussive research. Returning the cough reflex to a normal sensitivity without abolishing it would enable natural protection of the airways, a strategy unlike that used in the nonspecific downregulation of sensitivity seen with the inhalation of local anesthetics (32).

How Is the Cough Reflex Enhanced in Disease?

A number of different mediators have been suggested as the primary regulators of cough reflex sensitivity in disease. It is unlikely that a single agent is responsible and it is probable that in different clinical scenarios the importance of these mediators will vary. Interplay between the putative mediators to produce combined effects is the most likely paradigm.

Histamine

High levels of histamine have been demonstrated in induced sputum from patients with cough due to eosinophilic bronchitis (33). Levels were higher than a control population of matched asthmatics. Therapy with broad-spectrum antihistamines is advocated as an initial treatment for cough, and although the idea that this nonspecific therapy indicates a specific diagnosis of postnasal drip cannot be correct, there is a large body of experience mainly from United States suggesting efficacy in chronic cough (34). However, work in a guinea pig model indicates poor efficacy for H1 receptor antagonists in cough (35) and any activity in chronic cough may reside in other properties of these poorly characterized agents. Any effect of histamine is unlikely to be by a direct activation of the cough reflex since exogenous histamine does not enhance capsaicin cough challenge (36).

Nerve Growth Factor

The prolonged cough that sometimes accompanies upper respiratory tract infection continues after evidence of viral replication has disappeared. Nerve growth factor (NGF) is thought to sustain the hyperalgesia of inflammation by direct activation of the TRPV1 (VR1) (37). In addition, both bradykinin and NGF release TRPV1 from inhibition by phosphatidylinositol-4,5-biphosphate-induced suppression (38). In the airways of mice overexpressing NGF under control of a Clara cell promoter, there was unsurprisingly enhanced nerve density within the airways, which translated to heightened responses to inhaled capsaicin (39). Given the wide range of inflammatory cells and intrinsic lung tissue cells, including pulmonary fibroblasts (40), that express NGF, it is a prime candidate as a mediator of inflammation-induced enhanced cough reflex.

Peptides

That a peptide is an important regulator of the human cough reflex is demonstrated by the phenomenon of angiotensin converting enzyme (ACE) inhibitor cough. The heightened cough reflex is shown by the shift in the capsaicin dose–response curve (41). Since the condition is a class effect of ACE inhibition, the peptide substrates of ACE are implicated. Angiotensin II is an unlikely culprit since angiotensin II receptor antagonists do not enhance cough. Bradykinin has been suggested as the main mediator (42) but bradykinin has minimal protussive activity and does not alter capsaicin-induced cough (36). It may, however, release TRPV1 from inhibition, as does NGF (38). Substance P has recently been shown to have an important role in reflex regulation in inflamed airways (43). The prolonged resetting of the cough reflex that occurs with ACE inhibitors

(44) suggests that rather than a direct consequence of enzyme inhibition an alteration in reflex sensitivity occurs as is seen with substance P.

Prostaglandins

Inhaled prostaglandin (PG) E_2 enhances capsaicin induced cough (36). In sputum from patients with cough due to eosinophilic bronchitis, higher levels of PGD_2 were seen in comparison with normals and asthmatic controls (33). However, since levels of histamine were also elevated in this study it suggests that mast cell activation may be the common feature and PGD_2 may be merely a marker. Despite evidence of some effect of cyclooxygenase inhibition on the cough reflex (45), these agents have not been extensively tested in clinical practice.

Lipoxygenase Products

It has been suggested that the capsaicin-binding site represents the locus at which endogenous ligands derived from the lipoxygenase pathway modulate the opening probability of the TRPV1 ion channel (46). In this way, mediators of asthmatic inflammation can directly upregulate the cough reflex. The capsaicin cough response is unaffected by leukotriene receptor antagonists in classic asthma but a significant diminution of capsaicin-induced cough sensitivity is seen in cough-variant asthma (47).

Conclusion

Modulation of cough reflex sensitivity is fundamental to understanding how stimuli result in cough in health and disease. Knowledge of how the cough reflex is modulated will allow rational drug design to normalize rather than abolish the cough.

References

1. Fontana GA, Pantaleo T, Lavorini F, Benvenuti F, Gangemi S. Defective motor control of coughing in Parkinson's disease. Am J Respir Crit Care Med 1998; 158:458–464.
2. Smith Hammond CA, Goldstein LB, Zajac DJ, Gray L, Davenport PW, Bolser DC. Assessment of aspiration risk in stroke patients with quantification of voluntary cough. Neurology 2001; 56:502–506.
3. Morice AH, Kastelik JA, Thompson R. Cough challenge in the assessment of cough reflex. Br J Clin Pharmacol 2001; 52:365–375.
4. Dicpinigaitis PV. Short- and long-term reproducibility of capsaicin cough challenge testing. Pulm Pharmacol Ther 2003; 16:61–65.

5. Wong CH, Matai R, Morice AH. Cough induced by low pH. Respir Med 1999; 93:58–61.

6. Morice AH, Higgins KS, Yeo WW. Adaptation of cough reflex with different types of stimulation. Eur Respir J 1992; 5:841–847.

7. Lalloo UG, Fox AJ, Belvisi MG, Chung KF, Barnes PJ. Capsazepine inhibits cough induced by capsaicin and citric acid but not by hypertonic saline in guinea pigs. J Appl Physiol 1995; 79:1082–1087.

7a. Morice AH, Geppetti P. Cough. 5: The type 1 vanilloid receptor: a sensory receptor for cough. Thorax 2004; 59(3):257–258.

8. Fujimura M, Sakamoto S, Kamio Y, Matsuda T. Sex difference in the inhaled tartaric acid cough threshold in non-atopic healthy subjects. Thorax 1990; 45:633–634.

9. Fujimura M, Kasahara K, Yasui M, Myou S, Ishiura Y, Kamio Y, et al. Atopy in cough sensitivity to capsaicin and bronchial responsiveness in young females. Eur Respir J 1998; 11:1060–1063.

10. Dicpinigaitis PV, Rauf K. The influence of gender on cough reflex sensitivity. Chest 1998; 113:1319–1321.

11. Fujimura M, Kasahara K, Kamio Y, Naruse M, Hashimoto T, Matsuda T. Female gender as a determinant of cough threshold to inhaled capsaicin. Eur Respir J 1996; 9:1624–1626.

12. Morice A, Kastelik JA, Thompson RH. Gender differences in airway behaviour. Thorax 2000; 55:629.

13. Gibson GR. Enalapril-induced cough. Arch Intern Med 1989; 149:2701–2703.

14. Chang AB, Phelan PD, Sawyer SM, Del Brocco S, Robertson CF. Cough sensitivity in children with asthma, recurrent cough, and cystic fibrosis. Arch Dis Child 1997; 77:331–334.

15. Kastelik JA, Thompson RH, Aziz I, Ojoo JC, Redington AE, Morice AH. Sex-related differences in cough reflex sensitivity in patients with chronic cough. Am J Respir Crit Care Med 2002; 166:961–964.

16. Zhao XJ, McKerr G, Dong Z, Higgins CA, Carson J, Yang ZK, et al. Expression of oestrogen and progesterone receptors by mast cells alone, but not lymphocytes, macrophages or other immune cells in human upper airways. Thorax 2001; 56:205–211.

17. Brightling CE, Bradding P, Symon FA, Holgate ST, Wardlaw AJ, Pavord ID. Mast cell infiltration of airway smooth muscle in asthma. N Engl J Med 2002; 346:1699–1705.

18. Hutchings HA, Eccles R, Smith AP, Jawad MS. Voluntary cough suppression as an indication of symptom severity in upper respiratory tract infections. Eur Respir J 1993; 6:1449–1454.

19. Hutchings HA, Morris S, Eccles R, Jawad MS. Voluntary suppression of cough induced by inhalation of capsaicin in healthy volunteers. Respir Med 1993; 87:379–382.

20. Eccles R. The powerful placebo in cough studies? Pulm Pharmacol Ther 2002; 15:303–308.

21. Rostami-Hodjegan A, Abdul-Manap R, Wright CE, Tucker GT, Morice AH. The placebo response to citric acid-induced cough: pharmacodynamics and gender differences. Pulm Pharmacol Ther 2001; 14:315–319.

22. French CL, Irwin RS, Curley FJ, Krikorian CJ. Impact of chronic cough on quality of life. Arch Intern Med 1998; 158:1657–1661.
23. Ojoo JC, Kastelik JA, Morice AH. A boy with a disabling cough. Lancet 2003; 361:674.
24. Gordon SB, Curran AD, Fishwick D, Morice AH, Howard P. Respiratory symptoms among glass bottle workers—cough and airways irritancy syndrome? Occup Med (Oxford) 1998; 48:455–459.
25. Gordon SB, Curran AD, Turley A, Wong CH, Rahman SN, Wiley K, et al. Glass bottle workers exposed to low-dose irritant fumes cough but do not wheeze. Am J Respir Crit Care Med 1997; 156:206–210.
26. Dicpinigaitis PV. Cough reflex sensitivity in cigarette smokers. Chest 2003; 123:685–688.
27. O'Connell F, Thomas VE, Studham JM, Pride NB, Fuller RW. Capsaicin cough sensitivity increases during upper respiratory infection. Respir Med 1996; 90:279–286.
28. Benini L, Ferrari M, Sembenini C, Olivieri M, Micciolo R, Zuccali V, et al. Cough threshold in reflux oesophagitis: influence of acid and of laryngeal and oesophageal damage. Gut 2000; 46:762–767.
29. Ferrari M, Olivieri M, Sembenini C, Benini L, Zuccali V, Bardelli E, et al. Tussive effect of capsaicin in patients with gastroesophageal reflux without cough. Am J Respir Crit Care Med 1995; 151:557–561.
30. Nieto L, de Diego A, Perpina M, Compte L, Garrigues V, Martinez E, et al. Cough reflex testing with inhaled capsaicin in the study of chronic cough. Respir Med 2003; 97:393–400.
31. Ing AJ, Ngu MC, Breslin AB. Pathogenesis of chronic persistent cough associated with gastroesophageal reflux. Am J Respir Crit Care Med 1994; 149:160–167.
32. Choudry NB, Fuller RW, Anderson N, Karlsson JA. Separation of cough and reflex bronchoconstriction by inhaled local anaesthetics. Eur Respir J 1990; 3:579–583.
33. Brightling CE, Ward R, Woltmann G, Bradding P, Sheller JR, et al. Induced sputum inflammatory mediator concentrations in eosinophilic bronchitis and asthma. Am J Respir Crit Care Med 2000; 162:878–882.
34. Irwin RS, Boulet LP, Cloutier MM, Fuller R, Gold PM, Hoffstein V, et al. Managing cough as a defense mechanism and as a symptom. A consensus panel report of the American College of Chest Physicians. Chest 1998; 114(suppl 2):133S–181S.
35. Mcleod RL, Mingo G, O'Reilly S, Ruck LA, Bolser DC, Hey JA. Antitussive action of antihistamines is independent of sedative and ventilation activity in the guinea pig. Pharmacology 1998; 57:57–64.
36. Choudry NB, Fuller RW, Pride NB. Sensitivity of the human cough reflex: effect of inflammatory mediators prostaglandin E2, bradykinin, and histamine. Am Rev Respir Dis 1989; 140:137–141.
37. Shu X, Mendell LM. Nerve growth factor acutely sensitizes the response of adult rat sensory neurons to capsaicin. Neurosci Lett 1999; 274:159–162.

38. Chuang HH, Prescott ED, Kong H, Shields S, Jordt SE, Basbaum AI, et al. Bradykinin and nerve growth factor release the capsaicin receptor from PtdIns (4,5) P2-mediated inhibition. Nature 2001; 411:957–962.
39. Hoyle GW, Graham RM, Finkelstein JB, Nguyen KP, Gozal D, Friedman M. Hyperinnervation of the airways in transgenic mice overexpressing nerve growth factor. Am J Respir Cell Mol Biol 1998; 18:149–157.
40. Olgart C, Frossard N. Human lung fibroblasts secrete nerve growth factor: effect of inflammatory cytokines and glucocorticoids. Eur Respir J 2001; 18:115–121.
41. Morice AH, Lowry R, Brown MJ, Higenbottam T. Angiotensin converting enzyme and the cough reflex. Lancet 1987; 2:1116–1118.
42. Fox AJ, Lalloo UG, Belvisi MG, Bernareggi M, Chung KF, Barnes PJ. Bradykinin-evoked sensitization of airway sensory nerves: a mechanism for ACE-inhibitor cough. Nat Med 1996; 2:814–817.
43. Undem BJ, Carr MJ, Kollarik M. Physiology and plasticity of putative cough fibres in the guinea pig. Pulm Pharmacol Ther 2002; 15:193–198.
44. Ojoo JC, Kastelik JA, Morice AH. Duration of angiotensin converting enzyme inhibitor (ACEI) induced cough (abstract). Thorax 2002; 56(suppl III):72.
45. Foster G, Yeo WW, Ramsay LE. Effect of sulindac on the cough reflex of healthy subjects. Br J Clin Pharmacol 1991; 31:207–208.
46. Hwang SW, Cho H, Kwak J, Lee SY, Kang CJ, Jung J, et al. Direct activation of capsaicin receptors by products of lipoxygenases: endogenous capsaicin-like substances. Proc Natl Acad Sci USA 2000; 97:6155–6160.
47. Dicpinigaitis PV, Dobkin JB, Reichel J. Antitussive effect of the leukotriene receptor antagonist zafirlukast in subjects with cough-variant asthma. J Asthma 2002; 39:291–297.

21

Cough and Gender

MASAKI FUJIMURA

Kanazawa University, Graduate School of Medicine,
Kanazawa, Japan

Gender Distribution in Causes of Chronic Cough

A review of studies on chronic cough that report data on gender distribution (1–11) indicates that this condition appears to be more common in women, as shown in Table 1. The mean ratio of female to male patients with chronic cough is 1.8 [95% confidence interval (CI) 1.2–2.4] and this gender difference is significant ($p = 0.0128$). This suggests that the overall morbidity of chronic cough, without regard to its cause, is greater in females than in males.

Commonly reported causes of chronic cough include gastroesophageal reflux (GER) disease, postnasal drip (PND), cough-variant asthma, eosinophilic bronchitis without asthma, atopic cough, and angiotensin-converting enzyme (ACE) inhibitor therapy. Several large population-based studies (12–18) have clearly demonstrated that females are more susceptible to ACE inhibitor-induced cough when these agents are used for the treatment of hypertension (Table 2). However, comparable population studies have not been reported to examine gender differences in morbidity from other causes of chronic cough. Accordingly, reported clinical studies on

Table 1 Gender Distribution of Patients with Chronic Cough

Number of patients		Female/		
Male	Female	male	Investigators	Journals
43	59	1.3	Irwin et al. (1)	Am Rev Respir Dis 141: 640–647, 1990
17	28	1.6	Pratter et al. (2)	Ann Intern Med 119: 977–983, 1993
4	15	3.8	Boulet et al. (3)	Am J Respir Crit Care Med 149: 482–489, 1994
39	32	0.8	Smyrnios et al. (4)	Chest 108: 991–997, 1995
24	64	2.6	Mello et al. (5)	Arch Intern Med 156: 997–1003, 1996
37	85	2.3	Wongtim et al. (6)	Asian Pacific J Allergy Immunol 15: 9–14, 1997
18	12	0.6	Smyrnios et al. (7)	Arch Intern Med 158: 1222–1228, 1998
55	69	1.3	McGarvey et al. (8)	Int J Clin Pract 52: 158–161, 1998
27	51	1.9	Palombini et al. (9)	Chest 116: 279–284, 1999
12	23	1.9	McGarvey et al. (10)	Eur Respir J 13: 59–65, 1999
10	15	1.5	Lee et al. (11)	Chest 120: 1114–1120, 2001
Total 286	453	1.6		
Mean (95% CI)		1.8 (1.2–2.4, p = 0.0128)		

individual causes of chronic cough, which include data on sex distribution, are summarized as a reference. However, the existence of some bias cannot be excluded as most of the patients studied visited chest physicians for diagnosis and treatment. It is likely that females have a greater tendency to visit specialists and to participate in clinical studies.

In studies of GER-associated cough (19–34), as summarized in Table 3, the ratio of female to male patients is 2.4 (95% CI 1.6–3.4), which is significant. The ratio is 4.0 (95% CI 1.2–6.8, p = 0.0387) in atopic cough (35–41) (Table 4) and 2.4 (95% CI 0.5–4.3, p = 0.1126) in eosinophilic bronchitis without asthma (42–47) (Table 5). The latter is not statistically significant, but it seems that females are common in these conditions.

Table 2 Gender Difference in Incidence of ACE-Inhibitor-Induced Cough

Male		Female		Female/		
Number	%	Number	%	male	Investigators	Journals
10/256	0.4	23/2121	1.1	2.8	Coulter and Edwards (12)	Br Med J 294: 1521–1523, 1987
39/546	1.6	17/411	4.1	2.6	Coulter and Edwards (12)	Br Med J 294: 1521–1523, 1987
4/38	10.5	10/43	23.3	2.1	Yeo et al. (13)	Qward J Med 81: 763–770, 1991
10/39	25.6	12/50	24.0	0.9	Simon et al. (14)	Arch Intern Med 152: 1698–1700, 1992
4/58	6.9	4/62	6.5	0.9	Simon et al. (14)	Arch Intern Med 152: 1698–1700, 1992
19/398	4.8	49/494	9.9	2.1	Elliott (15)	Clin Pharmacol Ther 60: 582–588, 1996
9/207	4.4	26/205	12.6	2.9	Os et al. (16)	Lancet 339: 372–372, 1992
138/1557	8.9	286/2003	14.3	1.6	Moore et al. (17)	Lancet 341: 61–61, 1993
11/63	17.5	16/37	43.2	2.5	Adigun and Ajayi (18)	West Afr J Med 20: 46–47, 2001
Mean (95% CI)	9.0 (2.8–15.1)		15.4 (5.4–25.4)	2.0 (1.5–2.6, p = 0.0028)		

Cough reflex sensitivity has been shown to be increased in GER-associated cough, atopic cough, and eosinophilic bronchitis without asthma and to recover to the normal range when the cough is successfully treated. Thus, it is postulated that females more readily suffer from chronic cough when some pathogenesis operates to increase cough reflex sensitivity. The ratio of female to male adult patients diagnosed with cough-variant asthma is

Table 3 Gender Distribution of Patients with Gastroesophageal
Reflux-Associated Cough

Number of patients		Female/ male	Investigators	Journals
Male	Female			
4	5	1.3	Irwin et al. (19)	Am Rev Respir Dis 140: 1294–1300, 1989
2	10	5.0	Irwin et al. (20)	Chest 104: 1511–1517, 1993
3	7	2.3	Laukka et al. (12)	J Clin Gastroenterol 19: 100–104, 1994
11	11	1.0	Ing et al. (22)	Am J Respir Crit Care Med 149: 160–167, 1994
24	63	2.6	O'Connell et al. (23)	Am J Respir Crit Care Med 1 50: 374–380, 1994
6	21	3.5	Waring et al. (24)	Dig Dis Sci 40: 1093–1097, 1995
2	9	4.5	Vaezi and Richter (25)	South Med J 90: 305–311, 1997
10	20	2.0	Carney et al. (26)	Am J Respir Crit Care Med 156: 211–216, 1997
10	19	1.9	Kiljander et al. (27)	Eur Respir J 16: 633–638, 2000
3	5	1.7	Forsythe et al. (28)	Clin Exp Allergy 30: 225–232, 2000
5	6	1.2	Parameswaran et al. (29)	Can Respir J 8: 239–244, 2001
5	16	3.2	Novitsky et al. (30)	Surg Endosc 16: 567–571, 2002.
1	7	7.0	Irwin et al. (31)	Chest 121: 1132–1140, 2002.
5	7	1.4	Kastelik et al. (32)	Chest 122: 2038–2041, 2002.
21	16	0.8	Thoman et al. (33)	J Gastrointest Surg 6: 17–21, 2002
20	13	0.7	Kastelik et al. (34)	Am J Respir Crit Care Med 166: 961–964, 2002
Total				
132	235	1.8		
Mean (95% CI)		2.4 (1.6–3.4, p = 0.0039)		

Table 4 Gender Distribution of Patients with Atopic Cough

Number of patients		Female/ male	Investigators	Journals
Male	Female			
1	9	9.0	Fujimura et al. (35)	Intern Med 31: 447–452, 1992
3	9	3.0	Fujimura et al. (36)	J Asthma 31: 463–472, 1994
13	17	1.3	Fujimura et al. (37)	J Asthma 34: 119–126, 1997
1	7	7.0	Fujimura et al. (38)	Clin Exp Allergy 30: 41–47, 2000
12	6	0.5	Fujimura et al. (39)	Allergol Int 49: 135–142, 2000
19	63	3.3	Fujimura et al. (40)	Thorax 58: 14–18, 2003
2	8	4.0	Shirai et al. (41)	Clin Exp Allergy 33: 84–89, 2003
Total 51	119	2.3		
Mean (95% CI)		4.0 (1.2–6.8, $p = 0.0387$)		

2.9 (95% CI 1.7–4.2, $p = 0.0056$) (10,28,35–37,40,48–57) (Table 6). Increased cough reflex sensitivity is not a fundamental feature of either cough-variant asthma or typical asthma, although cough reflex sensitivity is increased in patients labeled as cough-variant asthma in some studies, possibly resulting in the higher frequency of females. No gender difference is apparent in children with cough-variant asthma (58–62) (Table 7).

In conclusion, females are more susceptible to chronic cough, especially ACE inhibitor-induced cough, GER-associated cough and atopic cough, and probably eosinophilic bronchitis without asthma, all of which are characterized by increased cough sensitivity.

Gender Difference in Cough Reflex Sensitivity

To explain the gender difference in morbidity of chronic cough, five studies have been reported. The first (63) was performed to elucidate the female preponderance in ACE inhibitor-induced cough and clearly showed that cough threshold to inhaled tartaric acid, defined as the lowest concentration to elicit five or more coughs, was significantly lower in nonsmoking nonatopic healthy young females (mean age 20 years) than in males (mean

Table 5 Gender Distribution of Patients with Eosinophilic Bronchitis Without Asthma

Number of patients				
Male	Female	Female/male	Investigators	Journals
3	4	1.3	Gibson et al. (42)	Lancet 0: 1346–1348, 1989
4	5	1.3	Gibson et al. (43)	Clin Exp Allergy 25: 127–132, 1995
2	10	5.0	Brightling et al. (44)	Am J Respir Crit Care Med 160: 406–410, 1999
6	5	0.8	Brightling et al. (45)	Eur Respir J 15: 682–686, 2000
3	5	1.7	Brightling et al. (46)	Am J Respir Crit Care Med 162: 878–882, 2000
2	9	4.5	Joo et al. (47)	Korean J Intern Med 17: 31–37, 2002
Total 20	38	1.9		
Mean (95% CI)		2.4 (0.5–4.3, $p=0.1126$)		

age 25 years). The same authors (64) further investigated the influence of gender and age on cough reflex sensitivity to inhaled capsaicin in 160 non-smoking nonatopic healthy subjects, consisting of 40 young males (mean age 24 years), 40 young females (mean age 22 years), 40 middle-aged males (mean age 48 years), and 40 middle-aged females (mean age 50 years). Cough threshold, defined as the lowest concentration of inhaled capsaicin causing five or more coughs, was used as an index of cough reflex sensitivity. The cough threshold was three- to fivefold lower in females than in males, both in young and in middle-aged subjects, but did not differ between young and middle-aged subjects of either sex (Fig. 1). Furthermore, when the middle-aged females were divided into premenopausal and postmenopausal groups, the capsaicin cough threshold was significantly lower in the latter group. These findings confirm a gender difference in cough reflex sensitivity, which is further enhanced in postmenopausal females, but suggest no influence of age on cough reflex sensitivity.

Dicpinigaitis and Rauf (65) also investigated the influence of gender on cough reflex sensitivity to inhaled capsaicin in healthy adult nonsmokers. The study population comprised 50 females of mean age 31.9 years and 50 males of mean age 30.8 years who had not experienced symptoms of

Table 6 Gender Distribution of Adult Patients with Cough-Variant Asthma

Number of patients		Female/ male	Investigators	Journals
Male	Female			
2	4	2.0	Corrao et al. (48)	N Engl J Med 22: 633–637, 1979
1	9	9.0	Fujimura et al. (35)	Intern Med 31: 447–452, 1992
4	6	1.5	Doan et al. (49)	Ann Allergy 69: 505–509, 1992
4	8	2.0	Fujimura et al. (36)	J Asthma 31: 463–472, 1994
6	6	1.0	Cherpiyan et al. (50)	Ann Allergy 73: 478–480, 1994
10	10	1.0	Shioya et al. (51)	Pul Pharmacol 9: 59–62, 1996
1	7	7.0	Fujimura et al. (37)	J Asthma 34: 119–126, 1997
6	8	1.3	Irwin et al. (52)	Arch Intern Med 157: 1981–1987, 1997
4	8	2.0	Niimi et al. (53)	Eur Respir J 11: 1064–1069, 1998
6	10	1.7	McGarvey et al. (10)	Eur Respir J 13: 59–65, 1999
2	10	5.0	Niimi et al. (54)	Lancet 356: 564–565, 2000
6	9	1.5	Forsythe et al. (28)	Clin Exp Allergy 30: 225–232, 2000
6	14	2.3	Shioya et al. (55)	Eur J Clin Pharmacol 58: 171–176, 2002
2	8	4.0	Cho et al. (56)	J Korean Med Sci 17: 616–620, 2002
8	6	0.8	Dicpinigaitis et al. (57)	J Asthma 39: 291–297, 2002
8	39	4.9	Fujimura et al. (40)	Thorax 58: 14–18, 2003
Total 76	162	2.1		
Mean (95% CI)		2.9 (1.7–4.2, $p = 0.0056$)		

Table 7 Gender Distribution of Childhood Patients with Cough Variant-Asthma

Number of patients		Female/		
Male	Female	male	Investigators	Journals
2	4	2.0	Koh et al. (58)	Clin Exp Allergy 23: 696–701, 1993
19	3	0.2	Tokuyama et al. (59)	J Asthma 35: 225–229, 1998
2	17	8.5	Koh et al. (60)	Eur Respir J 14: 302–308, 1999
34	5	0.1	Koh et al. (61)	J Asthma 39: 307–314, 2002
16	23	1.4	Koh et al. (62)	Allergy 57: 1165–1170, 2002
Total 73	52	0.7		
Mean (95% CI)		2.4 (−1.9 to 6.8, p = 0.4044)		

respiratory tract infection or seasonal allergy for at least 4 weeks prior to testing. They found that cough reflex sensitivity to inhaled capsaicin was 2.5-fold greater in females than in males. The same authors examined capsaicin cough sensitivity in 182 healthy males and females of three distinct ethnic groups: Caucasians, Indians, and Chinese. They confirmed the sex difference in cough reflex sensitivity to inhaled capsaicin but failed to find ethnic differences in cough sensitivity.

A sex difference in cough reflex sensitivity has also been demonstrated using citric acid as a tussive agent (66). Although atopy, which is indicated by positive specific IgE antibody in the serum, is a predictor of bronchial hyperresponsiveness, it has been shown not to be related to cough reflex sensitivity to inhaled capsaicin in asymptomatic young females (67). Thus, to date, only gender is an established factor determining cough reflex sensitivity of humans, whereas age, atopy, and ethnicity are not.

Possible Mechanism of Female Preponderance in Chronic Cough

Increased cough sensitivity in healthy women may explain why females more frequently suffer from chronic cough, especially that caused by ACE inhibitors, GER, atopic cough, and eosinophilic bronchitis without asthma, all of which are characterized by increased cough reflex sensitivity. Figure 2

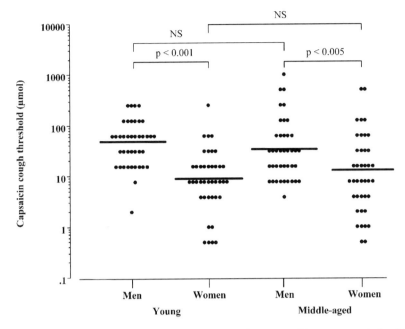

Figure 1 Cough threshold to inhaled capsaicin in nonsmoking nonatopic healthy subjects. Horizontal bars represent geometric mean cough threshold, defined as the lowest concentration of capsaicin solution causing five or more coughs. The capsaicin cough threshold was three- to fivefold lower in females than males, both in young and middle-aged subjects. The cough threshold was not significantly different between young and middle-aged subjects of either sex. (From Ref. 64.)

illustrates this possible mechanism. In response to the same intensity of a stimulus that modulates cough reflex sensitivity, such as airway inflammation, the cough sensitivity increases beyond the critical level for the onset of pathologic cough more frequently in females than in males. This concept may explain the gender difference in the number of patients with chronic cough.

To investigate the excess of females among chronic cough patients attending specialist cough clinics, Kastelik et al. (34) measured cough reflex sensitivity to inhaled capsaicin and citric acid in male and female patients with chronic cough. The authors showed that cough sensitivity to both tussigenic stimuli, defined as the concentrations causing two and five coughs, was significantly lower in female than in male patients with GER-associated cough and with asthma. They concluded that this sex difference in cough reflex sensitivity may explain the female preponderance in cough clinics. However, Choudry and Fuller (68) reported that cough reflex sensitivity

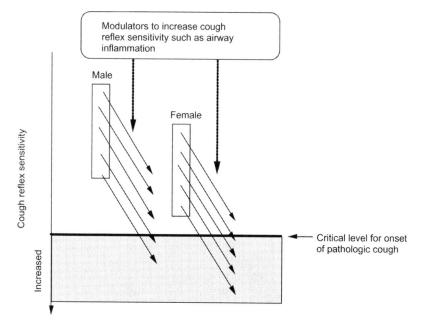

Figure 2   Possible mechanism of the gender difference in morbidity of chronic cough. Basal cough reflex sensitivity is nearly fourfold higher in normal females than in normal males. When the same intensity of a modulator that increases cough reflex sensitivity is added to normal cough reflex sensitivity in five females and five males, the cough sensitivity increases beyond the critical level for the onset of pathologic cough in four females but in only two males.

to inhaled capsaicin was not different between female and male patients with non-productive cough associated with GER or asthma.

Our experience (Fig. 3, unpublished data) is consistent with the investigation of Choudry and Fuller (68). Cough reflex sensitivity to capsaicin was not significantly different between female and male patients with atopic cough but was increased in female patients with asthma. Previous studies have established that cough reflex sensitivity is fundamentally within normal limits in stable asthma (69–74), although it is increased in acute asthma (75) and is correlated with intensity of daily coughing (76). Furthermore, cough reflex sensitivity in cough-variant asthma is not increased before treatment (37,40,77) and does not change following successful treatment (77). Thus, it is likely that the gender difference in cough reflex sensitivity in asthmatic patients directly reflects the difference in healthy subjects. Figure 3 may explain the gender difference in cough reflex sensitivity of patients with chronic cough shown by Kastelik and coworkers (34).

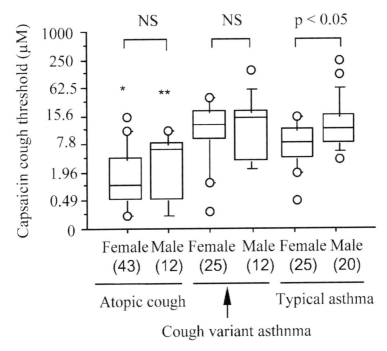

Figure 3 Capsaicin cough threshold at initial presentation in male and female patients with atopic cough and cough-variant asthma and under stable conditions in patients with typical asthma. $*p < 0.0001$ vs. female patients with cough-variant asthma and typical asthma. $**p < 0.01$ vs. male patients with cough-variant asthma and typical asthma.

References

1. Irwin RS, Curley FJ, French CJ. Chronic cough: the spectrum and frequency of causes, key components of the diagnostic evaluation, and outcome of specific therapy. Am Rev Respir Dis 1990; 141:640–647.
2. Pratter MR, Bartter T, Akers S, DuBois J. An algorithmic approach to chronic cough. Ann Intern Med 1993; 119:977–983.
3. Boulet L-P, Milot J, Boutet M, St, Georges F, Laviolette M. Airway inflammation in nonasthmatic subjects with chronic cough. Am J Respir Crit Care Med 1994; 149:482–489.
4. Smyrnios NA, Irwin RS, Curley FJ. Chronic cough with a history of excessive sputum production: the spectrum and frequency of causes, key components of the diagnostic evaluation, and outcome of specific therapy. Chest 1995; 108: 991–997.
5. Mello CJ, Irwin RS, Curley FJ. Predictive values of the character, timing, and complications of chronic cough in diagnosing its cause. Arch Intern Med 1996; 156:997–1003.

6. Wongtim S, Mogmeud S, Limthongkul S, Chareonlap P, Udompanich V, Nuchprayoon C, Chochaipanichnont L. The role of the methacholine inhalation challenge in adult patients presenting with chronic cough. Asian Pac J Allergy Immunol 1997; 15:9–14.
7. Smyrnios NA, Irwin RS, Curley F, French C. From a prospective study of chronic cough: diagnostic and therapeutic aspects in older adults. Arch Intern Med 1998; 158:1222–1228.
8. McGarvey LPA, Heaney LG, MacMahon J. A retrospective survey of diagnosis and management of patients presenting with chronic cough to a general chest clinic. Int J Clin Pract 1998; 52:158–161.
9. Palombini BC, Villanova CAC, Araújo E, Gastal OL, Alt DC, Stolz DP, Palombini CO. A pathogenic triad in chronic cough: asthma, postnasal drip syndrome, and gastroesophageal reflux disease. Chest 1999; 116:279–284.
10. McGarvey LPA, Forsythe P, Heaney LG, MacMahon J, Ennis M. Bronchoalveolar lavage findings in patients with nonproductive cough. Eur Respir J 1999; 13:59–65.
11. Lee SY, Cho JY, Shin JJ, Kim HK, Kang KH, Yoo SH, In KH. Airway inflammation as an assessment of chronic nonproductive cough. Chest 2001; 120: 1114–1120.
12. Coulter DM, Edwards IR. Cough associated with captopril and enalapril. Br Med J 1987; 294:1521–1523.
13. Yeo WW, Foster G, Ramsay LE. Prevalence of persistent cough during long-term enalapril treatment: controlled study versus nifedipine. Quart J Med 1991; 80:763–770.
14. Simon SR, Black HR, Moser M, Berland WE. Cough and ACE inhibitors. Arch Intern Med 1992; 152:1698–1700.
15. Elliott WJ. Higher incidence of discontinuation of angiotensin converting enzyme inhibitors due to cough in black subjects. Clin Pharm Ther 1996; 60:582–588.
16. Os I, Bratland B, Dahlof B, Gisholt K, Syvertsen JO, Tretli S. Female sex as an important determinant of lisinopril-induced cough. Lancet 1992; 339:332.
17. Moore N, Noblet C, Joannides R, Ollagnier M, Imbs JL, Lagier G. Cough and ACE inhibitors. Lancet 1993; 341:61.
18. Adigun AQ, Ajayi AA. Angiotensin converting enzyme inhibitor induced cough in Nigerians. West Afr J Med 2001; 20:46–47.
19. Irwin RS, Zawacki JK, Curley FJ, French CL, Hoffman PJ. Chronic cough as the sole presenting manifestation of gastroesophageal reflux. Am Rev Respir Dis 1989; 140:1294–1300.
20. Irwin RS, French CL, Curley FJ, Zawacki JK, Bennett FM. Chronic cough due to gastroesophageal reflux: clinical, diagnostic, and pathogenetic aspects. Chest 1993; 104:1511–1517.
21. Laukka MA, Cameron AJ, Schei AJ. Gastroesophageal reflux and chronic cough: which comes first? J Clin Gastroenterol 1994; 19:100–104.
22. Ing AJ, Ngu MC, Breslin AB. Pathogenesis of chronic persistent cough associated with gastroesophageal reflux. Am J Respir Crit Care Med 1994; 149:160–167.

23. O'Connell F, Thomas VE, Pride NB, Fuller RW. Capsaicin cough sensitivity decreases with successful treatment of chronic cough. Am J Respir Crit Care Med 1994; 150:374–380.

24. Waring JP, Lacayo L, Hunter J, Katz E, Suwak B. Chronic cough and hoarseness in patients with severe gastroesophageal reflux: diagnosis and response to treatment. Dig Dis Sci 1995; 40:1093–1097.

25. Vaezi MF, Richter JE. Twenty-four-hour ambulatory esophageal pH monitoring in the diagnosis of acid reflux-related chronic cough. South Med J 1997; 90:305–311.

26. Carney IK, Gibson PG, Murree-Allen K, Saltos N, Olson LG, Hensley MJ. A systematic evaluation of mechanisms in chronic cough. Am J Respir Crit Care Med 1997; 156:211–216.

27. Kiljander TO, Salomaa ER, Heitanen EK, Terho EO. Chronic cough and gastro-oesophageal reflux: a double-blind placebo-controlled trial with omeprazole. Eur Respir J 2000; 16:633–638.

28. Forsythe P, McGarvey LPA, Heaney LG, MacMahon J, Ennis M. Sensory neuropeptides induce histamine release from bronchoalveolar lavage cells in both nonasthmatic coughers and cough variant asthmatics. Clin Exp Allergy 2000; 30:225–232.

29. Parameswaran K, Allen CJ, Kamada D, Efthimiadis A, Anvari M, Hargreave FE. Sputum cell counts and exhaled nitric oxide in patients with gastroesophageal reflux, and cough or asthma. Can Respir J 2001; 8:239–244.

30. Novitsky YW, Zawacki JK, Irwin RS, French CT, Hussey VM, Callery MP. Chronic cough due to gastroesophageal reflux: efficacy of antireflux surgery. Surg Endosc 2002; 16:567–571.

31. Irwin RS, Zawacki JK, Wilson MM, French CL, Callery MP. Chronic cough due to gastroesophageal reflux disease: failure to resolve despite total/near-total elimination of esophageal acid. Chest 2002; 121:1132–1140.

32. Kastelik JA, Jackson W, Davies TW, Wright A, Redington AE, Wedgwood KR, Morice AH. Measurement of gastric emptying in gastroesophageal reflux-related chronic cough. Chest 2002; 122:2038–2041.

33. Thoman DS, Hui TT, Spyrou M, Phillips EH. Laparoscopic antireflux surgery and its effect on cough in patients with gastroesophageal reflux disease. J Gastrointest Surg 2002; 6:17–21.

34. Kastelik JA, Thompson RH, Aziz I, Ojoo JC, Redington AE, Morice AH. Sex-related difference in cough reflex sensitivity in patients with chronic cough. Am J Respir Crit Care Med 2002; 166:961–964.

35. Fujimura M, Sakamoto S, Matsuda T. Bronchodilator-resistive cough in atopic patients: bronchial reversibility and hyperresponsiveness. Intern Med 1992; 31:447–452.

36. Fujimura M, Kamio Y, Hashimoto T, Matsuda T. Cough receptor sensitivity and bronchial responsiveness in patients with only chronic nonproductive cough: in view of effect of bronchodilator therapy. J Asthma 1994; 31:463–472.

37. Fujimura M, Songür N, Kamio Y, Matsuda T. Detection of eosinophils in hypertonic saline-induced sputum in patients with chronic nonproductive cough. J Asthma 1997; 34:119–126.

38. Fujimura M, Ogawa H, Yasui M, Matsuda T. Eosinophilic tracheobronchitis and airway cough hypersensitivity in chronic non-productive cough. Clin Exp Allergy 2000; 30:41–47.
39. Fujimura M, Nishi K, Ohka T, Yasui M. Bronchial biopsy and sequential bronchoalveolar lavage in atopic cough: in view of the effect of histamine H_1-receptor antagonists. Allergol Int 2000; 49:135–142.
40. Fujimura M, Ogawa M, Nishizawa Y, Nishi K. Comparison of atopic cough with cough variant asthma: is atopic cough a precursor of asthma? Thorax 2003; 58:14–18.
41. Shirai T, Suzuki K, Inui N, Chida K, Nakamura. Th1/Th2 profile in peripheral blood in atopic cough ad atopic asthma. Clin Exp Allergy 2003; 33:84–89.
42. Gibson PG, Dolovich J, Denburg J, Ramsdale EH, Hargreave FE. Chronic cough: eosinophilic bronchitis without asthma. Lancet 1989; i:1346–1348.
43. Gibson PG, Hargreave FE, Girgis-Gabardo A, Morris M, Denburg JA, Dolovich J. Chronic cough with eosinophilic bronchitis: examination for variable airflow obstruction and response to corticosteroid. Clin Exp Allergy 1995; 25:127–132.
44. Brightling CE, Ward R, Goh KL, Wardlaw AJ, Pavord ID. Eosinophilic bronchitis is an important cause of chronic cough. Am J Respir Crit Care Med 1999; 160:406–410.
45. Brightling CE, Ward R, Wardlaw AJ, Pavord ID. Airway inflammation, airway responsiveness and cough before and after inhaled budesonide in patients with eosinophilic bronchitis. Eur Respir J 2000; 15:682–686.
46. Brightling CE, Ward R, Woltmann G, Bradding P, Sheller JR, Dworski R, Pavord ID. Induced sputum inflammatory mediator concentrations in eosinophilic bronchitis and asthma. Am J Respir Crit Care Med 2000; 162:878–882.
47. Joo JH, Park SJ, Park SW, Lee J, Kim Do J, Uh ST, Kim YH, Park CS. Clinical features of eosinophilic bronchitis. Korean J Intern Med 2002; 17:31–37.
48. Corrao WM, Braman SS, Irwin RS. Chronic cough as the sole presenting manifestation of bronchial asthma. N Engl J Med 1979; 300:633–637.
49. Doan T, Patterson R, Greenberger PA. Cough variant asthma: usefulness of a diagnostic-therapeutic trial with prednisone. Ann Allergy 1992; 505–509.
50. Cheriyan S, Greenberger PA, Patterson R. Outcome of cough variant asthma treated with inhaled steroids. Ann Allergy 1994; 73:478–480.
51. Shioya T, Ito N, Sasaki M, Kagaya M, Sano M, Shindo T, Kashima M, Miura M. Cough threshold for capsaicin increases by azelastine in patients with cough-variant asthma. Pulm Pharmacol 1996; 9:59–62.
52. Irwin RS, French CT, Smyrnios NA, Curley FJ. Interpretation of positive results of a methacholine inhalation challenge and 1 week of inhaled bronchodilator use in diagnosing and treating cough-variant asthma. Arch Intern Med 1997; 157:1981–1987.
53. Niimi A, Amitani R, Suzuki K, Tanaka E, Murayama T, Kuze F. Eosinophilic inflammation in cough variant asthma. Eur Respir J 1998; 11:1064–1069.
54. Niimi A, Matsumoto H, Minakuchi M, Kitaichi M, Amitani R. Airway remodelling in cough-variant asthma. Lancet 2000; 356:564–565.

55. Shioya T, Satake M, Sano M, Kagaya M, Watanabe A, Sato K, Ito T, Ito N, Sasaki M, Miura M. Effect of suplatast tosilate, a Th2 cytokine inhibitor, on cough variant asthma. Eur J Clin Pharmacol 2002; 158:171–176.
56. Cho YS, Lee C-K, Yoo B, Moon H-B. Cough sensitivity and extrathoracic airway responsiveness to inhaled capsaicin in chronic cough patients. J Korean Med Sci 2002; 17:616–620.
57. Dicpinigaitis PV, Dobkin JB, Reichel J. Antitussive effect of the leukotriene receptor antagonist zafirlukast in subjects with cough-variant asthma. J Asthma 2002; 39:291–297.
58. Koh YY, Chae SA, Min KU. Cough variant asthma is associated with a higher wheezing threshold than classic asthma. Clin Exp Allergy 1993; 23:696–701.
59. Tokuyama K, Shigeta M, Maeda S, Takei K, Hoshino M, Morikawa A. Diurnal variation of peak expiratory flow in children with cough variant asthma. J Asthma 1998; 35:225–229.
60. Koh YY, Jeong JH, Park Y, Kim CK. Development of wheezing in patients with cough variant asthma during an increase in airway responsiveness. Eur Respir J 1999; 14:302–308.
61. Koh YY, Park Y, Jeong JH, Kim CH, Kim JT. Relationship of wheezing to airflow obstruction in asthmatic children and a history of cough-variant asthma. J Asthma 2002; 39:307–314.
62. Koh YY, Park Y, Kim CK. The importance of maximal airway response to methacholine in the prediction of wheezing development in patients with cough-variant asthma. Allergy 2002; 57:1165–1170.
63. Fujimura M, Sakamoto S, Kamio Y, Matsuda T. Sex difference in the inhaled tartaric acid cough threshold in non-atopic healthy subjects. Thorax 1990; 45:633–634.
64. Fujimura M, Kasahara K, Kamio Y, Naruse M, Hashimoto T, Matsuda T. Female gender as a determinant of cough threshold to inhaled capsaicin. Eur Respir J 1996; 9:1624–1626.
65. Dicpinigaitis PV, Rauf K. The influence of gender on cough reflex sensitivity. Chest 1998; 113:1319–1321.
66. Rostami-Hodjegan A, Abdul-Manap R, Wright CE, Tucker GT, Morice AH. The placebo response to citric acid-induced cough: pharmacodynamics and gender differences. Pulm Pharmacol Ther 2001; 14:315–319.
67. Fujimura M, Kasahara K, Yasui M, Myou S, Ishiura Y, Kamio Y, Hashimoto T, Matsuda T. Atopy in cough sensitivity to capsaicin and bronchial responsiveness in young women. Eur Respir J 1998; 11:1060–1063.
68. Choudry NB, Fuller RW. Sensitivity of the cough reflex in patients with chronic cough. Eur Respir J 1992; 5:296–300.
69. Fujimura M, Sakamoto S, Kamio Y, Matsuda T. Cough receptor sensitivity and bronchial responsiveness in normal and asthmatic subjects. Eur Respir J 1992; 5:291–295.
70. Fujimura M, Sakamoto S, Kamio Y, Saito M, Miyake Y, Yasui M, Matsuda T. Cough threshold to inhaled tartaric acid and bronchial responsiveness to methacholine in patients with asthma and sino-bronchial syndrome. Intern Med 1992; 31:17–21.

71. Fujimura M, Sakamoto S, Kamio Y, Bando T, Kurashima K, Matsuda T. Effect of inhaled procaterol on cough receptor sensitivity to capsaicin in patients with asthma or chronic bronchitis and in normal subjects. Thorax 1993; 48: 615–618.
72. Fujimura M, Kamio Y, Kasahara K, Bando T, Hashimoto T, Matsuda T. Prostanoids and cough response to capsaicin in asthma and chronic bronchitis. Eur Respir J 1995; 8:1499–1505.
73. Schmidt D, Jorres RA, Magnussen H. Citric acid-induced cough thresholds in normal subjects, patients with bronchial asthma, and smokers. Eur J Med Res 1997; 2:384–388.
74. Fujimura M, Kamio Y, Hashimoto T, Matsuda T. Airway cough sensitivity to inhaled capsaicin and bronchial responsiveness to methacholine in asthmatic and bronchitic subjects. Respirology 1998; 3:267–272.
75. Chang AB, Phelan PD, Robertson CF. Cough receptor sensitivity in children with acute and non-acute asthma. Thorax 1997; 52:770–774.
76. Doherty MJ, Mister R, Pearson MG, Calverley PM. Capsaicin responsiveness and cough in asthma and chronic obstructive pulmonary disease. Thorax 2000; 55:643–649.
77. Fujimura M, Kamio Y, Hashimoto T, Matsuda T. Cough receptor sensitivity and bronchial responsiveness in patients with only chronic nonproductive cough: in view of effect of bronchodilator therapy. J Asthma 1994; 31:463–472.

22

Impact of Cough on Health Status

SURINDER S. BIRRING and IAN D. PAVORD

Department of Respiratory Medicine, Institute for Lung Health,
Glenfield Hospital, Leicester, U.K.

Introduction

Cough is one of the most common presenting symptoms to a general practitioner. Most cases are acute and self-limiting, although a significant minority with an isolated persistent cough are referred for a specialist opinion. The prevalence of chronic cough is variously estimated between 3% and 20% in the general population and is responsible for between 5% and 10% of respiratory outpatient referrals (1,2). These patients suffer considerable physical and psychological morbidity.

Chronic cough is often perceived as a trivial problem but can be a disabling symptom associated with significantly impaired quality of life (3,4). Until recently, there have been no tools with which to measure cough-specific quality of life. Indeed, there is a striking paucity of well-validated outcome measures in chronic cough. There is no consensus on the definition of quality of life as it is affected by health, but the definition of health proposed by the World Health Organization in 1948 as "a state of complete physical, mental, and social well-being, and not merely the absence of disease" (5) is widely quoted. Health status or health-related quality-of-life measurement is a means of quantifying the impact of disease on a patient's daily life and general well-being in a standardized and objective manner.

The assessment of health status has become increasingly important in respiratory disease, and various disease-specific quality-of-life question-naires have become standard end points in many randomized controlled trials and clinical studies. Health status has been studied most extensively in asthma and chronic obstructive pulmonary disease by the development of disease-specific questionnaires (6,7). Less is known about the effects of chronic cough on health status but the recent development of cough-speci-fic quality of life questionnaires has provided some new insights (3,4). This review will focus on the effects of chronic cough on health status and the measurement of quality of life in patients with chronic cough.

Adverse Impact of Cough on Health Status

Cough has wide-ranging effects on health status. The reasons why patients with chronic cough seek medical advice are poorly understood but may relate to worry about the cough, embarrassment, self-consciousness, and the presence of associated symptoms such as nausea and exhaustion (8). In acute cough, the adverse effects on health status result from physical symptoms and are transient. In contrast, the impact of chronic cough on health status is varied, being minimal in some patients who do not seek medical attention to disabling in others, associated with impairment of quality of life comparable to that in other chronic respiratory disorders such as chronic obstructive pulmonary disease. The most commonly affected domains of health are physical, psychological, and social (Table 1) (3). Patients with chronic cough frequently report musculoskeletal chest pains, sleep disturbance, and hoarse voice, but more marked symptoms such as blackouts, stress incontinence, and vomiting can occur. Psychological problems include worry about serious underlying diseases such as cancer and tuberculosis. The impact of cough on social well-being depends on indi-vidual circumstances. The cough may result in difficulties in relationships, avoidance of public places, disruption at work, and in severe cases, time off work. The wide-ranging and potentially profound effects of cough on health status highlight the importance of a detailed history of associated symptoms and concerns when assessing a patient with chronic cough.

Assessment of Health Status

Why Measure Quality of Life?

There are several reasons why quality of life measurement should be included in the clinical assessment of patients and in clinical trials. Quality

Table 1 Adverse Symptoms in Patients with Chronic Cough

Symptom

Physical
Musculoskeletal pains
Hoarse voice
Nausea and vomiting
Dizziness and syncope
Headaches
Sleep disturbance
Lack of energy
Stress incontinence

Psychological
Embarrassment
Anxiety
Depression
Fear of serious illness

Social
Avoidance of public places
Interrupted conversation
Relationship difficulties
Disturbance of partner's sleep
Interference with occupation or daily tasks
Interference with recreational activities

of life measures can be used to facilitate communication with patients and to establish information on the range of problems that affect them. The impact of the illness on health and treatment preferences often differs between patient and physician, and therefore quality of life considerations should take the patient's perspective into account. Quality of life measurement is particularly helpful when assessing treatments that are invasive or have significant adverse effects. Health status measures in clinical trials can be used to study changes in health after therapy and to compare treatments.

How to Measure Quality of Life

The simplest method to assess quality of life is to ask the patient (9). Drawbacks to this are that some observers are poor judges of patients' opinions. Assessment of patients with quality of life instruments is essentially similar to a structured clinical history, although the outcome parameter is an objective, validated, and quantifiable measurement. Quality of life domains are usually measured separately to assess emotional and psychological well-being as well as physical and practical aspects of daily life. Questionnaires may be divided into generic and disease specific.

Generic Vs. Disease-Specific Instruments

Generic instruments are intended for general use, irrespective of the illness, and have the advantage that quality of life scores from patients can be compared with other conditions and even healthy subjects (10). However, these instruments do not focus on issues related to patients with the condition and they lack responsiveness to specific interventions. This has led to the development of disease-specific quality of life questionnaires. Examples of generic and disease-specific instruments are given in Table 2.

Properties of a Quality-of-Life Measure

The properties of a quality of life questionnaire should satisfy the basic principles of any measure that is to be clinically useful. These are primarily validity, repeatability, sensitivity, responsiveness, and interpretability (16). Validation is an assessment of the extent to which the instrument measures quality of life. This usually involves comparison of the questionnaire with other objective parameters that may reflect disease severity and with other quality of life instruments in the intended population. Repeatability assesses the random variability of the measure. Ideally, the questionnaire should be repeatable over time in patients whose quality of life is unchanged. Sensitivity is the ability of an instrument to detect differences between patients and responsiveness is the ability to detect clinically meaningful changes within a patient, such as those that result from therapeutic intervention. The questionnaire scores must be clinically relevant if they are to be used in

Table 2 Examples of Generic and Disease-Specific Quality of Life Questionnaires

Questionnaire
Generic
Sickness Impact Profile (SIP) (11) 136 items
Nottingham Health Profile (NHP) (12) 38 items
Medical Outcomes Study 36-item Short Form (SF36) (13) 36 items
Respiratory disease
Asthma Quality of Life Questionnaire (AQLQ) (6) 32 items
St. Georges' Respiratory Questionnaire (SGRQ) (7) 76 items
Chronic Respiratory Disease Questionnaire (CRQ) (14) 20 items
Cystic Fibrosis Quality of Life Questionnaire (CFQoL) (15) 52 items
Cough
Cough-Specific Quality of Life Questionnaire (CQLQ) (4) 28 items
Leicester Cough Questionnaire (LCQ) (3) 19 items

clinical practice. Finally, the measure must be simple, brief, and easy to score if it is intended for clinical practice as well as research.

Cough-Specific Quality-of-Life Measures

Cough-Specific Quality-of-Life Questionnaire

Two cough-specific quality of life measures have been recently developed. The first is a 28-item questionnaire that has been developed and tested in North America (4). It is intended for use in adults with acute and chronic cough. The questionnaire is self-completed and has a four-point Likert response scale. The items are divided into six domains: physical complaints, extreme physical complaints, psychosocial issues, emotional well-being, personal safety fears, and functional abilities. Items for this questionnaire were selected by subjective methods and allocated to domains by factor analysis. This is a psychometric method used to select and allocate items to domains that is based largely on the structure of correlations between items, although the investigators must make a number of subjective decisions throughout the process. Although commonly used in the development of quality of life questionnaires, one weakness of factor analysis is that it does not take into account the perception of clinical relevance of items by the intended population. Concurrent validity is the assessment of an instrument against other standards that provide an indication of the true value for the measurement. This was assessed in a preliminary version of the Cough-Specific Quality of Life Questionnaire (CQLQ) called Adverse Cough Outcome Survey (ACOS), which correlated moderately with the Sickness Impact Profile (SIP) questionnaire (8). The CQLQ is both repeatable and responsive to change in patients with chronic cough but this has not been tested in patients with acute cough.

Leicester Cough Questionnaire

The Leicester Cough Questionnaire (LCQ) is a brief, easy to administer, and well-validated chronic cough health-related quality of life questionnaire developed in the United Kingdom (3). The LCQ comprises 19 items and 3 domains (physical, psychological, and social) (Tables 3 and 4). The questionnaire is self-completed and has a seven-point Likert response scale. One of the key differences between the LCQ and CQLQ is that items for the LCQ were chosen using the clinical impact factor method. This chooses items that patients label as a problem and ranks the importance that they associate with them. Items were categorized into domains using clinical sensibility. The LCQ was extensively validated against other quality of life questionnaires and measures of cough severity. The LCQ was repeatable and responsive in patients with chronic cough. Table 5 summarizes the

Table 3 Leicester Cough Questionnaire (LCQ)

This questionnaire is designed to assess the impact of cough on various aspects of your life. Read each question carefully and answer by *circling* the response that best applies to you. Please answer *all* questions as honestly as you can

1. *In the last 2 weeks, have you had chest or stomach pains as a result of your cough?*

1	2	3	4	5	6	7
All of the time	Most of the time	A good bit of the time	Some of the time	A little of the time	Hardly any of the time	None of the time

2. *In the last 2 weeks, have you been bothered by sputum (phlegm) production when you cough?*

1	2	3	4	5	6	7
Every time	Most times	Several times	Sometimes	Occasionally	Rarely	Never

3. *In the last 2 weeks, have you been tired because of your cough?*

1	2	3	4	5	6	7
All of the time	Most of the time	A good bit of the time	Some of the time	A little of the time	Hardly any of the time	None of the time

4. *In the last 2 weeks, have you felt in control of your cough?*

1	2	3	4	5	6	7
None of the time	Hardly any of the time	A little of the time	Some of the time	A good bit of the time	Most of the time	All of the time

5. *How often during the last 2 weeks have you felt embarrassed by your coughing?*

1	2	3	4	5	6	7
All of the time	Most of the time	A good bit of the time	Some of the time	A little of the time	Hardly any of the time	None of the time

6. *In the last 2 weeks, my cough has made me feel anxious*

1	2	3	4	5	6	7
All of the time	Most of the time	A good bit of the time	Some of the time	A little of the time	Hardly any of the time	None of the time

7. *In the last 2 weeks, my cough has interfered with my job, or other daily tasks*

1	2	3	4	5	6	7
All of the time	Most of the time	A good bit of the time	Some of the time	A little of the time	Hardly any of the time	None of the time

8. *In the last 2 weeks, I felt that my cough interfered with the overall enjoyment of my life*

1	2	3	4	5	6	7
All of the time	Most of the time	A good bit of the time	Some of the time	A little of the time	Hardly any of the time	None of the time

9. *In the last 2 weeks, exposure to paints or fumes has made me cough*

1	2	3	4	5	6	7
All of the time	Most of the time	A good bit of the time	Some of the time	A little of the time	Hardly any of the time	None of the time

10. *In the last 2 weeks, has your cough disturbed your sleep?*

1	2	3	4	5	6	7
All of the time	Most of the time	A good bit of the time	Some of the time	A little of the time	Hardly any of the time	None of the time

11. *In the last two weeks, how many times a day have you had coughing bouts?*

1	2	3	4	5	6	7
All the time (continuously)	Most times during the day	Several times during the day	Sometimes during the day	Occasionally through the day	Rarely	None

12. *In the last 2 weeks, my cough has made me feel frustrated*

1	2	3	4	5	6	7
All of the time	Most of the time	A good bit of the time	Some of the time	A little of the time	Hardly any of the time	None of the time

13. *In the last 2 weeks, my cough has made me feel fed up*

1	2	3	4	5	6	7
All of the time	Most of the time	A good bit of the time	Some of the time	A little of the time	Hardly any of the time	None of the time

14. *In the last 2 weeks, have you suffered from a hoarse voice as a result of your cough?*

1	2	3	4	5	6	7
All of the time	Most of the time	A good bit of the time	Some of the time	A little of the time	Hardly any of the time	None of the time

15. *In the last 2 weeks, have you had a lot of energy?*

1	2	3	4	5	6	7
None of the time	Hardly any of the time	A little of the time	Some of the time	A good bit of the time	Most of the time	All of the time

(Continued)

Table 3 Leicester Cough Questionnaire (LCQ) (Continued)

16. *In the last 2 weeks, have you worried that your cough may indicate a serious illness?*

1	2	3	4	5	6	7
All of the time	Most of the time	A good bit of the time	Some of the time	A little of the time	Hardly any of the time	None of the time

17. *In the last 2 weeks, have you been concerned that other people think something is wrong with you, because of your cough?*

1	2	3	4	5	6	7
All of the time	Most of the time	A good bit of the time	Some of the time	A little of the time	Hardly any of the time	None of the time

18. *In the last 2 weeks, my cough has interrupted conversation or telephone calls*

1	2	3	4	5	6	7
All of the time	Most of the time	A good bit of the time	Some of the time	A little of the time	Hardly any of the time	None of the time

19. *In the last 2 weeks, I feel that my cough has annoyed my partner, family, or friends*

1	2	3	4	5	6	7
Every time I cough	Most times when I cough	Several times when I cough	Sometimes when I cough	Occasionally when I cough	Rarely	Never

Thank you for completing this questionnaire.

Table 4 Scoring of LCQ

1. Domains (questions):	Physical: 1, 2, 3, 9, 10, 11, 14, 15
	Psychological: 4, 5, 6, 12, 13, 16, 17
	Social: 7, 8, 18, 19
2. Domain scores:	Total score from items in domain/ number of items in domain (range 1–7)
3. Total scores:	Addition of domain scores (range 3–21)

repeatability and responsiveness of the LCQ compared to other measures of cough severity.

Both questionnaires are intended for use in an adult chronic cough population and have a number of potential applications. First, they would be useful in measuring longitudinal changes that take place in patients with chronic cough. They can be used to identify aspects of health affected by cough and how these change over time. Finally, they can be used in clinical trials evaluating new treatments for cough. Further work is necessary to compare the LCQ and CQLQ in the assessment of chronic cough in European and North American populations.

Table 5 Repeatability and Responsiveness of Outcome Measures Used to Assess Patients with Chronic Cough

	Repeatability		Responsiveness
Outcome measure	Within-subject SD	Between-subject SD	Effect size
LCQ (range 3–21)	0.9	3.4	1.7
CQLQ (range 28–112)	—	13.9	2.4
Cough VAS (0–100 mm) (17)	7.8 mm	26.5 mm	3.2
C2 (doubling dose, dd) (18)	0.5 dd	1.5 dd	1.7
C5 (doubling dose, dd) (18)	1.7 dd	3.1 dd	1.2
Cough monitor (coughs per 24 hr) (19)	NK	Range (64–3639)	NK

Abbreviations: SD, standard deviation; effect size, difference in mean measurement pre- and postintervention/SD of measurement preintervention (effect size > 0.4 indicates responsive instrument); LCQ, total Leicester Cough Questionnaire score; CQLQ, total Cough-Specific Quality of Life Questionnaire score; cough VAS, visual analog score (worst cough: 100 mm); C2, concentration of capsaicin that causes two coughs; C5, concentration of capsaicin that causes five coughs; NK, not known.

Pitfalls in Measuring Quality of Life

Quality of life is a highly individual concept. There are clearly patients who have a severe and troublesome cough but report quality of life scores that are inconsistent with their level of disability. There is also the possibility that questionnaires may not cover the most important issues relevant to an individual patient and the weighting of domain scores may differ between patients. Quality of life instruments are not an alternative to communicating with patients and should not be considered a substitute for disease outcome measures such as cough frequency. Instead they should be used to supplement objective markers of disease severity, assess the effectiveness of interventions, and in cost utility analysis.

Health Status in Chronic Cough

Little is known about the effects of chronic cough on health status. Preliminary data from studies investigating the health status in patients with chronic cough using quality of life measures suggest that quality of life is impaired to the same degree as in chronic obstructive pulmonary disease, is worse in female patients compared with males, and is not related to the age of the patient or duration of cough (8,20). Health status improves significantly with improvement in cough after specific therapy for the underlying disorder (3,4). Further studies are required to investigate the relationship between quality of life, cough frequency, and cough reflex sensitivity in patients with chronic cough.

Conclusions

Chronic cough has profound effects on quality of life. Its management should include an assessment of health status. The use of well-validated cough-specific quality of life measures should complement other objective measures of chronic cough such as cough recording and measurement of cough reflex sensitivity in the clinical setting and in the evaluation of new antitussive therapies in clinical trials.

References

1. Janson C, Chinn S, Jarvis D, Burney P. Determinants of cough in young adults participating in the European Community Respiratory Health Survey. Eur Respir J 2001; 18:647–654.
2. Fuller RW, Jackson DM. Physiology and treatment of cough. Thorax 1990; 45:425–430.

3. Birring SS, Prudon B, Carr AJ, Singh SJ, Morgan MDL, Pavord ID. Development of a symptom specific health status measure for patients with chronic cough: Leicester Cough Questionnaire (LCQ). Thorax 2003; 58:339–343.
4. French CT, Irwin RS, Fletcher KE, Adams TM. Evaluation of a cough-specific quality-of-life questionnaire. Chest 2002; 121:1123–1131.
5. World Health Organisation. Constitution of the World Health Organisation. Geneva: WHO, 1947.
6. Juniper EF, Guyatt GH, Ferrie PJ, Griffith LE. Measuring quality of life in asthma. Am Rev Respir Dis 1993; 147:832–838.
7. Jones PW, Quirk FH, Baveystock CM, Littlejohns P. A self-complete measure of health status for chronic airflow limitation: the St. George's Respiratory Questionnaire. Am Rev Respir Dis 1992; 145:1321–1327.
8. French CL, Irwin RS, Curley FJ, Krikorian CJ. Impact of chronic cough on quality of life. Arch Intern Med 1998; 158:1657–1661.
9. Fayers PM, Machin D. Quality of Life: Assessment, Analysis and Interpretation. 1st ed. New York: Wiley, 2000.
10. Juniper EF. Health-related quality of life. In: Barnes PJ, Grunstein MM, Leff AR, Woodcock AJ, eds. Asthma. Philaldelphia: Lippincott-Raven Publishers, 1997:1487–1497.
11. Gilson BS, Gilson JS, Bergner M, Bobbit RA, Kressel S, Pollard WE, et al. The sickness impact profile: development of an outcome measure of health care. Am J Public Health 1975; 65:1304–1310.
12. Hunt SM, McKenna SP, McEwen J, Williams J, Papp E. The Nottingham Health Profile: subjective health status and medical consultations. Soc Sci Med A 1981; 15:221–229.
13. Brazier JE, Harper R, Jones NMB, O'Cathain A, Thomas KJ, Usherwood T, Westlake L. Validating the SF-36 health survey questionnaire: new outcome measure for primary care. Br Med J 1992; 305:160–164.
14. Guyatt GH, Berman LB, Townsend M, Pugsley SO, Chambers LW. A measure of quality of life for clinical trials in chronic lung disease. Thorax 1987; 42: 773–778.
15. Gee L, Abbott J, Conway SP, Etherington C, Webb AK. Development of a disease specific health related quality of life measure for adults and adolescents with cystic fibrosis. Thorax 2000; 55:946–954.
16. Higginson IJ, Carr AJ. Measuring quality of life: using quality of life measures in the clinical setting. Br Med J 2001; 322:1297–1300.
17. Brightling CE, Monterio W, Green RH, Parker D, Morgan MDL, Wardlaw AJ, Pavord ID. Induced sputum and other outcome measures in chronic obstructive pulmonary disease: safety and repeatability. Respir Med 2001; 95:999–1002.
18. Prudon B, Birring SS, Vara DD, Pavord ID. Repeatability of capsaicin cough reflex sensitivity measurement (abstract). Thorax 2002; 57(suppl III):iii23.
19. Hsu JY, Stone RA, Logan-Sinclair RB, Worsdell M, Busst CM, Chung KF. Coughing frequency in patients with persistent cough: assessment using a 24 hour ambulatory recorder. Eur Respir J 1994; 7:1246–1253.
20. Birring SS, Patel RB, Prudon B, Singh SJ, Morgan MDL, Pavord ID. Quality of life in chronic cough. Am J Respir Crit Care Med 2002; 167:A135.

23

Chronic Cough in Children

JULIE M. MARCHANT and ANNE B. CHANG

Royal Children's Hospital, Herston Road,
Herston, Queensland, Australia

Introduction

Cough is the most common presenting symptom to general practitioners
and has significant direct cost to the community (1). In the United States,
approximately \$2 billion per year is spent on cough and cold over-the-
counter medications (2). A U.S. survey showed that 35% of preschool-aged
children had used over-the-counter medications in the previous month for
cough (2). The additional cost to families of sleep disturbance and school
and work absenteeism should be considered (3). A recent study of children
aged 7–11 years showed a lifetime prevalence of bronchitis of 55.9% (4).
Cough without wheeze has been reported at 12.8% in a longitudinal U.K.
study (5) and that of recurrent cough without colds at 21.8% (6). In accept-
ing that cough is a common problem in children it must be stated that prevalence data are generally gathered from epidemiologic studies and the true
incidence of cough, particularly chronic cough, in the pediatric population
is unknown.

The most widely accepted definition of chronic cough is a cough of
>3 weeks' duration (7,8), although this definition varies from 3 to as long

as 12 weeks in the literature (9,10). Cough due to an acute upper respiratory tract infection (URTI) is generally self-limited and resolves within 1–3 weeks in most children (11). The data that exist on the natural history of cough due to an acute URTI suggest that 5–10% of preschool-aged children still cough 3 weeks after a URTI (12). Whether this relates to the initial URTI, or complications such as bronchitis, remains debatable as cough may be present with both (12).

Major Conceptual Differences in Children and Adults with Chronic Cough

There are important differences when considering chronic cough in children. These include:

1. The etiology of childhood chronic cough is different to that of adults. A retrospective study shows the diagnoses differ significantly to the most common adult diagnoses (13). Other examples of the clear differences in pediatric versus adult respiratory disease include respiratory syncytial virus (RSV) which causes a simple URTI in adults but can cause significant, even life-threatening, disease in the form of bronchiolitis in children (14). Another example is found in lung cancer and chronic obstructive pulmonary disease which are serious causes of adult chronic cough but very rarely occur in the pediatric population (1). These examples illustrate why the adult protocol for investigation and management of chronic cough (7) should not be applied to children.
2. Is the cough reflex different in children? Children differ from adults in their respiratory responses and other physiological parameters (15). In adults cough receptor sensitivity (CRS) to capsaicin shows a gender bias, with women being more sensitive (16). This difference is not present in children and instead CRS is influenced by age (17). Plasticity of the cough reflex has been shown (18) and one can speculate that the cough reflex has maturational differences also.
3. The cough reflex may be of increased importance in children due to developmental differences in lung anatomy. For example, the pores of Kohn (small epithelium-lined openings in alveolar walls) that act as collateral channels in obstructed airways are minimally present in infancy and continue to develop postnatally (19–21). In the event of mucous plugging associated with a weak cough reflex, such as in a myopathy (22), the atelectasis would be more significant in children as the collateral channels of ventila-

tion are poorly developed and so there is little communication between alveoli.

4. The use of airway hyperresponsiveness (AHR) to methacholine challenge (MHC) as an aid to diagnosis of cough associated with asthma in adults cannot be applied to children as the data on direct AHR challenge in children are arguably different to adults (23). Also children 6–7 years—the age group where cough is most prevalent—are unable to perform MHC.

5. In evaluating cough in children readers should also be cognizant that:

   a. isolated cough (cough in the absence of other respiratory symptoms) is a poorly repeatable respiratory symptom in children with kappa values (chance-corrected measure of repeatability) of 0.14–0.38 (6,24);

   b. nocturnal cough is reported unreliably when compared to objective measures, such as cough meter recording (25–27). Kappa values comparing reported nocturnal cough with objective measures vary from –0.3 to 0.3 (28);

   c. many clinical studies on cough have utilized nonvalidated scoring systems; and

   d. the reporting of cough is dependent on the population (29) and setting (30) studied.

The remainder of this chapter deals with the issues specific to chronic cough in children.

Causes of Chronic Cough in Children

Chronic cough in children can be classified in various ways. A commonly used framework is the duration of cough which divides cough into acute (<2 weeks), subacute (2–4 weeks), and chronic (>3–4 weeks). Figures 1–3 illustrate this type of approach to cough in children (9).

A second classification is to categorize cough according to etiology. This divides cough into "expected" cough, nonspecific cough, and specific cough (Fig. 4). Specific cough is cough with a clearly definable and often serious cause elicited from history and examination. There is certain to be some overlap between nonspecific cough and both "expected" and specific cough, given the nature of nonspecific cough. In contrast, specific cough is clearly distinct from "expected" cough (31).

A third classification places children with chronic cough in a number of categories:

1. Expected cough in a normal child
2. Chid with serious illness such as cystic fibrosis or tuberculosis

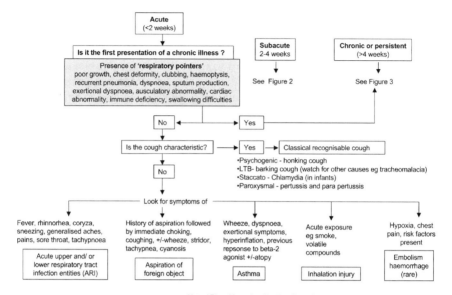

Figure 1   Coughing child and length of cough. (From Ref. 9.)

3.   Child with nonserious but treatable cause of cough and wheeze, e.g., gastroesophageal reflux or postnasal drip
4.   Child with an asthma syndrome
5.   Overestimation of symptoms for psychological reasons in either child or family
6.   A nonrespiratory cause such as habit cough, medications (e.g., ACE inhibitors) (31,32).

We will use this framework to discuss relevant recent literature as it pertains to chronic cough in children.

Expected Cough in a Normal Child

The "medicalization" of an otherwise "expected symptom" can be an issue with cough (33). All children cough at some point, as a normal child may have up to 10 coughing illnesses associated with URTIs in a year (10). The frequency of URTIs and associated cough is heightened when children first attend a day-care facility and averages about every 3 weeks at this time (32). As discussed, cough due to an URTI should have resolved by 3 weeks and coughing beyond this is considered abnormal (11,12). In the absence of an URTI in the preceding 4 weeks healthy children have a cough frequency average of 11.3 cough episodes per 24 hr, with a range of 1–34. However, nocturnal coughing or prolonged coughing episodes were not seen in these

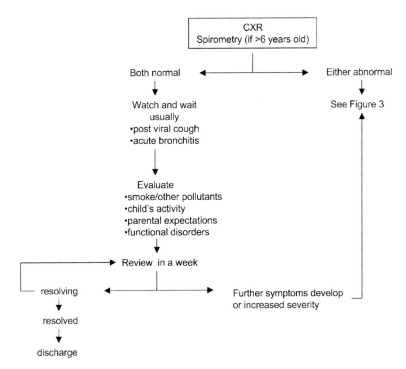

Figure 2 Subacute cough not associated with other symptoms. (From Ref. 9.)

children (34). When children with URTIs were not excluded, age-, sex-, and season-matched normal controls have 0–141 (median 10) coughs per 24 hr (29). It must be remembered for a child to fulfill the criteria of "expected cough in a normal child" the child should be otherwise well and all symptoms in Table 1 absent. It is the role of the physician to define which children cough abnormally.

Specific Cough Due to Serious Illness

Children who present with these diseases generally have abnormal pointers in their history or examination which alert the physician to them. These pointers are listed in Table 1. Complete discussion of these diseases are beyond the scope of this chapter and can be found in standard pediatric respiratory textbooks (35,36). Specific cough descriptions are, however, discussed where data are available.

Chronic Suppurative Lung Disease

Chronic suppurative lung disease is used to describe children who present with a chronic moist cough with sputum production, including cystic fibro-

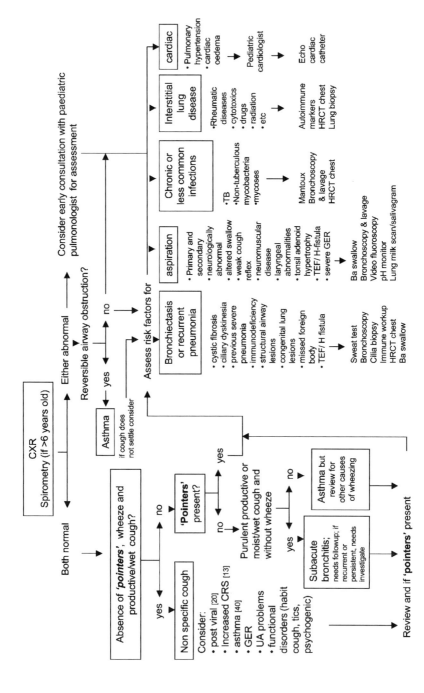

Figure 3 Chronic/persistent cough (>4 weeks) or acute/subacute cough associated with other symptoms. (From Ref. 9.)

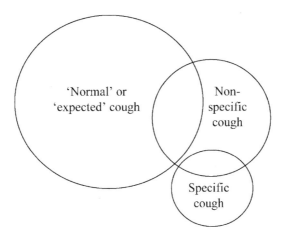

Figure 4 Causes of cough in children. (From Ref. 31.)

sis, bronchiectasis, and primary ciliary dyskinesia, although this term is poorly defined in standard pediatric respiratory textbooks (36–38). A high resolution computed tomography (CT) scan is necessary to exclude or confirm the presence of radiological bronchiectasis. Historically, there is often a worsening of their cough first thing in the morning and no seasonal variation (39). Despite this classic definition, children with these conditions may present with a dry cough and cardinal signs (such as clubbing and failure to thrive) may not be present (40).

In a small study of 14 children with cystic fibrosis admitted to hospital for a respiratory exacerbation cough epochs per hour were 18.2 ± 8.4 (mean $\pm$ SD) during the day and 5.8 ± 2.9 during the night. Cough frequency did not correlate with subjective patient scoring of their cough either during the day or night (41). However, these findings are limited by

Table 1 Pointers to Specific Cause of Cough

Daily moist cough
Failure to thrive
Clubbing
Hemoptysis
Recurrent pneumonia
Chronic dyspnea
Exertional dyspnea
Auscultatory findings
Cardiac abnormalities
Immune deficiency

(From Ref. 31.)

the very small sample size and it is possible that a correlation would be found if a larger sample size was recruited (calculated power of the study was inadequate at only 48.5% for α of 0.05).

Children with cystic fibrosis have a lower cough sensitivity to capsaicin challenge when compared to controls and children with asthma (17). It was also found although these children have an increased threshold to cough, once this is reached they cough multiple times. This increased cough threshold is possibly related to the pathology of thickened airway mucus and bacterial colonization (17).

Cough may be underreported in some situations, such as indigenous groups with bronchiectasis (42). This highlights the fact that cough history is not always reliable and emphasizes the need for suspicion when assessing the child with cough to ensure that no children with these specific causes are missed.

Primary Aspiration

Primary pulmonary aspiration is typically seen in children who are neurologically impaired and results from laryngopalatal discoordination or discoordinated swallowing (31). These children typically cough with feeds and have patchy changes on chest x-ray (43). This disorder must also be considered in neurologically normal infants as Sheikh et al. (44) reported a group of otherwise healthy infants with documented primary aspiration due to swallowing dysfunction. Cough, however, may be minimal when the condition is chronic possibly related to a downregulation of the cough reflex.

Endobronchial Foreign Body

An acute history of choking and cough should prompt clinicians to think of foreign body aspiration (39). However, a child with an inhaled foreign body may present with a chronic cough if the acute episode was not noticed. Around 20% of children in whom an endobronchial foreign body is found do not have a history of choking (45). Chest x-rays are normal in approximately 20–40% of children who are found to have a foreign body on bronchoscopy (45). Cough is found in approximately 80% of children with an airway foreign body so a high index of suspicion must remain for this diagnosis, especially in those aged under 3 years (45). An undiagnosed foreign body can have serious complications including bronchiectasis and bronchial hyperresponsiveness with ongoing symptoms of cough and wheeze (46).

Cardiac Causes of Chronic Cough

Although children with heart disease usually present with cyanosis, dyspnea, or failure to thrive they can also present with chronic cough. Cough can result from pulmonary edema, an enlarged left atrium, or pulmonary hypertension causing bronchial constriction (8). These patients often have cardiomegaly on chest x-ray. Examination findings may include a cardiac murmur or loud P2 and right ventricular heave. These will often be a history of exertional dyspnea (43).

Post Childhood Cancer

Chronic cough has been reported as a feature in children who survived childhood cancer (47). This most likely relates to intrapulmonary processes such as interstitial lung disease but whether an alteration in cough reflex and sensitivity is also contributory is unknown.

Specific Infections

Pulmonary tuberculosis (TB) presents typically with a chronic cough, fever, and chest x-ray changes. A study which looked at tuberculosis in the pediatric population in a developed country found that only 50% cases were identified due to case contact identification. The remainder came to medical attention due to an ill child (48). There are no specific cough data on chronic cough and TB. Some infections are associated with a characteristic cough that may become chronic. Whooping cough (*Bordetella pertussis*) infection is usually associated with paroxysmal coughing. It can be diagnosed on nasopharyngeal swab using culture, polymerase chain reaction (PCR), or via serology. In older children typical cough with paroxysms may not be present. Parapertussis presents with a similar characteristic cough. *Chlamydia pneumoniae* infection in infancy presents with a staccato cough. *Mycoplasma pneumoniae* infection can cause prolonged cough and can be confirmed with serology for complement fixing antibodies (10). More specific details of respiratory infections causing chronic cough can be found in standard texts (49).

Nonspecific Cough—Nonserious Causes of Cough in Children

Nonspecific cough refers to cough which is dry and where none of the pointers of specific cough listed in Table 1 are found. Adults and children with a nonspecific dry cough, normal examination, no other symptoms on history, and a normal chest x-ray have increased cough receptor sensitivity (50,51). The diagnoses discussed in the preceding pages must all be considered and explored if history, examination, or chest x-ray warrant this. In children, in contrast to adults, a postviral cough with temporal increase in cough receptor sensitivity (52) is perhaps the most likely diagnosis (9). Unfortunately due to inadequate prospective longitudinal studies of cough in children the natural history of nonspecific cough is unknown. In Powell and colleagues' study (53), 42.9% of children with frequent nocturnal cough had a reduced frequency of cough when surveyed 2 years later, and 14.2% had stopped coughing. One can postulate that the natural history of non-specific cough is therefore one of natural resolution with time but this awaits further study.

Some authors suggest that children with nonspecific chronic cough follow the same anatomical pathway of investigation and management as adults (8). This involves therapies added sequentially and additionally when cough does not resolve fully (8). It is the opinion of the authors and others (10) that this approach is not valid in children. Certainly the literature contains few pediatric studies that would support this (9,54). Occasionally the history will support a trial of asthma therapy, low-dose inhaled corticosteroids, but if this is the case close follow-up and cessation of therapy must be done if it is ineffective (9).

The following nonserious causes of cough fall into the category of nonspecific cough. We present here only a summary of issues as they pertain to children highlighting that the etiology and management of chronic cough is different to adults.

Cough and Gastroesophageal Reflux Disease

In children, the complex relationship between gastroesophageal reflux disease (GERD) and cough is unclear. GERD can cause cough in a number of ways which include: microaspiration of reflux materials (so-called laryngopharyngeal reflux), reflex cough from distal esophageal acidification and stimulation of cough receptors and non-acid volume reflux (1,55). Similarly cough can cause GERD. Laukka et al. (56) found that cough more often occurred before reflux events than after. Further research is needed to delineate the temporal relationship between the two. GERD has been identified in the adult literature as a common cause of chronic cough (7,8). The treatments for GERD involve medical therapy and surgical intervention with Nissen fundoplication (57,58), and are not always benign. This treatment has failed to improve cough symptoms in some adult studies (59) and the opinion that GERD is one of the commonest causes of cough in adults is also being questioned by some (56). There are limited studies which look at the causes of chronic cough in children prospectively but those available suggest that GERD is infrequently the sole cause of pediatric cough. One prospective study of the causes of chronic cough in children found only one child with GERD out of a series of 38 (60). A more recent retrospective study found GERD in 4 of 49 children with chronic cough, although this may not have been the sole diagnosis of their cough (13). There is no convincing evidence that GERD is a common cause of cough in children.

Cough and Upper Airway Disorders

Postnasal drip syndrome is frequently quoted as one of the most common causes of chronic cough in adults (8,61). This syndrome encompasses sinusitis and rhinitis of various causes (61). Dry cough can be associated with allergic rhinitis (62). How postnasal drip causes cough is unclear. The pharynx is innervated by the glossopharyngeal nerve, not the vagal nerve which makes up the afferent limb of the cough reflex (63). Although adult studies have found that cough resolved with treatment of chronic sinusitis or rhinitis (64) it is possible that the medication used also treated infection lower in the respiratory tract (54). Currently none of the available data has proven that cough can be directed attributed to sinus disease (54). The additional factor that must be considered in diagnosis of sinusitis in children is the poor correlation of abnormal sinus x-rays and CT scans with symptomatology, which has been confirmed in numerous studies (65,66). Diament et al. (66) found that 50% of asymptomatic children had CT scans consistent with sinusitis. The Tucson Children's Respiratory Group (67) found that, although sinusitis was associated with cough in children, when skin test reactivity and allergic rhinitis were adjusted for this was no longer the case. A recent study by Turktas et al. (68) has used extrathoracic airway hyperresponsiveness (EAHR) to methacholine as an objective measure of upper airway disease in a group of children presenting with cough. There was a significantly higher probability of finding EAHR, without bronchial hyperresponsiveness, in the children with cough as a sole symptom. Other studies have linked EAHR to sinusitis and rhinitis (69,70). Although indicating that upper airway disease was present in this select group of children, the link between upper and lower airway disease is still unclear and needs further exploration.

Airway Malformations and Cough

Congenital airway malformations, which include laryngomalacia, tracheomalacia, bronchomalacia, tracheal stenosis, and tracheoesophageal fistula, typically all present with symptoms in early childhood. Despite this, they are often misdiagnosed or remain undiagnosed for many years (71–73). Clinically the majority of these patients have chronic cough, although stridor and wheeze may also be features. A recent prospective data review of patients with these malacia disorders showed that 70% presented with cough (71), which has been confirmed in other studies (72). This cough is typically "brassy" in nature. Thomson et al. (13) found that 23 of 49 children who presented for tertiary hospital review of chronic cough had a lower airway malacia disorder. These studies indicate a clear relationship between cough and malacia disorders in children which is different to findings in adult patients where none of 24 adults with tracheomalacia complained of cough (74). The pathogenesis of cough in malacia disorders remains poorly understood but one can speculate that the abnormal airway anatomy impairs mucociliary clearance (75) thus allowing a chronic bronchitic picture to develop.

Chronic Bronchitis and Children

Currently, standard pediatric respiratory textbooks do not have a definition for chronic bronchitis in children (38). Certainly there is a group of children who present with chronic moist cough who do not have chronic suppurative lung disease, as per current clinical definitions discussed previously. Generally, their parents will describe a "rattly" breathing pattern perhaps referring to the sound of secretions in large airways as they are cleared. Occasionally these children will have crepitations on auscultation but more often examination is normal (43). These children may have normal chest x-rays but will often have bilateral peribronchial thickening (43). It is vital to exclude bronchiectasis in this group with a high-resolution CT scan. Bronchoscopy can be performed to exclude foreign body and airway malformations and to confirm visually the bronchitis. We have found that 25% of children with chronic cough have bacterial bronchitis defined by culture of $\geq 10^5/\text{mL}$ organisms and neutrophilia on bronchoalveolar lavage (BAL) fluid (76).

Environmental

It is recognized that intrauterine exposure to cigarette smoke causes alterations in pulmonary development (77). A recent review looking at the effects of smoke exposure showed a statistically significant increase in cough in schoolchildren whose fathers smoked but whose mothers did not, suggesting that postnatal exposure must also play a significant part (78). Another study used objective overnight recording of cough compared with cough diary data in smoking and nonsmoking households and found significant under-reporting in smoking parents compared with nonsmoking parents (79). This perhaps indicates that the odds ratios quoted which relate childhood cough to environmental tobacco smoke (ETS) are underestimated (78). Outdoor particulate pollution is also associated with an increased cough in children (80). Cook and Strachan (78) have suggested that chronic cough associated with ETS exposure is due to decreased mucociliary clearance and goblet cell hypertrophy or hypersecretion. Whilst there is no doubt that ETS is associated with increased cough in children the mechanisms remain to be elucidated.

Asthma and Cough

The relationship between asthma and childhood cough is complex and a detailed discussion is beyond the scope of this chapter but can be found in a number of excellent reviews (9,81). Some children with asthma present with cough (82,83), and some will have cough as a major symptom during exacerbations (84). However, cough-variant asthma is overdiagnosed in the community (81,85,86). We have recently shown an overdiagnosis of asthma in a group of children with persistent cough. Of the 49 children reviewed for chronic cough, 61% had a pre-existing diagnosis of asthma at referral but none had a sole final diagnosis of asthma (13). Of this group 12.9% had significant steroid side effects due to overuse of asthma medications (13).

Initial studies of cough-variant asthma described groups of patients with evidence of airway obstruction (either spirometric or clinically) and AHR to methacholine (83,87). These patients responded to asthma medications of the time (oral theophylline) within 48 hr and cough returned on cessation of medications. Many doctors now use long-term steroid medication for the treatment of isolated cough (8,88), despite evidence in the literature suggesting that this is inappropriate (89,90). A randomized placebo-controlled study in children with nonspecific recurrent cough showed inhaled beta-agonists and corticosteroids no more effective in reducing objectively measured cough than placebo (89).

Further evidence supporting the difference between isolated cough and asthma can be found in studies that look at airway inflammation. Fitch and colleagues (91) found that only a small number of children with persistent cough have asthma-type airway inflammation. Gibson and colleagues (92) found in a community-based survey that children with cough but not wheeze did not have the same airway cytology (as defined by induced sputum) as children with asthma and so should not be considered a variant of asthma.

The relationship between AHR and cough and asthma is complex and will be discussed later in the chapter.

Overestimation of Cough for Psychological Reasons

Subjective scoring of cough is variable and reporting of nocturnal cough is unreliable (27). The comparison of the objective scoring of cough meter and subjective scoring of cough diary assumes parents equate severity with frequency. This may not be the case. Parental anxiety may lead to increased medical consultation for a child, as has been found in childhood asthma (93). The effect of the illness on the child must also be explored, as what the cough means to the child in school and home environments can perpetuate the problem, leading to a "sick child" syndrome.

Nonrespiratory Causes of Cough

There is a spectrum of habitual cough ranging from a minor motor/vocal tic to severe psychogenic honking cough (94,95). Over 90% of cases of psychogenic cough are in children and adolescents (96). Characteristically, cough secondary to habit does not occur in sleep but can be present for much of the child's waking hours. In correctly diagnosing this condition one must remember that nocturnal cough reporting correlates poorly with objective measurements of cough (27). A degree of clinical suspicion must remain for this condition, as underlying psychological problems for the child may not be evident during the initial consultation (97). This form of cough often responds to psychological intervention including behavior modification therapy (95,97).

Apart from psychogenic cough other nonrespiratory causes of cough, such as angiotensin converting enzyme (ACE) inhibitor-induced cough, are rare in children but should be remembered when history and clinical features suggest.

Assessment and Management of Childhood Chronic Cough

In all children who cough for >3 weeks a chest x-ray and spirometry (if over 6 years) are considered minimal investigations necessary. A suggested pathway of investigation is shown in Figures. 1–3. These are only suggested pathways based on clinical experience and available literature. There is no level A evidence-based approach to cough in children.

A child with a cough can be assessed in a number of ways including duration of cough or dry versus moist. A number of questions should be asked when assessing the child:

1.   Is it a symptom of an underlying problem?
2.   Are there possible modifiers of exacerbation and/or contributing factors?
3.   How does the cough affect the parents and child?
4.   Is it necessary to investigate?
5.   Are any treatment modalities available or necessary? (31)

In managing cough in children regardless of the cause exacerbating factors which can increase coughing illnesses and respiratory illnesses must be addressed (98,99). An attempt to reduce all exacerbating factors, particularly ETS, becomes an important part of the management of a child with chronic cough. A frank discussion with parents about how cigarette smoke affects children is essential early in a clinician's management of this problem. Parental concerns must be addressed as these often differ from those of the treating physician (3). Perhaps the most common presentation in a community setting will be the child with a dry cough and normal chest x-ray and spirometry and this will be discussed in the following text.

Dry Cough and Otherwise Normal History and Examination

If a child presents with a dry cough and no other abnormal features on history or examination and a chest x-ray and spirometry are normal one can assume the diagnosis of nonspecific cough or cough with nonserious cause, such as asthma, GERD, or habit cough. In the setting of a history of wheeze, family history of reactive airways disease, or personal history of atopy a trial of low dose inhaled corticosteroids (400 µg budesonide or beclomethasone dipropionate or equivalent) for a short period (2–4 weeks) is appropriate. If after the trial there has been no improvement in cough they must be stopped. Cough from asthma in children should be markedly improved in 1–2 weeks (100,101). One should always review a diagnosis of asthma in children with cough based on response to a therapeutic trial as cough tends to resolves spontaneously (period effect) (9). There is evidence in the pediatric literature of significant side effects from corticosteroid medication being used unnecessarily for prolonged periods in children with chronic cough (13).

The adult literature suggests these patients then be investigated for GERD with a 24 hr pH probe (102). The pediatric literature on GERD has yet to confirm or rebut this suggestion, but available data suggest GERD is not a frequent a cause of chronic cough in children (13,60). Consideration of habitual cough must always be made as it can often be successfully treated by psychological intervention. Again the history is suggestive of this diagnosis as there is no cough in sleep. Dry cough has been described in the presence of allergic rhinitis (62). Data in adult patients have shown that treatment with intranasal corticosteroids results in significant improvement in the cough when compared with placebo (64). No pediatric data are available but in a child with allergic rhinitis symptoms and a dry cough a trial of intranasal corticosteroids is appropriate. Whether this is treating nasal disease alone or rhinitis and a lower airway inflammation remains to be elucidated, although it has been shown that administration of intranasal corticosteroids does result in some intrapulmonary deposition (54).

If all of these are excluded then increased cough receptor sensitivity (CRS) seems most likely and a watch-and-wait approach would be most appropriate (Fig. 3). Increased CRS can be confirmed in the research setting using capsaicin challenge but this is not currently used in a clinical setting. Initially, patients who fall into this final category should be reviewed regularly to ensure that none of the specific pointers of cough (Table 1) become apparent. Our current understanding of cough would suggest that the natural history of nonspecific childhood cough is one of natural resolution. Without another apparent diagnosis, the physician's role is that of review of clinical changes, reassurance, and support for the child and family.

**Moist Cough or Abnormalities Present in History
and Examination**

A moist and/or productive cough is always abnormal and thus this group of children are most likely to have specific cough as discussed above. Diagnoses may include diseases such as bronchiectasis, aspiration lung disease, or respiratory infections, e.g., tuberculosis (Fig. 3). The presence of any pointers to specific cough (Table 1) indicates that further investigations are necessary as suggested by clinical findings. These investigations are included in Figure 3 (most commonly used but not a comprehensive list). The investigation of these children with abnormal features and chronic cough should be done where expertise is available, with access to bronchoscopy and high-resolution CT scanning. The approach is involved and beyond the scope of this chapter but we will review the controversial issues pertaining to investigation of childhood cough in the following text.

Investigation of Childhood Chronic Cough

There are a number of investigations that are now considered standard care in children with specific chronic cough. These are outlined in the following text with respect to their use and what literature is available as to findings in populations of children with cough.

High-Resolution Computed Tomography Scan

A recent study by Coren et al. (103) looked at the use of high-resolution CT (HRCT) in a tertiary pediatric center and found chronic productive cough the most common indication for referral. Of the 48 patients referred for HRCT, 21 (43%) had bronchiectasis confirmed by this investigation. Importantly, it should be noted that two of these patients had normal chest x-rays. HRCT scans expose the patient to one-seventh dose of radiation when compared with conventional CT scans (104). Additionally, these high resolution scans provide increased accuracy and sensitivity in diagnosing respiratory diseases when compared with conventional scans (105).

Bronchoscopy and Bronchoalveolar Lavage

Flexible bronchoscopy can confirm or exclude anatomic airway lesions and an inhaled foreign body. Combined with BAL, microbiology can aid in organism identification in infective states and cytology can be helpful in the diagnosis of many lung diseases (106). Certainly its use in the setting of chronic cough, both clinically and as a research tool, is increasing. A small study looked at nonbronchoscopic BAL findings in children with chronic cough and found that the group had a statistically significant increase in both eosinophils (0.28% vs. 0.10%, $p = 0.01$) and neutrophils

(5.85% vs. 3.21%, $p = 0.03$) when compared with normal controls. The results reflect the heterogeneity of children with chronic cough, as three of the children had eosinophils above the normal range and four patients had neutrophils above the normal range (91). Other studies, with smaller coughing groups, have found no characteristic pattern of airway inflammation again suggesting the heterogeneity of this group and the difference in pathology of this group compared with an asthma cohort (107,108). The analysis of airway markers from BAL fluid is not yet useful clinically and will be discussed later with other markers of airway inflammation used in the research setting.

Other Standard Investigations

There are a number of other investigations which are used in the investigation of chronic cough. We will not discuss them all in detail here but they include:

    a. cilial biopsy to exclude abnormalities of cilial structure and function which can present with chronic cough;

    b. sweat chloride test to exclude cystic fibrosis;

    c. serology for *Mycoplasma pneumoniae* and *Bordetella pertussis*;

    d. blood work-up for immunological disorders;

    e. barium swallow and videofluoroscopy for suspected aspiration; and

    f. Mantoux test for suspected mycobacterial infection.

This list is not fully inclusive of all investigations but the most commonly used.

Other Tools for Cough Monitoring and Investigation

Cough Diary and Cough Meter

Objective measurement of cough using an ambulatory cough meter is arguably the best method to monitor cough frequency (25). Nonetheless, due to the expense and expertise required to read the cough meter results this method of cough monitoring is currently limited to research. A cough diary, the verbal category descriptive score, completed by children with parental assistance is the most valid subjective measure of cough (27). It has a use in research protocols and clinical settings when an estimation of coughing severity is needed.

Markers of Airway Inflammation

When a patient can expectorate sputum it can be used clinically for microbiological and cytological examination. In cases of children who cannot produce sputum spontaneously, sputum induction using hypertonic saline can be used. This has become a reliable and safe tool for use in children, although it is still used primarily in the research setting in pediatrics (109). Induced sputum can identify children with eosinophilic or neutrophilic inflammation which can guide therapy, as eosinophilic inflammation will more likely respond to steroid therapy (110). Studies that have looked at induced sputum cytology in children with chronic cough have found only a small minority with airway eosinophilia compared with children with asthma (92,111).

Several of these research groups have looked at inflammatory markers as well as cytology in assessing airway inflammation. Gibson et al. (92) looked at sputum eosinophilic cationic protein (ECP) in children with wheeze, cough, colds and controls and found no difference between the groups in ECP levels. Another study which looked at the levels of soluble intercellular adhesion molecule 1 (sICAM-1) in BAL fluid found an increased level in those with severe chronic cough, but no characteristic inflammatory profile in the whole group with chronic cough (107). Although inflammatory markers may be useful in the research setting to define the differences between groups with chronic cough and others their usefulness in individual cases has yet to be proved. Another method of looking at airway inflammation is via exhaled gases, such as nitric oxide, or breath condensate measurements, such as nitrite (112). Malmberg and colleagues (113) found an increase in exhaled nitric oxide levels in children with chronic cough, although the levels remained less then in children with wheeze. Other studies have contradicted this, finding no significant difference between nitric oxide levels in children with cough and controls (114,115), perhaps indicating the heterogeneity of the group of children who present with chronic cough. These techniques are currently used only in the research setting.

Airways Resistance by the Interrupter Technique (RINT)

This technique has been used to measure bronchodilator responsiveness. McKenzie and colleagues (116) showed that a group of children with recurrent or persistent cough had an intermediate mean bronchodilator responsiveness when compared with a group of known wheezers and controls. These children had normal IgE levels which separated them from the wheezing group. This application of airways resistance has shown that children with cough form a separate diagnostic group to those with asthma. Despite its usefulness in the research setting intersubject variability has limited its use clinically (117).

Cough Receptor Sensitivity Testing

CRS testing has been described using capsaicin, which has good repeatability in children (118). In children with asthma and recurrent cough, cough sensitivity returns to normal with successful treatment (50,84). This has not been shown in chronic cough. The individual usefulness of the CRS test has not been shown.

Airway Hyperresponsiveness

The literature on the usefulness of AHR in children suggests that it is not necessarily representative of asthma, as it is in an adult population (83,119). The prevalence of AHR in asymptomatic children varies from 6.7% to 33% (120,121). Galvez and colleagues (122) found that the demonstration of AHR in children with cough was unhelpful in predicting the later development of asthma. Nishimura et al. (123) found a relationship between dose of methacholine required to induce a fall in PO_2 (used as a measure of AHR) and the later development of asthma in a group of children with cough, but they did not control for confounders such as atopy. The relationship between AHR and cough is even less well defined. Studies have found that cough did not relate to AHR to methacholine when wheeze was controlled for (89).

Future Research

Chronic cough in children differs from cough in adults (9). Large gaps in the pediatric literature on the management of cough currently exist. Prospective studies looking at the causes of cough are needed. Further exploration of the complex relationship between gastroesophageal reflux and cough in children is also necessary. A clinical definition of chronic bronchitis as it applies to children is required and the management and natural history of this condition need to be defined. The pathophysiology of cough in airway lesions also remains poorly understood and needs further research. Only after the causes of cough in children and the pathophysiology of these conditions are understood can appropriate and effective treatment options be explored.

References

1. Morice AH. Epidemiology of cough. Pulm Pharmacol Ther 2002; 15:253–259.
2. Kogan MD, Pappas G, Yu SM, Kotelchuck M. Over-the-counter medication use among preschool-age children. J Am Med Assoc 1994; 272:1025–1030.
3. Fuller P, Picciotto A, Davies M, McKenzie SA. Cough and sleep in inner-city children. Eur Respir J 1998; 12:426–431.
4. Leonardi GS, Houthuijs D, Nikiforov B, Volf J, Rudnai P, Zejda J, et al. Respiratory symptoms, bronchitis and asthma in children of Central and Eastern Europe. Eur Respir J 2002; 20:890–898.
5. Clough JB, Williams JD, Holgate ST. Effect of atopy on the natural history of symptoms, peak expiratory flow, and bronchial responsiveness in 7- and

8-year-old children with cough and wheeze. Am Rev Respir Dis 1991; 143:755–760.

6. Luyt DK, Burton PR, Simpson H. Epidemiological study of wheeze, doctor diagnosed asthma, and cough in preschool children in Leicestershire. Br Med J 1993; 306:1386–1390.

7. Irwin RS, Curley FJ, French CL. Chronic cough. The spectrum and frequency of causes, key components of the diagnostic evaluation, and outcome of specific therapy. Am Rev Respir Dis 1990; 141:640–647.

8. Irwin RS, Boulet LP, Cloutier MM, Fuller R, Gold PM, Hoffstein V, et al. Managing cough as a defense mechanism and as a symptom. A consensus panel report of the American College of Chest Physicians. Chest 1998; 114(2 suppl):133S–181S.

9. Chang AB, Asher MI. A review of cough in children. J Asthma 2001; 38: 299–309.

10. Phelan PD, Asher MI. Recurrent and persistent cough in children. New Ethicals J 1999; June:41–45.

11. Faniran AO, Peat JK, Woolcock AJ. Measuring persistent cough in children in epidemiological studies: development of a questionnaire and assessment of prevalence in two countries. Chest 1999; 115:434–439.

12. Hay AD, Wilson AD. The natural history of acute cough in children aged 0 to 4 years in primary care: a systematic review. Br J Gen Pract 2002; 52:401–409.

13. Thomson F, Masters IB, Chang AB. Persistent cough in children–overuse of medications. J Paediatr Child Health 2002; 38:578–581.

14. Couriel J. Infection in children. In: Ellis M, ed. Infectious Diseases of the Respiratory Tract. Cambridge: Cambridge University Press, 1998:406–429.

15. Gratas-Delamarche A, Mercier J, Ramonatxo M, Dassonville J, Prefaut C. Ventilatory response of prepubertal boys and adults to carbon dioxide at rest and during exercise. Eur J Appl Physiol Occup Physiol 1993; 66:25–30.

16. Fujimura M, Kasahara K, Kamio Y, Narusse M, Hashimoto T, Matsuda T. Female gender as a determinant of cough threshold to inhaled capsaicin. Eur Respir J 1996; 9:1624–1626.

17. Chang AB, Phelan PD, Sawyer SM, Del Brocco S, Robertson CF. Cough sensitivity in children with asthma, recurrent cough, and cystic fibrosis. Arch Dis Child 1997; 77:331–334.

18. Undem BJ, Carr MJ, Kollarik M. Physiology and plasticity of putative cough fibres in the Guinea pig. Pulm Pharmacol Ther 2002; 15:193–198.

19. Bastacky J, Goerke J. Pores of Kohn are filled in normal lungs: low-temperature scanning electron microscopy. J Appl Physiol 1992; 73:88–95.

20. Menkes H, Traystman R, Terry P. Collateral ventilation. Fed Proc 1979; 38:22–26.

21. Van Meir F. The alveolar pores of Kohn in young postnatal rat lungs and their relation with type II pneumocytes. Histol Histopathol 1991; 6:55–62.

22. Schramm CM. Current concepts of respiratory complications of neuromuscular disease in children. Curr Opin Pediatr 2000; 12:203–207.

23. Wilson N, Silverman M. Bronchial responsiveness and its measurement. In: Silverman M, ed. Childhood Asthma and Other Wheezing Disorders. London: Chapman & Hall, 1995:142–174.

24. Brunekreef B, Groot B, Rijcken B, Hoek G, Steenbekkers A, de Boer A. Reproducibility of childhood respiratory symptom questions. Eur Respir J 1992; 5:930–935.

25. Hsu JY, Stone RA, Logan-Sinclair RB, Worsdell M, Busst CM, Chung KF. Coughing frequency in patients with persistent cough: assessment using a 24 hour ambulatory recorder. Eur Respir J 1994; 7:1246–1253.

26. Archer LNJ, Simpson H. Night cough counts and diary card scores in asthma. Arch Dis Child 1985; 60:473–474.

27. Chang AB, Newman RG, Carlin J, Phelan PD, Robertson CF. Subjective scoring of cough in children: parent-completed vs child-completed diary cards vs an objective method. Eur Respir J 1998; 11:462–466.

28. Falconer A, Oldman C, Helms P. Poor agreement between reported and recorded nocturnal cough in asthma. Pediatr Pulmonol 1993; 15:209–211.

29. Chang AB, Phelan PD, Robertson CF, Newman RG, Sawyer SM. Frequency and perception of cough severity. J Paediatr Child Health 2001; 37:142–145.

30. Rietveld S, Van BI, Everaerd W. Psychological confounds in medical research: the example of excessive cough in asthma. Behav Res Ther 2000; 38:791–800.

31. Chang AB. Causes of cough, assessment and measurement in children. In: Widdicombe JG, Chung F, Boushey H, eds. Cough: Mechanisms, Causes and Therapy. London: Blackwell Science, 2003. In press.

32. Bush A. Paediatric problems of cough. Pulm Pharmacol Ther 2002; 15: 309–315.

33. Bonaccorso SN, Sturchio JL. For and against: direct to consumer advertising is medicalising normal human experience: Against. Br Med J 2002; 324: 910–911.

34. Munyard P, Bush A. How much coughing is normal? Arch Dis Child 1996; 74:531–534.

35. Phelan PD, Landau LI, Olinsky A, eds. Respiratory Illness in Children. Oxford: Blackwell, 1990.

36. Chernick V, Boat TF, eds. Kendig's Disorders of the Respiratory Tract in Children. Philadelphia: W.B. Saunders, 1998.

37. Chang AB, Boyce NC, Masters IB, Torzillo PJ, Masel JP. Bronchoscopic findings in children with non-cystic fibrosis chronic suppurative lung disease. Thorax 2002; 57:935–938.

38. Taussig LM, Landau LI, eds. Pediatric Respiratory Medicine. St. Louis: Mosby Inc., 1999.

39. Bush A. The child with chronic cough- diagnosis, management and outlook. Respir Med 1997; 11:35–39.

40. Williams H. Bronchiectasis: its multiple clinical and pathological features. Arch Dis Child 1959; 2:192–201.

41. Hamutcu R, Francis J, Karakoc F, Bush A. Objective monitoring of cough in children with cystic fibrosis. Pediatr Pulmonol 2002; 34:331–335.

42. Chang AB, Grimwood K, Mulholland EK, Torzillo PJ. Bronchiectasis in indigenous children in remote Australian communities. Med J Aust 2002; 177: 200–204.

43. Chang AB, Powell CV. Non-specific cough in children: diagnosis and treatment. Hosp Med 1998; 59:680–684.

44. Sheikh S, Allen E, Shell R, Hruschak J, Iram D, Castile R, et al. Chronic aspiration without gastroesophageal reflux as a cause of chronic respiratory symptoms in neurologically normal infants. Chest 2001; 120:1190–1195.

45. Ayed AK, Jafar AM, Owayed A. Foreign body aspiration in children: diagnosis and treatment. Pediatr Surg Int 2003.

46. Karakoc F, Karadag B, Akbenlioglu C, Ersu R, Yildizeli B, Yuksel M, et al. Foreign body aspiration: what is the outcome? Pediatr Pulmonol 2002; 34:30–36.

47. Mertens AC, Yasui Y, Liu Y, Stovall M, Hutchinson R, Ginsberg J, et al. Pulmonary complications in survivors of childhood and adolescent cancer. A report from the Childhood Cancer Survivor Study. Cancer 2002; 95:2431–2441.

48. Starke JR, Taylor-Watts KT. Tuberculosis in the pediatric population of Houston, Texas. Pediatrics 1989; 84:28–35.

49. Ellis M. Infectious Diseases of the Respiratory Tract. 1st ed. Cambridge: Cambridge University Press, 1998.

50. Chang AB, Phelan PD, Sawyer SM, Robertson CF. Airway hyperresponsiveness and cough-receptor sensitivity in children with recurrent cough. Am J Respir Crit Care Med 1997; 155:1935–1939.

51. Choudry NB, Fuller RW. Sensitivity of the cough reflex in patients with chronic cough. Eur Respir J 1992; 5:296–300.

52. Shimizu T, Mochizuki H, Morikawa A. Effect of influenza A virus infection on acid-induced cough response in children with asthma. Eur Respir J 1997; 10:71–74.

53. Powell CVE, Primhak RA. Stability of respiratory symptoms in unlabelled wheezy illness and nocturnal cough. Arch Dis Child 1996; 75:385–391.

54. Campanella SG, Asher MI. Current controversies: sinus disease and the lower airways. Pediatr Pulmonol 2001; 31:165–172.

55. Corrado G, Pacchiarotti C, Cavaliere M, Rea P, Cardi E. Esophageal disorders and chronic cough in children. Chest 1998; 114:659.

56. Laukka MA, Cameron AJ, Schei AJ. Gastroesophageal reflux and chronic cough: which comes first? J Clin Gastroenterol 1994; 19:100–104.

57. Poe RH, Kallay MC. Chronic cough and gastroesophageal reflux disease: experience with specific therapy for diagnosis and treatment. Chest 2003; 123:679–684.

58. Novitsky YW, Zawacki JK, Irwin RS, French CT, Hussey VM, Callery MP. Chronic cough due to gastroesophageal reflux disease: efficacy of antireflux surgery. Surg Endosc 2002; 16:567–571.

59. Teichtahl H, Kronborg IJ, Yeomans ND, Robinson P. Adult asthma and gastro-oesophageal reflux: the effects of omeprazole therapy on asthma. Aust NZ J Med 1996; 26:671–676.

60. Holinger LD. Chronic cough in infants and children. Laryngoscope 1986; 96:316–322.

61. Irwin RS, Madison JM. Diagnosis and treatment of chronic cough due to gastro-esophageal reflux disease and postnasal drip syndrome. Pulm Pharmacol Ther 2002; 15:261–266.

62. Lack G. Pediatric allergic rhinitis and comorbid disorders. J Allergy Clin Immunol 2001; 108(1 suppl):S9–S15.

63. Widdicombe JG. Neurophysiology of the cough reflex. Eur Respir J 1995; 8: 1193–1202.
64. Gawchik S, Goldstein S, Prenner B, John A. Relief of cough and nasal symptoms associated with allergic rhinitis by mometasone furoate nasal spray. Ann Allergy Asthma Immunol 2003; 90:416–421.
65. Shopfner CE, Rossi JO. Roentgen evaluation of the paranasal sinuses in children. Am J Roentgenol 1973; 118:176–186.
66. Diament MJ, Senac MO, Gilsanz V, Baker S, Gillespie T, Larsson S. Prevalence of incidental paranasal sinuses opacification in pediatric patients: a CT study. J Comput Assist Tomogr 1987; 11:426–431.
67. Lombardi E, Stein RT, Wright AL, Morgan WJ, Martinez FD. The relation between physician-diagnosed sinusitis, asthma, and skin test reactivity to allergens in 8-year-old children. Pediatr Pulmonol 1996; 22:141–146.
68. Turktas I, Dalgic N, Bostanci I, Cengizlier R. Extrathoracic airway responsiveness in children with asthma-like symptoms, including chronic persistent cough. Pediatr Pulmonol 2002; 34:172–180.
69. Bucca C, Rolla G, Brussino L, De Rose V, Bugiani M. Are asthma-like symptoms due to bronchial or extrathoracic airway dysfunction? Lancet 1995; 346:791–795.
70. Rolla G, Colagrande P, Scappaticci E, Bottomicca F, Magnano M, Brussino L, et al. Damage of the pharyngeal mucosa and hyperresponsiveness of airway in sinusitis. J Allergy Clin Immunol 1997; 100:52–57.
71. Masters IB, Chang AB, Patterson L, Wainwright C, Buntain H, Dean BW, et al. Series of laryngomalacia, tracheomalacia, and bronchomalacia disorders and their associations with other conditions in children. Pediatr Pulmonol 2002; 34:189–195.
72. Gormley PK, Colreavy MP, Patil N, Woods AE. Congenital vascular anomalies and persistent respiratory symptoms in children. Int J Pediatr Otorhinolaryngol 1999; 51:23–31.
73. Wood RE. Localised tracheomalacia or bronchomalacia in children with intractable cough. J Paediatr 1997; 116:404–406.
74. Grathwohl KW, Afifi AY, Dillard TA, Olson JP, Heric BR. Vascular rings of the thoracic aorta in adults. Am Surg 1999; 65:1077–1083.
75. Finder JD. Primary bronchomalacia in infants and children. J Paediatr 1997; 130:59–66.
76. Marchant JM, Masters IB, Chang AB. Chronic cough in children—understanding the spectrum of disease. ERS 13th Annual Congress, Vienna, Austria, Sept 27–Oct 1, 2003.
77. Stick S. Pediatric origins of adult lung disease. 1. The contribution of airway development to paediatric and adult lung disease. Thorax 2000; 55:587–594.
78. Cook DG, Strachan DP. Health effects of passive smoking-10: summary of effects of parental smoking on the respiratory health of children and implications for research. Thorax 1999; 54:357–366.
79. Dales RE, White J, Bhumgara C, McMullen E. Parental reporting of children's coughing is biased. Eur J Epidemiol 1997; 13:541–545.
80. Lewis PR, Hensley MJ, Wlodarczyk J, Toneguzzi RC, Westley-Wise VJ, Dunn T, et al. Outdoor air pollution and children's respiratory symptoms in the steel cities of New South Wales. Med J Aust 1998; 169:459–463.

81. Chang AB. State of the Art: cough, cough receptors, and asthma in children. Pediatr Pulmonol 1999; 28:59–70.
82. Hannaway PJ, Hopper GDK. Cough variant asthma in children. J Am Med Assoc 1982; 247:206–208.
83. Cloutier MM, Loughlin GM. Chronic cough in children: a manifestation of airway hyperreactivity. Pediatrics 1981; 67:6–12.
84. Chang AB, Phelan PD, Robertson CF. Cough receptor sensitivity in children with acute and non-acute asthma. Thorax 1997; 52:770–774.
85. Henry RL. All that coughs is not asthma [editorial]. Pediatr Pulmonol 1999; 28:1–2.
86. McKenzie S. Cough-but is it asthma? Arch Dis Child 1994; 70:1–2.
87. Corrao WM, Braman SS, Irwin RS. Chronic cough as the sole presenting manifestation of bronchial asthma. N Engl J Med 1979; 300:633–637.
88. Picciotto A, Hubbard M, Sturdy P, Naish J, McKenzie SA. Prescribing for persistent cough in children. Respir Med 1998; 92:638–641.
89. Chang AB, Phelan PD, Carlin J, Sawyer SM, Robertson CF. Randomised controlled trial of inhaled salbutamol and beclomethasone for recurrent cough. Arch Dis Child 1998; 79:6–11.
90. Davies MJ, Fuller P, Picciotto A, McKenzie SA. Persistent nocturnal cough: randomised controlled trial of high dose inhaled corticosteroid. Arch Dis Child 1999; 81:38–44.
91. Fitch PS, Brown V, Schock BC, Taylor R, Ennis M, Shields MD. Chronic cough in children: bronchoalveolar lavage findings. Eur Respir J 2000; 16:1109–1114.
92. Gibson PG, Simpson JL, Chalmers AC, Toneguzzi RC, Wark PAB, Wilson A, et al. Airway eosinophilia is associated with wheeze but is uncommon in children with persistent cough and frequent chest colds. Am J Respir Crit Care Med 2001; 164:977–981.
93. Mellis CM. Can we reduce acute asthma attendances to hospital emergency departments? Aust NZ J Med 1997; 27:275–276.
94. Matthews LH, Leibowitz JM, Matthews JR. Tics, habits and mannerisms. In: Walker CE, Roberts MC, eds. Clinical Child Psychology. New York: John Wiley & Sons, 1992:283–286.
95. Lokshin B, Lindgren S, Weinberger M, Koviach J. Outcome of habit cough in children treated with a brief session of suggestion therapy. Ann Allergy 1991; 67:579–582.
96. Riegel B, Warmoth JE, Middaugh SJ, Kee WG, Nicholson LC, Melton DM, et al. Psychogenic cough treated with biofeedback and psychotherapy. A review and case report. Am J Phys Med Rehabil 1995; 74:155–158.
97. McGarvey LP, Warke TJ, McNiff C, Heaney LG, MacMahon J. Psychogenic cough in a schoolboy: evaluation using an ambulatory cough recorder. Pediatr Pulmonol 2003; 36:73–75.
98. Wu-Williams AH, Samet JM. Environmental tobacco smoke: exposure–response relationships in epidemiologic studies. Risk Anal 1990; 10:39–48.
99. Couriel JM. Passive smoking and the health of children [editorial]. Thorax 1994; 49:731–734.

100. Chang AB, Harrhy VA, Simpson JL, Masters IB, Gibson PG. Cough, airway inflammation and mild asthma exacerbation. Arch Dis Child 2002; 86: 270–275.
101. Chang AB, Gibson PG. Relationship between cough, cough receptor sensitivity and asthma in children. Pulm Pharmacol Ther 2002; 15:287–291.
102. Irwin RS, Corrao WM, Pratter MR. Chronic persistent cough in the adult: the spectrum and frequency of causes and successful outcome of specific therapy. Am Rev Respir Dis 1981; 123:413–417.
103. Coren ME, Ng V, Rubens M, Rosenthal M, Bush A. The value of ultrafast computed tomography in the investigation of pediatric chest disease. Pediatr Pulmonol 1998; 26:389–395.
104. Mayo JR, Jackson SA, Muller NL. High-resolution CT of the chest: radiation dose. AJR Am J Roentgenol 1993; 160:479–481.
105. Copley SJ, Bush A. Series: imaging. HRCT of paediatric lung disease. Paediatr Respir Rev 2000; 1:141–147.
106. de Blic J, Midulla F, Barbato A, Clement A, Dab I, Eber E, et al. Bronchoalveolar lavage in children. ERS Task Force on bronchoalveolar lavage in children. European Respiratory Society. Eur Respir J 2000; 15:217–231.
107. Marguet C, Dean TP, Warner JO. Soluble intercellular adhesion molecule-1 (sICAM-1) and interferon-gamma in bronchoalveolar lavage fluid from children with airway diseases. Am J Respir Crit Care Med 2000; 162:1016–1022.
108. Marguet C, Jouen Boedes F, Dean TP, Warner JO. Bronchoalveolar cell profiles in children with asthma, infantile wheeze, chronic cough, or cystic fibrosis. Am J Respir Crit Care Med 1999; 159:1533–1540.
109. Jones PD, Hankin R, Simpson J, Gibson PG, Henry RL. The tolerability, safety, and success of sputum induction and combined hypertonic saline challenge in children. Am J Respir Crit Care Med 2001; 164:1146–1149.
110. Jayaram L, Parameswaran K, Sears MR, Hargreave FE. Induced sputum cell counts: their usefulness in clinical practice. Eur Respir J 2000; 16:150–158.
111. Zimmerman B, Silverman FS, Tarlo SM, Chapman KR, Kubay JM, Urch B. Induced sputum: comparison of postinfectious cough with allergic asthma in children. J Allergy Clin Immunol 2000; 105:495–499.
112. Gibson PG, Henry RL, Thomas P. Noninvasive assessment of airway inflammation in children: induced sputum, exhaled nitric oxide, and breath condensate. Eur Respir J 2000; 16:1008–1015.
113. Malmberg LP, Pelkonen AS, Haahtela T, Turpeinen M. Exhaled nitric oxide rather than lung function distinguishes preschool children with probable asthma. Thorax 2003; 58:494–499.
114. Leuppi JD, Downs SH, Downie SR, Marks GB, Salome CM. Exhaled nitric oxide levels in atopic children: relation to specific allergic sensitisation, AHR, and respiratory symptoms. Thorax 2002; 57:518–523.
115. Formanek W, Inci D, Lauener RP, Wildhaber JH, Frey U, Hall GL. Elevated nitrite in breath condensates of children with respiratory disease. Eur Respir J 2002; 19:487–491.
116. McKenzie SA, Mylonopoulou M, Bridge PD. Bronchodilator responsiveness and atopy in 5–10-yr-old coughers. Eur Respir J 2001; 18:977–981.

117. Klug B, Nielsen KG, Bisgaard H. Observer variability of lung function measurements in 2–6-yr-old children. Eur Respir J 2000; 16:472–475.
118. Chang AB, Phelan PD, Roberts RGD, Robertson CF. Capsaicin cough receptor sensitivity test in children. Eur Respir J 1996; 9:2220–2223.
119. Salome CM, Peat JK, Britton WJ, Woolcok AJ. Bronchial hyperresponsiveness in two populations of Australian children.I. Relation to respiratory symptoms and diagnosed asthma. Clin Allergy 1987; 17:271–281.
120. Clifford RD, Radford M, Howell JB, Holgate ST. Prevalence of respiratory symptoms among 7 and 11 year old schoolchildren and association with asthma. Arch Dis Child 1989; 64:1118–1125.
121. Lombardi E, Morgan WJ, Wright AL, Stein RT, Holberg CJ, Martinez FD. Cold air challenge at age 6 and subsequent incidence of asthma. Am J Respir Crit Care Med 1997; 156:1863–1869.
122. Galvez RA, McLaughlin FJ, Levison H. The role of the methacholine challenge in children with chronic cough. J Allergy Clin Immunol 1987; 79: 331–335.
123. Nishimura H, Mochizuki H, Tokuyama K, Morikawa A. Relationship between bronchial hyperresponsiveness and development of asthma in children with chronic cough. Pediatr Pulmonol 2001; 31:412–418.

Index